QUANTITATIVE METHODS IN BONE DENSITOMETRY

QUANTITATIVE METHODS IN BONE DENSITOMETRY

ALAN L. HUDDLESTON, PH.D.
Chief, Medical Physics
Baylor University Medical Center
Charles A. Sammons Cancer Center
Division of Radiation Oncology
Dallas, Texas 75246

KLUWER ACADEMIC PUBLISHERS
BOSTON/DORDRECHT/LONDON

Kluwer Academic Publishers, 101 Philip Drive, Assinippi Park, Norwell, MA 02061

PRINTED IN THE UNITED STATES

Distributors

for the United States and Canada: Kluwer Academic Publishers, 101 Philip Drive, Assinippi Park, Norwell, MA 02061

for the UK and Ireland: Kluwer Academic Publishers, Falcon House, Queen Square, Lancaster LA1 1RN, UK

for all other countries: Kluwer Academic Publishers Group, Distribution Centre, P.O. Box 322, 3300 AH Dordrecht, The Netherlands

---

Library of Congress Cataloging-in-Publication Data

Huddleston, Alan.
Quantitative methods in bone densitometry.
Includes index.
1. Osteoporosis — Diagnosis. 2. Bone densitometry.
1. Title. [DNLM: 1. Bone and Bones — radiography.
2. Densitometry — methods. 3. Osteoporosis — radiography.
4. Tomography, X-Ray Computed-methods. WE 200 H884q]
RC931.073H83 1988 616.7'10754 87-35241
ISBN 0-89838-362-5

To the memory of my brother, Gary Lee Huddleston, M.D.

CONTENTS

PREFACE

Interest in bone densitometry methods has recently experienced a resurgence within the medical community. Physicians have become more interested than ever before in the diagnosis and treatment of degenerative diseases of bone such as osteoporosis. The public perception of osteoporosis and its prevention has been recently heightened. Because osteoporosis is widespread, especially in women, and leads to an increase in fractures in our population, many researchers and clinicians are strongly motivated in their search for more sensitive and accurate methods of diagnosis.

This book was written for physicians, scientists, engineers, medical physicists, and others desiring an introduction or further understanding of this exciting field. Beginning with the early development of x-ray film methods for assessing bone status, the field has steadily grown throughout the years. Novel and interesting devices have been designed for the measurement of bone mass, bone density, cortical thickness, and other parameters of bone changes. Both qualitative and quantitative bone methods are described. The techniques include imaging devices such as CT and radiography as well as fixed point methods in which bone characteristics of a region of interest are analyzed.

Clinical applications of these bone densitometry methods are included as an indication of the usefulness of the various techniques, although the complete analysis of clinical data was not exhaustive nor intended in this work. However, it is intended that an appreciation of the extensive efforts of the many researchers who have worked to develop these techniques and an understanding of the basic physical principles will be realized by this book. Further development of the field of bone densitometry will require new insights for the integration of technology and biomedical knowledge. Further investigation of the methodology is necessary to increase the sensitivity, precision, and accuracy with which bone parameters may be assessed by noninvasive means in the human body. It is hope that this work may inspire others to meet this challenge.

ACKNOWLEDGMENTS

Grateful acknowledgment is made for the interest and appreciation expressed by the many authors of published works in this field. Special thanks are conveyed to those authors who have granted permission to reproduce or extract information from their published works and to the publishers of the many referenced journals and books on the subject. In particular, I would like to acknowledge Moses A. Greenfield, Ph.D., my mentor and adviser as a graduate student, without whose encouragement and enthusiasm this work would not have been written. Appreciation is expressed for the patience of my wife, Diane, and my daughters, Lisa and Katherine, and for the encouragement of my family and friends.

Alan L. Huddleston

QUANTITATIVE METHODS IN BONE DENSITOMETRY

1. INTRODUCTION

Osteoporosis has been described as the commonest of all diseases (Jackson, 1955). In this disease the skeletal mass decreases and bones become more susceptible to fracture. In the nineteenth century, several physicians noted the unusual frequency of fractures in the elderly population, but they were not aware of the disease process, osteoporosis, as the underlying cause (Davies and Saha, 1985). Senile osteoporosis was first described in 1926 by Alwens. The first report on postmenopausal osteoporosis was published by Albright et al. (1941), who first clearly defined the crush fracture syndrome.

On an annual basis, about 1.3 million fractures attributable to osteoporosis occur in the United States in people aged 45 years and older. Of the more than one million fractures occurring annually in women of this age, 70% are sustained by women with osteoporosis. The National Institutes of Health have estimated that in people who live to be 90 years old, 32% of women and 17% of men will suffer a fracture of the hip, most of which will be caused by osteoporosis. The cost of osteoporosis in the United States has been estimated at $3.8 billion annually.

Loss of bone mineral with advancing age is generally accepted as the main risk factor in the pathogenesis of osteoporotic fractures (Newton-John and Morgan, 1970; Doyle, 1972; Smith et al., 1975; Riggs, 1982). The clinical syndrome of osteoporosis consists of a reduced amount of bone tissue per unit volume of anatomic bone (osteopenia) and fractures of the vertebrae, femoral neck, or the distal forearm after minor trauma (Krolner, 1985). The bone tissue itself is considered to be normal (Nordin, 1970; Frost, 1970; Riggs, 1981). Osteoporosis is becoming a growing health problem because of the growing number of elderly persons in our society. These circumstances may be regarded as an epidemic for which there are now preventative measures (Gordan, 1984).

The most common problem for older women is osteoporosis. About one in four white women over 60 years of age suffer the pain, stiffness, and deformity of osteoporosis over the latter 10 to 20 years of life (Harrison, 1984). The problem has been neglected and considered to be an inevitable part of aging that cannot be prevented. However, we now know that osteoporotic bone loss is not inevitable and that treatment methods can be found through further research and the availability of valid tests for the diagnosis of bone loss.

Decreased bone density of the skeleton may result from osteoporosis, osteomalacia, hyperparathyroidism, renal osteodystrophy, metastatic disease, or multiple myeloma. Primary osteoporosis is an age-related disorder characterized by decreased bone mass and by increased susceptibility to fractures in the absense of other recognizable causes of bone loss (Avioli, 1984). Immobilization and prolonged bed rest may also produce rapid bone loss. Osteomalacia, on the other hand, is primarily characterized by abnormalities of the peripheral skeleton, which are more common than spinal abnormalities (Chalmers et al., 1967).

Osteoporosis is characterized by the decreased formation of bone matrix, which may be localized or distributed throughout the skeleton. Osteomalacia is characterized by the decreased mineralization of bone tissue. Bone resorption and bone apposition represent dynamic competing processes, which ultimately determine the amount of bone mineral that is present in the skeleton. Hyperparathyroidism is characterized by excessive bone resorption (figure 1). Renal osteodystrophy is characterized by excessive bone resorption and by decreased mineralization of bone matrix. The term *osteopenia* is often used to describe these conditions in which the amount of bone tissue is decreased. It may not be possible to distinguish between the causes of osteopenia by the use of non-invasive radiological methods, and the diagnosis requires the use of clinical or laboratory tests or bone biopsy.

Senile and postmenopausal osteoporosis usually start and are most severe in the spine, and are later evident with less severe effects in the peripheral skeleton. Most patients presenting with a compression fracture of the spine will be found to fall into the primary osteoporosis classification; 95% of these will have postmenopausal or senile osteoporosis (Gruber and Baylink, 1981). Women have more fractures than men, and they have accelerated bone loss after menopause, unlike the gradual bone loss experienced by men. In women, bone mass is lost rapidly during the 3 to 7 year period following menopause (Avioli, 1984). Early menopause increases the chances of women developing osteoporosis. American women live 40% of their lives after menopause (32 years), and, by age 70, these susceptible women have, on the average, lost

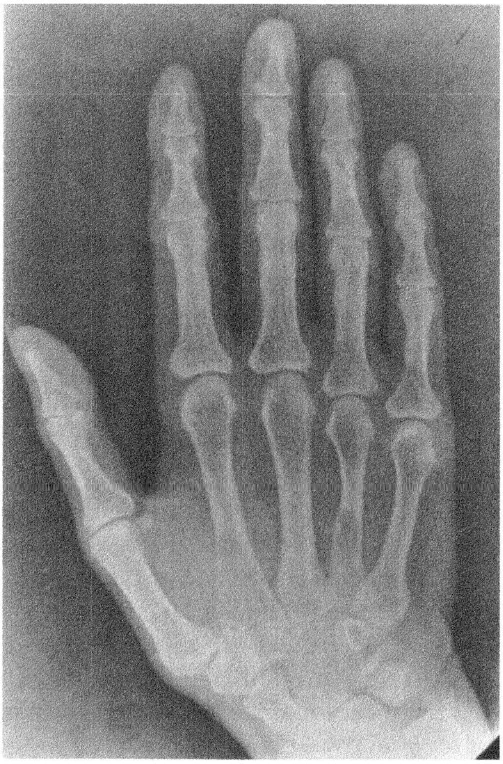

Figure 1. Bone resorption of middle phalanges as a result of primary hyperparathyroidism (Courtesy: R Schneider)

50% of their peripheral cortical bone mass. In women, bone loss in the lumbar spine (L2-L4), which consists of approximately 60% trabecular bone, is about 0.8% per year. This rate of loss is accelerated to 3 to 8% per year during menopause and decreases to less than 1% in old age. Bone diminution at menopause appears to be greater in the lumbar spine than elsewhere in trabecular bone (Mazess, 1981). It has been stated that the majority of evidence suggests that the decrease of trabecular bone density begins during young adulthood (20 to 40 years) in both sexes and thereafter decreases at similar rates of 6% to 8% per decade (Mazess, 1982).

In women, bone loss in the radius (which is predominantly cortical bone) does not occur until menopause, and this loss is accelerated until about age 65 and then decelerates somewhat in old age. In men, age-related bone loss is a linear decrease from the age at which maximum bone mass occurs (Wahner, 1985). Women are at higher risk for osteoporosis than men, since the bone mass of men is approximately 30% higher than that of wmen. In addition, white women are at much higher risk for osteoporosis than black women, and white men are at higher risk than black men.

Osteoporosis is linked with significant morbidity and mortality in our society. Vertebral fractures occur most frequently in 55- to 75-year-old women during the accelerated loss of trabecular bone. Hip fractures occur most frequently in older men and women who have slowly lost trabecular and cortical bone mass (Avioli, 1984). It is estimated that 25% of all white women over 60 years of age have radiological evidence of vertebral crush fracture, which contributes to a loss of weight and may progress to spinal deformity (Heaney, 1976). Women in their 80s have a 40% chance of having sustained one or more hip fractures (Genant, 1983). Of the estimated 190,000 hip fractures that occur each year, two-thirds are due to osteoporosis. Acute care for these patients costs $1.4 billion annually. More importantly, half of the patients who survive hip fractures are unable to live independently after the fracture (Davies and Saha, 1985). Hip fractures have an associated mortality rate of 12% to 15% and are the second leading cause of death among people 47 to 74 years of age. It has been reported in England and Wales that the mortality associated with sustained fracture of the femur in women over age 45 years was 16.8%, representing a 20-fold increase in the expected mortality for this age group (Lewis, 1981).

Three factors determine the likelihood of fractures: (1) the magnitude, direction, and duration of applied forces, (2) the dissipation of forces by muscle contraction and soft-tissue absorption, and (3) the bone strength. The reduction in bone mass is the most important reason for the increased frequency of bone fractures in postmenopausal women and in the elderly (Avioli, 1984).

Krolner and Nielsen (1982) suggested that exercise can inhibit the involutional bone loss from the axial skeleton in middle-aged women and may even lead to a net gain in axial bone mass. Osteoporosis is being treated with various therapeutic agents including calcium, vitamin D, sodium fluoride, and estrogen; and it is essential that accurate and reliable methods for diagnosing and following the course of the disease be found (Briancon and Meunier, 1981; Riggs et al., 1982).

COMPOSITION OF BONE TISSUE

Bone consists of a collagen-rich organic matrix upon which a crystalline mineral phase (primarily calcium and phosphate) is deposited. The mineral phase deposited within the organic matrix contains 99% of the body's calcium, 80% to 85% of the body's phosphate, and most of the magnesium. Bone is, therefore, the repository for these minerals, which are used to maintain ions in the extracellular fluid and are required for stabilizing the electrical potential of neural membranes (Chesney, 1981).

There are two major forms of bone: (1) compact (or cortical) bone and (2) trabecular (or cancellous or medullary) bone (figure 2). Cortical bone forms the external envelopes of the skeleton; trabecular bone forms plates that traverse the internal cavities of the skeleton. The proportions of trabecular and

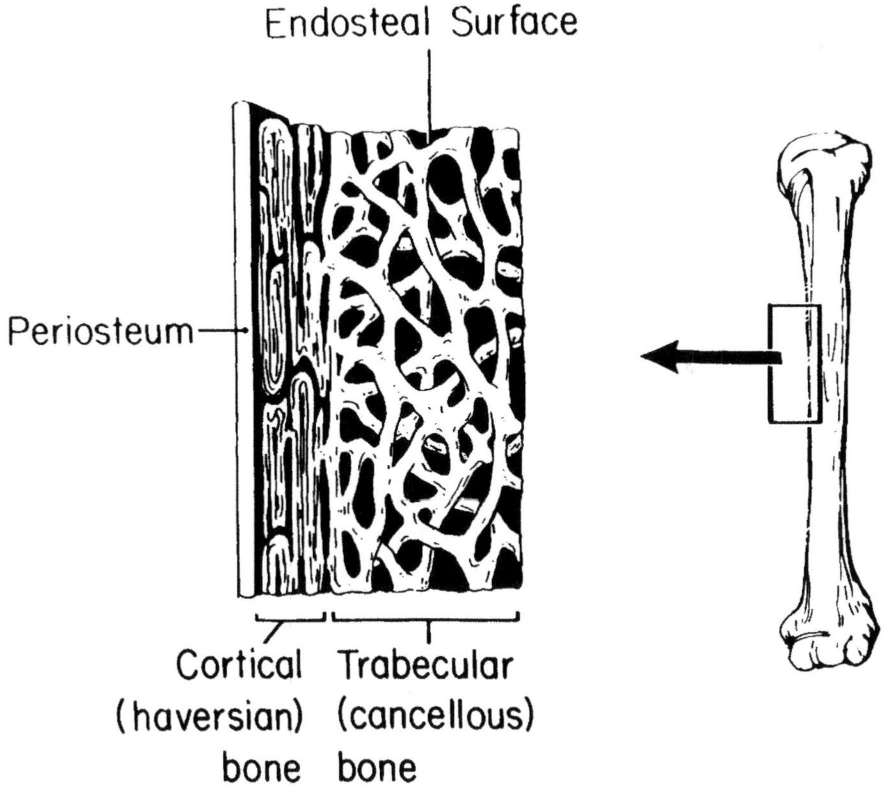

Figure 2. Structure of bone (Courtesy: CYC Pak)

cortical bone vary from one site to another in the skeleton. Vertebral bodies of the spine contain principally trabecular bone, whereas the peripheral skeleton (arms and legs) contains predominantly cortical bone.

Bone is continuously remodeling (turnover) throughout life. Osteoclasts resorb bone in microscopic cavities within the bones, whereas osteoblasts rebuild the bone surfaces and refill the cavities. The remodeling process is influenced by mechanical and electrical forces, hormones, and other factors. The maximum amount of bone is attained at about age 35 and decreases thereafter. Bones lose both mineral and organic matrix, but they retain their basic structural organization.

The bone substance itself has variable composition. Typically, bone tissue represents only 15% to 25% of the total volume in the trabecular areas of the skeleton, whereas the marrow represents 75% to 85% of the total volume. Marrow consists of hematopoietic cells and adipose cells. Water represents 50% of the total mass. The exact composition of the bone marrow is variable, and these marrow changes can introduce errors in clinical bone measurements (Mazess, 1983).

Trabecular bone volume, expressed as a percentage of total volume, was investigated using iliac crest biopsy specimens obtained from cadavers (Nordin et al., 1984). The mean bone volume was lower in the old than in the young controls and significantly lower in the osteoporotic specimens. It was concluded that age-related (simple) osteoporosis in men appears to be a result of reduced bone formation, whereas pathological (accelerated) osteoporosis is due to increased bone resorption.

Bone mass can be evaluated with histomorphometry, usually performed on a bone biopsy from the iliac crest. Osteomalacia and certain forms of secondary osteoporosis can be excluded by this method. Bone biopsy is a safe technique, but it requires specialized equipment and expert analysis, which are not widely available. Other data obtained from the histomorphometric characterization of osteoporosis have not been found to be of routine clinical value. The most critical parameter for assessing osteopenia is the trabecular bone volume (TBV) (Jaworski, 1976; Meunier, 1977). The TBV is about 20% (±5%) in young adults of both sexes. In older females it is about 14% (±4%); the relative loss of trabecular bone volume is about 10% per decade. The TBV in symptomatic female osteoporotics is about 11% (±3%) (Meunier et al., 1975).

Trabecular bone volume of the iliac crest, although it may not reflect the status of trabecular bone in other parts of the body, does appear to be correlated with the amount of trabecular bone present in the spine (Bell et al., 1967; Meunier, 1981). Some investigations have shown poorer correlations between measurements in the iliac crest (biopsy) and the vertebral mass, density, or strength (Mazess, 1979). Meunier et al. (1979), using the iliac crest biopsy, defined a *TBV fracture threshold* of 11% (±3%) at which vertebral collapse appears in the patient, independent of age and sex.

Bone loss affects dense cortical bone to a different degree than the less dense trabecular bone. Trabecular bone is found mainly in the axial skeleton (e.g., spine), whereas cortical bone is found mainly in the appendicular skeleton (arms and legs). The skeleton consists of approximately 80% cortical bone and 20% trabecular bone. In the appendicular skeleton, the long bones consist of cortical and trabecular bone, whereas the ends of these bones are primarily trabecular bone. The spine consists of individual vertebrae containing primarily trabecular bone; however, the end plates and the posterior regions of the vertebrae contain cortical bone. Trabecular bone is distinquished from cortical bone by its higher *turnover rate* (resorption and apposition of bone). The exact mechanism of osteoporosis at the cellular level is unknown, but it is believed to be directly related to the predominant process of resorption during the osteoclastic-osteoblastic activities in bone tissues.

BONE STRENGTH AND BONE MASS

Bone mineral content (BMC) is a major determinant of the strength or the fragility of bone (Weaver and Chalmers, 1966; Bell et al., 1967; Chalmers,

1973; Hansson et al., 1980). It has been shown that the breaking strength of bone is linearly related to mineral content (Riggs et al., 1981). However, it has been noted that three factors prevent a complete dependence of bone strength on bone mass (density): (1) Geometric changes affect the modulus of elasticity of bone, such as the increased circumference of long bones with age, (2) smaller changes in the trabecular bone mass may be required to reduce bone strength than changes in compact bone mass; and (3) fat content increases with age and changes the mechanical behavior of bone (Mazess, 1982).

BONE MASS MEASUREMENTS

The measurement of bone mass or bone density has been the subject of intensive research over the years. This book describes the physical principles and the utilization of these methods. The development of appropriate techniques has been complicated by the complexities associated with the disease process itself, namely, which physical parameter should be measured? The physical quantities — mass, density, calcium concentration, and other parameters — may only partially characterize the bone loss associated with a disease such as osteoporosis. In addition, the degree of instrumental accuracy and precision obtainable from the measurement of these physical parameters is a challenge that medical science has not successfully conquered. Yet, progress has been made toward the achievement of successful noninvasive bone measurements. Quantitative methods of bone mineral determination are becoming more readily available for widespread clinical use, but many of these quantitative methods are available only in centers where treatments for osteoporosis are being invesigated.

In evaluating densitometric methods, it is necessary to determine the (1) precision and (2) accuracy of the measurement. The precision is a measure of the reproducibility of the method and is given by the coefficient of variation for repeated measurements. The precision is important in longitudinal studies, and it describes the ability to distinquish changes in the density values over time or as a result of therapy. Accuracy is a measure of the degree to which the density measurement agrees with an accepted or "true" value. True values are generally determined by performing measurements on removed bone or other tissue specimens. Since all bone measurements have some degree of error associated with them, it is difficult to determine the "true" density or bone mineral concentration. Accuracy is important in cross-sectional studies in which it is desired to separate patients with osteopenia from normal patients (Schneider, 1984).

Although a diagnostic index need not be a physical quantity in nature, it must provide a sensitive measure with which to discriminate the diseased individual or population from the healthy population. However, it is desirable that the measured quantity be a physical quantity (such as density or mass), which may be measured or calculated and compared with the true value. Bone measurements have tended to be made in both of these categories, that is, both morphological indices as well as physical quantities have been investigated for clinical applications.

For monitoring the natural course of bone loss (osteopenia) or therapy for osteopenia, a measurement method must have high precision. This is necessary since the aging bone loss in females from 45 to 75 years of age is about 1% per year; for females following oophorectomy bone loss is 2% to 3% annually (Newton-John and Morgan, 1970). The systematic errors associated with bone mineral measurements should be minimal. The accuracy of the method is critical, and there must be standards for comparison and calibration.

When assessing the sensitivity and accuracy of various bone densitometry methods, we are faced with the uncertainties associated with defining and diagnosing the disease states. Osteoporosis is not always manifested in the same manner or to the same degree from one individual to another and from one skeletal site to another. The usual clinical criterion of multiple compression fractures of the vertebrae may be inadequate (Mazess, 1979). Some individuals with osteopenia do not manifest fractures, while, on the other hand, some "normal" individuals will have fractures (Iskrant and Smith, 1969). This inability to exactly identify the osteoporotic population, combined with the measurement errors of any bone mineral method, decreases our ability to discriminate between normal subjects and osteoporotic individuals.

Some of these quantitative methods have not been fully developed for clinical use but are of potential value. They vary widely in cost, availability, and radiation dose. The semiquantitative methods, which are based upon changes in certain radiographic indicators such as the visibility of the trabeculae in radiographs of bone, have also been suggested for clinical use, although with little success. Unfortunately, there are no blood or urine tests for establishing specifically the diagnosis of primary osteoporosis, although such tests may exclude the secondary causes of osteoporosis (Avioli, 1984).

The requirements for a good diagnostic procedure for bone mineral measurement include: (1) high precision or reproducibility for longitudinal studies, (2) low cost, (3) low radiation dose, and (4) minimal inconvenience for the patient. The accuracy of the method is very important for the detection of osteopenia, in which the patient's measured bone mineral status is compared with the data for a normal population. In addition, the densitometry method must be sufficiently sensitive for the clinical detection of significant bone loss on the order of 1% to 3%. For patients whose bone loss is on the order of 25% to 30%, there is little need for the quantification of bone loss, since the deficiency of bone mineral is probably evident from radiographic films of the skeleton.

The radiologic methods for evaluation of osteopenia are either (1) qualitative or (2) quantitative. Qualitative methods involve the use of standard radiographic films or nuclear medicine scans. Quantitative methods include the following:

A. Radiogrammetry
B. Radiographic photodensitometry

C. Single-photon absorptiometry (SPA)
D. Dual-photon absorptiometry (DPA)
E. Quantitative computed tomography (QCT)
F. Compton scattering
G. Coherent/Compton scattering
H. Positron emission, muonic x-ray emission
I. Neutron and proton activation

It is often stated that all of the densitometry techniques measure the same properties of bone. However, it is not clear whether they actually represent the same properties or whether the measured quantities are comparable. Efforts have been made to compare measurement procedures in different laboratories and to calibrate instruments with the same or comparable standards (Moore and Wahner, 1974). For the present, standard clinical procedures are not a reality in densitometry, making it difficult to confirm the findings or to transfer patients to other centers for follow-up measurements.

The quantities that are measured by densitometry differ in their physical units. *Density* (mass per unit volume) is obtained only by the Compton-scattering method or by the analysis of excised bone samples. The *cortical index* is related to bone mass and is usually related to the total bone diameter or the cross-sectional area. The *bone mineral content* (mass per centimeter is measured by the single-photon absorptiometric method. The *area density* (mass per square centimeter) is determined by dual-photon absorptiometry.

The capability for accurately documenting bone mineral changes at the skeletal sites in which fractures have been demonstrated would be of considerable importance in identifying the risk of subsequent fracture. Radiogrammetry and radiographic photodensitometry are methods that can provide this type of measurement, but only in the appendicular skeleton, such as in the radius or femur. The single-photon absorptiometry (SPA) method is unable to provide measurements of bone mineral in the spine and hips, sites where most clinically important fractures occur (Fogelman, 1985). Many studies have been reported in which forearm measurements have been used; however, SPA has shown poor discrimination between osteoporotic and normal women (Christiansen et al., 1981), limiting the usefulness of the technique. Bone mineral content (BMC) of the radius as determined by single-photon absorptiometry has been useful in identifying appendicular osteopenia (Johnston et al., 1979). However, a normal BMC value of the radius does not exclude osteopenia of the axial skeleton.

By comparison, dual-photon absorptiometry (DPA) is regarded as a major advance in bone mineral measurement (Wahner et al., 1983). At the present time, experience with dual-photon absorptiometry comes largely from the United States and Scandinavia (Riggs et al., 1981; Krolner and Nielsen, 1982; Gotfredsen, 1984). Dual-photon absorptiometry has been used to obtain rectilinear scans of the lumbar vertebrae and femoral neck. The measured areal density represents a measure of both cortical and trabecular bone (Mazess,

1983). These studies have shown that DPA is highly accurate and reproducible. Most of the studies have been cross-sectional studies, however, and there is a clear need to document bone mineral changes in longitudinal studies in normal subjects. In addition, total-body bone mineral content (TBBM) has been determined by dual-photon absorptiometry. However, this relatively new measurement is used at only a few centers in the world (Peppler and Mazess, 1981). The advantages and disadvantages of both the SPA and DPA methods are discussed later.

Quantitative computed tomography has been developed as a viable procedure for the clinical determination of bone mineral density of the spinal vertebrae. Because CT is an accepted diagnostic tool in most radiology departments in this country and abroad, most clinicians have potential access to the CT procedures. The primary advantages of QCT are its applicability in the central skeleton and its ability to provide separate evaluations for the trabecular and the compact bone. QCT can also be used for densitometry of the appendicular skeleton if the equipment modifications are made available. A discussion of the QCT method is included in Chapter 5.

Although scattering methods are perhaps the least clinically developed procedures in densitometry, such methods offer the potential for additional quantitative information regarding the status of bone. No other method assesses directly the physical density of bone. The coherent-scatter methods provide information regarding the effective atomic number of tissues within the scattering volume as well as electron density information. Various Compton-scatter imaging methods have been developed with limited success for body imaging. These methods, as well as the fixed-point Compton-scatter methods, are discussed and compared with the most popular clinical densitometry methods.

Because the skeleton functions both for mechanical support and as a calcium reservoir, it is desirable to determine the strength and the calcium content of bones. In order to estimate the local bone strength, an assessment of the local bone itself must be made. Alternatively, the bone mineral content of another part of the skeleton may be assessed, provided there is a correlation between the two skeletal sites in terms of bone strength. In order to assess the total bone mineral (or calcium) in the body, a local bone mineral content measurement must be highly correlated with the total-body bone mineral content. The standard method for determination of total-body calcium is the method of in vivo neutron activation analysis (Cohn et al., 1970; Nelp et al., 1970). This method represents a direct measure of total skeletal mass, since 98% to 99% of the human body's calcium is stored in the skeleton (Chesnut et al., 1977). A study by Cohn et al. (1976) evaluated total-body calcium in 79 human subjects aged 30 to 90 years. It was determined that in females the average rate of loss of total-body calcium was 0.4% per year prior to menopause and 1.1% per year after menopause. This study supports the contention that bone loss in females is accelerated following the onset of menopause. In males, the average rate of TBCa loss was 0.7% per year after the age of 50. Females were found to lose approximately 28% of their maximum (age 30) TBCa by age 80, whereas males were found to lose only 20% of their maximum TBCa by age 80. In vivo neutron activation analysis techniques have provided a basis for comparison and testing of other noninvasive methods, and, in addition, they have yielded unique information about calcium metabolism in the body. However, the use of total body NAA is restricted by the relatively high radiation doses received by the patient (Krolner, 1985).

A qualitative method, which has been less successful in the assessment of osteoporosis, is radionuclide scanning. One approach has been the normal bone scintigram, in which markedly increased uptake is seen in the skull, mandible, ends of the femurs, and the proximal ends of the tibias (listed in order of the frequency of occurrence in metabolic bone disease). Radioisotopes of calcium, strontium, chlorine, phosphorus, sodium, and other elements have been used as tracers in studies of the skeleton (Bauer, 1968). ^{85}Sr, ^{87}Sr, and ^{18}Cl have been used for bone scanning; ^{99m}Tc-labeled phosphorus complexes have become widely used. Clinical imaging with ^{99m}Tc is done 24 hours after the intravenous injection of 10 to 20 millicuries. The radiation dose to the whole body is less than 0.2 rads. Bone takes up 30% to 40% of the injected ^{99m}Tc, and the rest of the isotope is excreted or taken up by soft tissues or blood (Holder, 1982). The radionuclide accumulates in regions of high bone blood flow and high bone turnover such as fractures, malignant tumors, and myositis ossificans, and these areas appear as "hot spots" in the scan image. The 24-hour whole-body retention study (^{99m}Tc-labeled phosphates) has been shown to be a more sensitive indicator than the qualitative bone scan or the regional bone-to-soft tissue ratio in differentiating normals and osteoporotics from patients with metabolic disease (Fogelman, 1978). However, the whole-body retention studies do not provide differentiation between normals and osteoporotics. In addition, these studies require the use of a whole-body counter, which is not generally available in the clinic.

Bone scans can be used to determine whether fractures are new or old, recent fractures demonstrating high uptake of the radionuclide. Approximately 24 months after the occurrence of a fracture, the radionuclide uptake is normal or only slightly elevated. Bone scans are not specific for osteopenic compression fractures, because the increased uptake can be seen in many conditions such as malignancies and infections. Stress fractures can be detected by bone scans approximately 2 weeks before these fractures can be demonstrated using standard radiographs. Osteopenia results in stress fractures of the femoral neck, ribs, calcanei, and pubis. In senile or postmenopausal osteoporosis, radionuclide bone scans demonstrate poor uptake of the radionuclide. The bone-to-soft tissue uptake ratio is low in these scans. However, in patients with known osteopenia, bone scans may be used to demonstrate metabolic bone diseases (high bone-to-soft tissue ratio), such as osteomalacia or renal osteodystrophy, in which there is a high turnover of bone tissue.

Bone densitometry methods have evolved over the years through various developmental stages. The current state-of-the-art in clinical densitometry is represented by the QCT and DPA methods, although research is continuing in other areas. The progress and development of this technology is slowed by the requirements for clinical testing of the sensitivity, accuracy, and precision of each new method. The in vivo discrimination of small changes in bone mass or density are necessary for the early detection of osteoporosis and other bone-related diseases. These requirements place stringent demands upon the design of noninvasive densitometry intrumentation.

2. RADIOGRAPHIC FILM METHODS

Osteoporosis remained an undetected and unmentioned disease until the 1920s. It was not until x-ray film methods came into widespread use in the 1920s that there was a means of visualizing the disease. As the life expectancy in humans increased in the early decades of the twentieth century, more people were living long enough to manifest the disease. In the 1930s and 1940s, routine x-ray film methods were used to detect osteoporosis (Davies and Saha, 1985). Today, the most widely available technique for the diagnosis of osteoporosis is the use of standard radiographs of the spine and other areas of the skeleton.

Radiographs are, however, insensitive indicators of bone loss; the bone density must have decreased by at least 30% (Lachman, 1955) before a significant reduction can be observed in the radiographic image. Radiographs can be used for establishing the diagnosis of osteoporosis only if secondary causes are excluded either clinically or roentgenographically. Other radiographic information may also be used to aid in the diagnosis, including the measurement of the cortical thickness of long bones and the use of the trabecular indices.

Roentgenographic methods for the evaluation of osteopenia are divided into three types: (1) qualitative, (2) semi-quantitative, and (3) quantitative. The qualitative methods include plain film radiography and radionuclide bone scanning, and are usually the initial techniques used in the clinical diagnosis of osteopenia. Semiquantitative methods are those that are based upon a grading system for osteopenia, such as the Singh index, and may include the evaluation of selected parameters in radionuclide bone scanning. Semiquantitative methods often lack the sensitivity, precision, and accuracy of the quantitative methods. Quantitative methods include radiogrammetry and radiographic photodensitometry.

Radiographs are helpful in excluding focal bone disorders and in detecting advanced diffused disease of the skeleton. Therefore, standard radiographs should be the first test, including unilateral radiographs of the thoracic spine, biplanar views of the lumbar spine, and occassionally radiographs of the pelvis and hips with internal rotation of the feet. The spine and hips are searched for signs of osteopenia — a vertical striation picture frame appearance, visibility of iliac crest through L4 and L5 on the lateral spine film, a general density decrease — and then for evidence of ballooning, wedging, or collapse of the vertebrae. The radiographs of the hips are inspected for trabecular changes of the femoral neck and head, and thickness of the calcor femorale (cortical thicknesses of both minor trochanter). This method may be satisfactory for the diagnosis of bone loss in advanced cases of osteoporosis when compression fractures have already occurred.

RADIOGRAPHIC DIAGNOSIS (RADIOSCOPY)

The criteria for diagnosing osteopenia from standard radiographs are: (1) radiolucency, (2) trabecular pattern changes with loss of trabeculae, (3) cortical thinning, and (4) fractures of vertebral bodies, femoral necks, intertrochanteric regions, humeri, distal radii, ribs, and ischial and public rami. Because of the subjective nature of the diagnosis, the course of osteopenia is difficult to follow using standard radiographs (Schneider, 1984). The more quantitative methods may therefore be useful.

Qualitative morphometry may be performed by observing the vertebral density from a lateral radiograph of the lumbar spine. It is important that the selected vertebra is nondeformed. The radiolucency of the radiographic image of the spine is produced by loss of trabecular bone in the vertebral bodies. Bone loss in the spine may be observed by the presence of vertical trabeculae appearing as vertical striations. During the process of skeletal atrophy the transverse trabeculae waste more rapidly than the vertical ones. If the trabeculae are resorbed, the vertebral body demonstrates a hollow appearance. A grading system based upon the appearance of these vertical trabeculae has been used (Aitken, 1984). However, this type of assessment is highly subjective, and variations in the radiographic technique may produce serious artifacts.

The most useful diagnostic criterion for osteopenia observed in standard radiographs is the compression fracture of the vertebral body. Anterior wedging (loss of height on the anterior aspect of the vertebral body) may be observed. Both anterior and posterior compression may also be found; the height of the vertebrae may be compared to their normal adjacent vertebrae. However, other conditions that may present or appear as deformities may be mistaken for osteopenic vertebral deformities. Biconcavity of the vertebral endplates may signal weakness of the vertebral body and loss of bone mineral (Schneider,

1984). Osteoporosis in children is more likely to reveal biconcavity in several vertebrae, but compression fractures are more common in adults (Pitt, 1983).

Horsman (1976) presented a method for the determination of the number and severity of vertebral compressions from spinal radiographs. A semiquantitative method using an index of biconcavity of the lumbar vertebrae has not proved to be sufficiently accurate for diagnosing osteopenia (Doyle et al., 1967). Virtama et al. (1962) found no correlation between the biconcavity index and the actual vertebral bone density. In the assessment of osteopenia and skeletal status, the degree of biconcavity of the vertebral bodies is now largely discounted as being neither reliable nor diagnostic. The biconcavity index does not change with age in normal females and does not reliably discriminate osteoporotics, although it is related to the number and extent of vertebral fractures (Mazess, 1979).

Factors that influence the diagnosis from a radiographic image include: (1) radiographic technique, (2) film-screen combination, (3) film processing, (4) overlying tissue thickness, and (5) patient positioning. The use of high kilovoltage techniques can increase the latitude on the film, making the bony regions appear more grey (less dense), whereas low kilovoltage techniques make the bone appear more white (more dense) in the radiographs. Radiographic changes in the spine provide the best evidence for osteoporosis (Siegelman, 1970).

The radiographic technique used in the procedure is another significant factor in the potential diagnosis of osteopenia in the vertebral bodies. If the x-ray beam is not parallel to the vertebral endplates, the endplates will not overlap, and it may be difficult to determine if a deformity is present, especially in patients with scoliosis. Positioning of the patient, therefore, may have a strong influence upon the ability to reproduce the deformity or to find new deformities of the vertebrae in subsequent radiographs taken at a later date (Schneider, 1984).

A qualitative method for viewing the cortical bone resorption patterns of the hand has been used in which fine detailed radiographic films are analyzed with a magnification eyepiece (7X). Microradioscopy is helpful in differentiating the possible causes of osteopenia but is not common in clinical practice. Thinning of the cortex in the metacarpals may be detected by this method, in which bone resorption may be observed as suggested by irregularities on the endosteal surface. When striations or longitudinal lucencies appear in the intracortical region, high bone turnover as well as cortical thinning may indicate conditions such as hyperparathyroidism, osteomalacia, and hyperthyroidism (Meema and Meema, 1975; Meema and Schatz, 1970).

TRABECULAR INDICES

Changes in the trabecular pattern of the upper end of the femur (Singh index) and of the calcaneus represent semiquantitative methods of diagnosing and rating osteopenia (Jhamaria et al., 1983; Singh et al., 1970). A simple grading

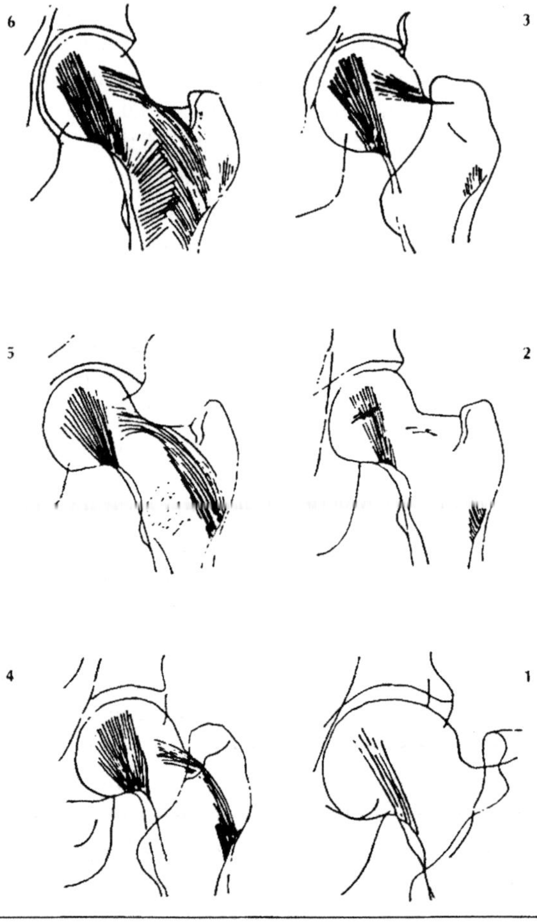

Figure 3. Singh Index. Severe osteoporosis (1,2) represented by loss of trabeculae (Courtesy: HR Fish)

system has been applied following the taking of radiographs in which the hips were viewed using a 15° internal rotation (Singh et al., 1972). The assumption was made that bone loss is more rapid in trabecular bone than in cortical bone and that the trabecular pattern indicated the degree of vertebral osteoporosis (figure 3). Singh suggested that the trabecular index was superior to the cortical thickness measurements for detecting vertebral osteoporosis (Singh, 1976). Later studies by other investigators supported his suggestion (Wahner et al., 1977), while other studies were unable to verify that superiority of the Singh Index (Aloia et al., 1977). Dequeker et al. (1974) have suggested that the Singh Index is valuable in identifying patients who are particularly susceptible to femoral neck fractures (Dequeker et al., 1974).

The striated patterns that can be observed in radiographs of the upper end of

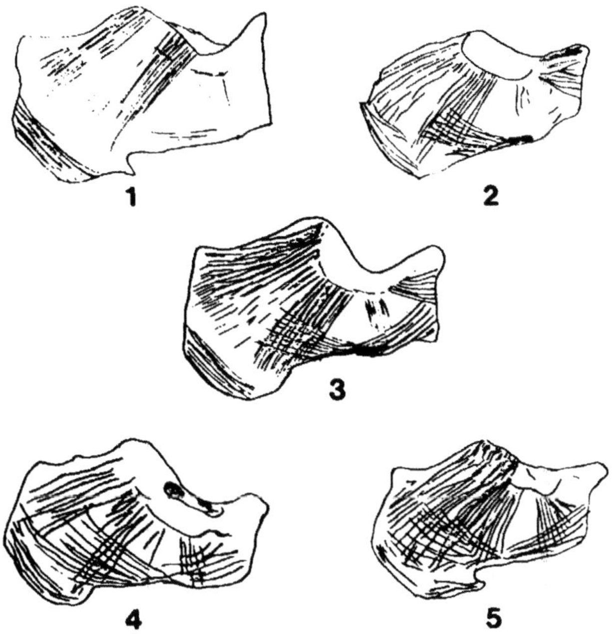

Figure 4. Calcaneal osteoporotic index given by Jhamaria, 1983 (Courtesy: WP Cockshott)

the femur are the trabeculae of the weight-bearing cancellous bone. The appearance of these trabeculae depends upon the compressive and tensile stresses to which the femur is subjected. The tensile trabeculae are generally lost earlier than the compressive trabeculae. The degree to which trabeculae are lost produces a pattern that is identifiable in different stages. It has been stated that intraobserver variation and lack of sensitivity in diagnosing early osteoporosis limit the usefulness of this technique (Schneider, 1984).

The trabecular pattern of the femoral neck was found to be poorly correlated with forearm bone mineral content (Kranedonk et al., 1972; Khairi et al., 1976) as determined by single-photon absorptiometry and with lumbar spine scores (Dalen and Lamke, 1974). In addition, the femoral trabecular index was poorly correlated with total-body calcium (Aloia et al., 1975). Roh (1973) found that 49% of patients with vertebral collapse had normal values for the trabecular index.

A calcaneal morphologic index was investigated by Cockshott et al. (1984) in which the trabecular patterns of the os calcis (heel) were evaluated. Using lateral radiographs of the foot, the method of Jhamaria et al. (1983) was used to score the trabecular patterns on a five-point scale (figure 4). The grading system was reported to fail, however, as it showed no correlation with the actual bone density of the os calcis. The bone density was determined by the Compton scattering method described by Webber and Kennett (1976).

PRINCIPLES OF RADIOGRAMMETRY

Radiogrammetry is the measurement of the thickness of the cortex of the metacarpal or other tubular bones using standard antero-posterior roentgenograms. This method is noninvasive but it involves minimal radiation exposures of the extremities, with negligible bone marrow and gonadal radiation. The method generally provides information on the relative changes in bone volume of an individual, but it is not useful for evaluation of the axial skeleton (American College of Physicians, 1984). Radiogrammetry is applicable only in the appendicular skeleton for sites including the radius, humerus, femur, clavicle, and tibia. Radiogrammetry does not provide the absolute bone mineral content measurement, and it does not measure intracortical bone mineral porosity.

Radiogrammetry is a simple and inexpensive method for evaluating bone loss. Because the method utilizes standard radiographic equipment, it is easily performed in the radiology department. During the aging process of the human skeleton, the long bones become larger in diameter, while the cortex becomes thinner. The medullary (marrow) cavity width (M) increases in diameter, although at a faster rate than the bone width (W). Radiogrammetry provides a method for obtaining information on perosteal bone remodeling (outer diameter of the cortex) and endosteal resorption (inner diameter of the cortex) (Garn et al., 1967). Several indices have been defined for studying the behavior and interactions of these parameters.

Fine detailed radiographs, in which the thicknesses of the cortices of bones are measured with calipers, provides an index for bone density or bone mass (Bloom and Libson, 1983; Evans et al., 1978; Horsman and Simpson, 1975). Radiogrammetry is a reliable procedure when utilized by trained personnel who ensure the consistency of the technique and accurate results. It has also been stated that radiogrammetry is well correlated with densitometric measurements in the radius (Meema and Meema, 1972).

However, conflicting results have been noted by other investigators, who have found that radiogrammetric values are only moderately correlated with the bone mineral content by photon absorptiometry (Mazess et al., 1970). This moderate correlation makes it difficult to predict the radius BMC or other BMC values from parameters such as the cortical area. Furthermore, the correlations between radiogrammetric values and the total-body calcium by neutron activation are generally far poorer than those obtained with absorptiometry (Aloia et al., 1977; Manzke et al., 1975). More recent studies have shown that radiogrammetric methods reflect fairly well the changes in bone mass (e.g., in involutional osteoporosis). Conventional radiogrammetry permits quite accurate measurement of cortical bone volume or thickness (Meema and Meema, 1981).

Radiogrammetry methods are based upon the assumptions that the measured bone (1) is of cylindrical shape on the outer and inner surfaces, (2) contains uniformity of the cortex, (3) has reproducible positioning for radiography, (4) has minimal surrounding tissue, and (5) is well correlated with skeletal bone mass. Some believe that the best single parameter for separation of normal and osteoporotic women is the cortical thickness index used by Barnett and Nordin (Dequeker, 1982). The normalization of the measured parameters has been proposed to account for variations in skeletal size; however, longitudinal studies are best performed without this correction.

COMBINED CORTICAL THICKNESS

The combined cortical thickness is given by $C = W - M$ and has been shown to be correlated ($r = 0.68$) with bone mass (Horsman and Kirby, 1972). This index is thought by some investigators to be a good indicator of age-related bone loss (Virtama and Helela, 1969; Helela, 1970; Morgan, 1973). The cortical thickness as measured by the metacarpal index correlates moderately well with both regional and total skeletal osteopenia; this index also correlates well with compression fractures of the spine (Wahner, 1984).

BARNETT-NORDIN INDEX

This parameter may be obtained from the radiographic image of a long bone in which the combined cortical thickness (C) and total width (W) have been measured with calipers. The Barnett-Nordin Index is computed: $C/W \times 100$. It has been assumed that the cortical thickness is a measure of bone mass and that the ratio of cortical-to-total width is a measure of bone density (Garn, 1970; Kivilaasko and Palolampi, 1965).

CORTICAL AREA

Another indicator is the cross-sectional cortical area ($CA = 0.785\,[W^2 - M^2]$), which is moderately well correlated ($r = 0.78$ to 0.85) with the absolute bone mass (Horsman and Kirby, 1972; Gryfe et al., 1972). However, CA is rarely used in clinicial studies, because it is more dependent upon the bone width W than on the marrow cavity width M and is therefore not a sensitive measure of endosteal bone resorption and loss of bone mass (Meema and Meema, 1981). Some investigators believe that the cross-sectional area of long bones, when calculated using the assumption that bone is cylindrical at the site of the measurement, is more closely related to the mass than the density; but there is considerable variability in this relationship (Horsman and Kirby, 1972). Mazess (1979) has stated that the compact bone area correlates only moderately with the actual bone mass, the error being 10% to 20%. In addition, the compact bone areas at different skeletal locations are only moderately intercorrelated ($r = 0.5 - 0.7$). Thus, the choice of a measurement site is important, since the cortical area measured at one site cannot be used to accurately predict the cortical area at another site.

PERCENT CORTICAL AREA

The percent cortical area is determined:

$$\%CA = \frac{W^2 - M^2}{W^2} \cdot 100$$

This index has a high diagnostic sensitivity for the detection of bone loss resulting from endosteal resorption.

EXTON-SMITH INDEX

The Exton-Smith index is defined as the ratio of the cortical area to the surface area ($[W^2 - M^2]/WL$), where L is the length of the bone. This index is more applicable to studies in children, because the bone mass is normalized to WL, which compensates for growth (Gryfe et al., 1971).

PRINCIPLES OF METACARPAL MEASUREMENTS

Radiogrammetry of the midshaft of the second metacarpal is the most common bone measurement performed in clinical practice. It was first used by Barnett and Nordin (1960); other investigators further studied the method (Garn, 1970; Dequeker, 1972; Smith and Frame, 1965; Morgan et al., 1967).

Usually, the second metacarpal of the nondominant hand or several metacarpals from one or both hands are investigated (figure 5). This method requires a high quality radiograph taken under standardized conditions. The palm of the hand must be firmly flattened against the film cassette for better visualizing the periosteal margins of the metacarpal in the image; this position is highly reproducible and lends itself to repeated studies. Industrial fine-grain film is required with the x-ray generator set for approximately 50 kVp and 20 mAs. The focus-film distance is 100 cm, and the films are processed in an automatic processor. The outer and inner diameters of the metacarpal cortex are measured with an accuracy of 0.1 mm using high precision needle-tipped calipers; the measurement is performed at the midpoint of the second metacarpal, as determined by measurement of its total length (figure 6). The thickness of the cortex is measured along the line through the midpoint and perpendicular to the long axis of the metacarpal bone. The radiation dose to the patient's hands as measured using an electrometer and ionization chamber is about 40 mrem (Aitken, 1984).

The following indices are derived from measurements of the total width (TW) and the medullary width (MW) on the second metacarpal (Aitken, 1984):

The metacarpal index (MI) is defined:

$$MI = \frac{TW - MW}{TW}$$

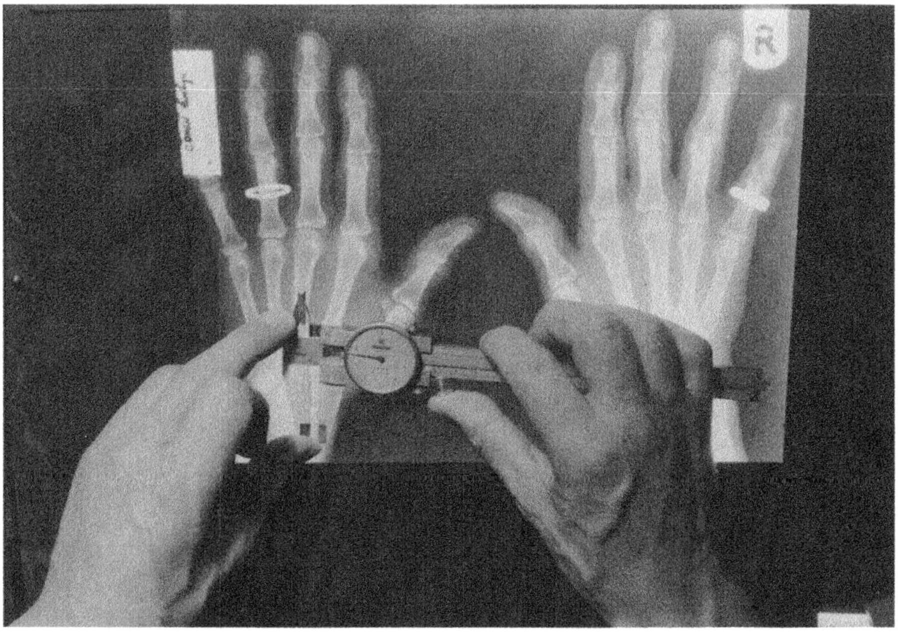

Figure 5. Measurement of metacarpal dimensions (Courtesy: M Aitken)

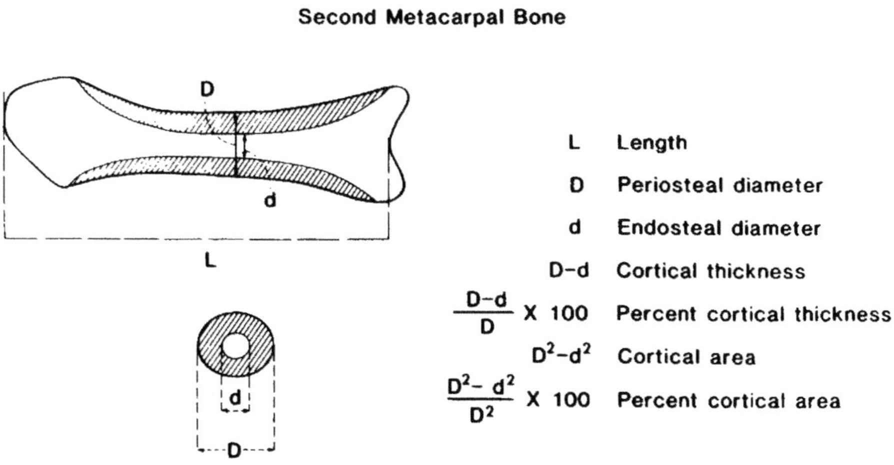

Figure 6. Basic measurements in radiogrammetry (Courtesy: HW Wahner)

The percentage cortical thickness (hand score, HS) is defined:

$$HS = MI \cdot 100$$

The percentage cortical area (%CA) is defined:

$$\frac{(TW^2 - MW^2)}{TW^2} \cdot 100$$

The cortical area (CA) is defined:

$$CA = \frac{\pi}{4}(TW^2 - MW^2).$$

The cortical area/surface area (CA/SA) is defined:

$$\frac{CA}{SA} = \frac{TW^2 - MW^2}{4L \cdot TW}$$

where L is the metacarpal length, introduced to provide a correction of the cortical area for body size. Unfortunately, the measurement of the metacarpal length introduces another source of error when using the index CA/SA.

The %CA is thought to be as accurate and reproducible as CA/SA. Measurements of the medullary and total widths for the six middle metacarpals of both hands are combined to calculate the six-metacarpal hand score (6MHS) and the six-metacarpal percentage cortical area (6M%CA). The volume of cortical bone may be calculated from the cortical area by employing the simplistic assumption that the metacarpal is cylindrical in shape at the site of the measurement. The time required for the measurement is minimal, and it takes about 10 minutes for the technician to calculate the 6MHS index.

The following objections to the use of metacarpal measurements have included: (1) This bone rarely fractures, and (2) it is composed primarily of cortical bone. These facts make it difficult to extrapolate these peripheral assessments to critical areas of the skeleton such as the vertebral bodies, distal radius, and the proximal femur, where fractures commonly occur (Aitken, 1984). In vitro experiments have shown that the mineral content per unit volume of whole bone at the metacarpal midshaft and the mineral content per unit volume of the body of the third lumbar vertebra yield a good correlation ($r = 0.67$).

MAGNIFICATION TECHNIQUES

Magnification radiogrammetry improves the ability to detect intracortical porosity, which cannot be observed using the standard technique (Meema and Schatz, 1970). This technique utilizes stereoscopic microscopes or high-power magnifiers with up to 10X magnification, using fine-grain industrial films. Abnormal intracortical resorptive processes can be observed with this procedure, such as thyrotoxicosis, hyperparathyroid disease, and acromegaly. These disease processes may be differentiated from low bone-turnover diseases, such as osteoporosis and Cushing's Syndrome.

VERTEBRAL MEASUREMENTS

Barnett and Nordin (1960) investigated the use of the *lumbar spine score*. Micrometer measurements were made from lateral radiographs of the vertebrae, in which the heights AB and CD of the vertebrae were measured at the anterior and midsections of the vertebrae, respectively. The lumbar spine score was defined by:

$$\frac{AB}{CD} \cdot 100.$$

However, in a later study of excised vertebrae (Hanson and Roos, 1980), the lumbar spine score (radiographic method) showed no correlation with the bone mineral content (dual-photon absorptiometry method). It was found that the highest precision of the lumbar spine score was obtained when the measurements of the actual heights of the vertebrae were made from lateral tomograms. Hanson and Roos (1980) concluded that the radiographic method does not adequately reflect the bone mineral content of the vertebrae.

RADIUS MEASUREMENTS

Cortical bone measurements at the proximal end of the radius are well suited for radiogrammetric evaluation because of the nearly cylindrical cross section of the radial shaft at this site (Meema, 1962). The combined cortical thickness (C) is determined by standard lateral radiography of the elbow with the hand supinated. In the radiographic image, the cortical thickness is measured in the region of parallel cortices distal to the tuberosity. Positioning of the proximal radius may not be as reproducible as the metacarpal of the hand, because of possible rotation of the arm. The use of a horizontal x-ray beam and a vertical film cassette with fine detail screens (industrial film) improves the radiographic detail and reduces geometrical distortion since the proximal radius is positioned closer to the image receptor (Meema and Meema, 1981).

The combined cortical thickness C of the proximal radius was shown to be significantly correlated ($r = 0.61$) with the fat-free dry weight of the iliac crest biopsy (Saville, 1965). However, the correlation between the radius and the spine is not good; for men, $r = 0.59$ and for women, $r = 0.34$. The correlation between the metacarpal and the spine is worse ($r = 0.1$) (Horsman, 1976).

Meema suggested the measurement of the "minimum" combined cortical thickness (Min CCT) for the diagnosis of maximum endosteal resorption.

Table 1. Bone mineral mass (M), and density (D) in the proximal radial shaft in normal men and women according to age (Courtesy: HE Meema)

		M (g/cm)		D (g/cm^3)	
Decade	n*	Men	Women	Men	Women
20–29	46/56	1.314 ± 0.237	0.956 ± 0.140	1.134 ± 0.112	1.186 ± 0.104
30–39	37/58	1.364 ± 0.228	0.940 ± 0.148	1.147 ± 0.104	1.179 ± 0.098
40–49	42/62	1.292 ± 0.198	0.929 ± 0.174	1.132 ± 0.106	1.166 ± 0.115
50–59	46/48	1.251 ± 0.248	0.875 ± 0.161	1.074 ± 0.125	1.105 ± 0.144
60–69	63/37	1.161 ± 0.240	0.685 ± 0.132	1.004 ± 0.158	0.984 ± 0.170
70–79	42/30	1.056 ± 0.226	0.559 ± 0.168	0.977 ± 0.156	0.899 ± 0.189
80–89	16/11	0.949 ± 0.260	0.610 ± 0.083	0.937 ± 0.195	1.033 ± 0.163

* number of men/women

The measurement site was selected on the basis of the size of the head of the radius; a distance of 2.5 times the diameter of the head of the radius; a distance of 2.5 times the diameter of the head of the radius was measured from the capitulum humeri and marked on the radiograph. A 5-mm long region of the radius at this distance was used for the CCT measurement. The smallest cortical thicknesses within the region were measured on both sides of the marrow cavity and summed (A + B). Normal ranges for Min CCT have been given for men and women (Meema and Meema, 1967; Meema and Meema, 1976).

Meema and Meema (1978) published normal ranges of bone mineral mass (g/cm), bone mineral density (g/cc), combined cortical thickness C, and external width W in the proximal radial shaft for men and women according to age (tables 1 and 2). The bone mineral mass per unit length of bone M_2 was calculated by the equation (Meema et al., 1976):

$$M_2 = \frac{\pi}{4} \cdot M_1 \cdot (2W - C),$$

where M_1 is the bone mineral mass expressed as mineral thickness in g/cm^2. M_2 is an expression of the mineral content of a cross-sectional slice of bone 1 cm in length. This quantity is consistent with the bone mineral mass as determined by the Cameron-Sorenson method. Meema has noted that the separate determination of the combined cortical thickness and bone mineral density provide greater insight into the resorptive processes in cortical bone than the single-photon absorptiometric measurements (g/cm) alone. Measurement of bone mineral density was thought be the only way to diagnose intracortical porosity in the bones of the forearm and leg. The coefficient of variation for bone mineral density measurements was given as 9% for women and 9.4% for men (aged 20 to 49 years), whereas the coefficients for the cortical thickness measurements were approximately 10% and 11%, respectively. The coefficient

Table 2. Combined cortical thickness (C), and external width (W) in the proximal radial shaft in normal men and women according to age (Courtesy: HE Meema)

		C (cm)		W (cm)	
Decade	n*	Men	Women	Men	Women
20–29	46/56	0.71 ± 0.08	0.61 ± 0.06	1.39 ± 0.10	1.15 ± 0.09
30–39	37/58	0.72 ± 0.08	0.60 ± 0.06	1.42 ± 0.13	1.15 ± 0.09
40–49	42/62	0.70 ± 0.08	0.60 ± 0.06	1.40 ± 0.11	1.15 ± 0.11
50–59	46/48	0.69 ± 0.09	0.58 ± 0.06	1.42 ± 0.11	1.15 ± 0.08
60–69	63/37	0.68 ± 0.10	0.48 ± 0.10	1.43 ± 0.09	1.18 ± 0.08
70–79	42/30	0.64 ± 0.09	0.41 ± 0.10	1.40 ± 0.13	1.18 ± 0.09
80–89	16/11	0.59 ± 0.15	0.39 ± 0.07	1.41 ± 0.14	1.17 ± 0.08

* number of men/women

of variation for bone mineral mass measurements (g/cm) were said to be higher.

PRECISION AND ACCURACY (RADIOGRAMMETRY)

The disadvantages of the radiogrammetric methods include errors in patient repositioning and errors in the precision and accuracy of the caliper measurements. The method is limited because it reflects changes in cortical bone but not in trabecular bone. In addition, intracortical resorption of bone, which is found in osteopenia, causes high bone turnover, porosity, and decreased bone density, which may not be reflected by the cortical thickness measurement (Schneider, 1984). Technical problems limit the precision and accuracy of the method, such as beam hardening, scattered radiation, variations in the thickness of overlying tissues, subtle changes in the kVp or mA of the x-ray machine, and variations in film development.

Van Gerven et al. (1969) have shown that the measured widths from radiographs do not yield the actual bone widths. It has been shown that the bone width is systematically overestimated in radiographs (Roh, 1973). Divergence of the x-ray beam inevitably causes the consistent overestimation of these widths. However, the determination of the ratio of the cortical-to-total width eliminates the effect of the slight magnification of these dimensions in the radiograph, rendering the effect insignificant in patient studies. Tilting of the hand leads to significant errors due to the triangular cross section of the metacarpal. Aitken (1984) has stated that about 25% of radiographs of the second metacarpal alone were not amenable to reproducible measurements, whereas only 11% of radiographs used to measure the 6MHS (six-metacarpal hand score) were not amenable to reproducible measurements. The mean percentage difference between pairs of films on 100 consecutive patients for 6MHS was 2.99%.

The errors associated with measurements of the cortical thickness at the center of the second metacarpal, as measured by radiogrammetry, have been reported to be in the range of 3% to 10% (intraobserver error) and 8% to 11% (interobserver error) (Adams et al., 1969; Morgan et al., 1967; Dequeker, 1977). The primary difficulty in the cortex measurement is the determination of the inner diameter adjacent to trabecular bone; the inner diameter is more difficult to define as bone loss progresses. Under the best of circumstances, radiogrammetry can detect only advanced stages of osteoporosis and is not useful for early detection of the disease. Cortical thickness is not well correlated with risk factors for spinal compression fractures. The method, however, is useful for epidemiological studies in advanced diseases. The range of overlap between osteoporotic and normal populations is significant. Some investigations have shown that less than 5% of the cases with osteoporosis lie beyond two standard deviations from the normal cortical thickness index. Radiogrammetry has shown that the cortical thickness is greater in men than in women at all bone sites and decreases with age in both men and women; the cortical thickness decreases more rapidly in women for 10 to 15 years after menopause (Wahner, 1984).

Radiogrammetry in the elderly population and in patients with bone disease is less accurate and less precise than in the healthy young population (Arnold, 1970; Meema and Meema, 1969; Atkinson and Weatherall, 1967). The inaccuracy and imprecision are the result of the inability of radiogrammetry to take into account the intracortical porosities and endosteal erosion of cortical bone. The precision error of the compact bone area measurements is about 5 to 10% (Adams et al., 1969; Naor et al., 1972). The precision error can be reduced to 1 to 2% by making measurements of several bones at the same time (Dequeker, 1977; Horsman, et al., 1977).

CLINICAL MEASUREMENTS

The following characteristics of cortical bone have been confirmed using metacarpal measurements: (1) MW increases with age and is consistent with an aging effect, (2) the total width of the second metacarpal does not change in respect to age, time, or cohort, (3) the length of the second metacarpal does not change once adulthood has been reached in males, (4) CT decreases with increasing age, (5) since TW remains unchanged with age, the MW increase is responsible for the decrease in cortical thickness, and (6) PCA decreases with increasing age and is a result of the decrease in cortical area.

Radiogrammetry was utilized in a recent study of postmenopausal osteoporosis (Elias et al., 1985). The method described by Garn (1970) was used to determine metacarpal cortical thickness ($C = T - M$, where T = total metacarpal diameter and M = medullary diameter). Cortical thicknesses from three metacarpal measurements were summed. In addition, cortical and medullary diameters of the radius were measured at the site determined as one-third the distance from the distal end. Finally, the left femur was measured at a location one-fourth the distance from the greater trochanter.

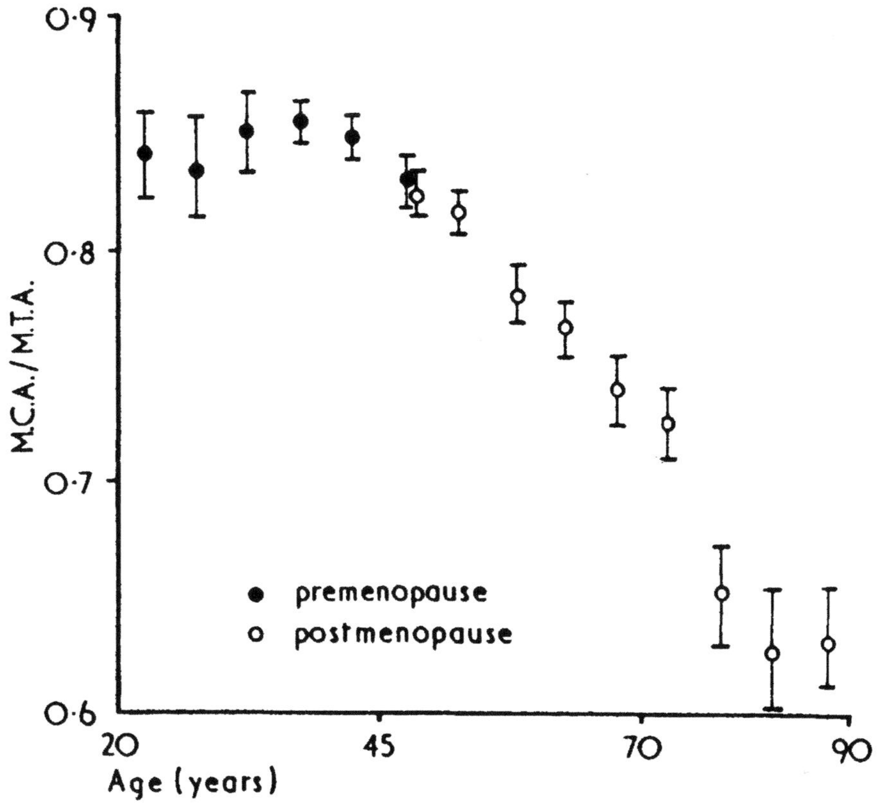

Figure 7. Metacarpal cortical/total area ratios for females (Courtesy: BEC Nordin)

Fox et al. (1986) reported on a longitudinal study (Baltimore Longitudinal Study of Aging) of bone loss in males from 1958 to 1981. Hand-wrist radiographs (left hand) were obtained and were evaluated for total width (TW), medullary width (MW), and length of the second metacarpal. The hand-wrist (AP) radiographs were taken using Kodak RP/S X-Omat film (60 kVp and 100 mAs). Measurements of TW, MW, and length of the second metacarpal were made at the midshaft of the bone using calipers with an accuracy of 0.5 mm. The cortical thickness (CT) was derived from the measurments (TW − MW). The percent cortical area (PCA) was defined as the ratio of cortical area (CA) to the total area (TA) of the bone (PCA = TA/CA × 100).

The largest data base for cortical thickness measurements was accumulated in the Finnish population (Virtama and Helela, 1969). Mean bone widths and mean combined cortical thicknesses versus age for this large population were tabulated for the clavicle, radius, ulna, humerus, metacarpals, phalanges, femur, tibia, fibula, and metatarsals for adults. Mean values for normal populations in different countries (different races) are expected to vary (Virtama,

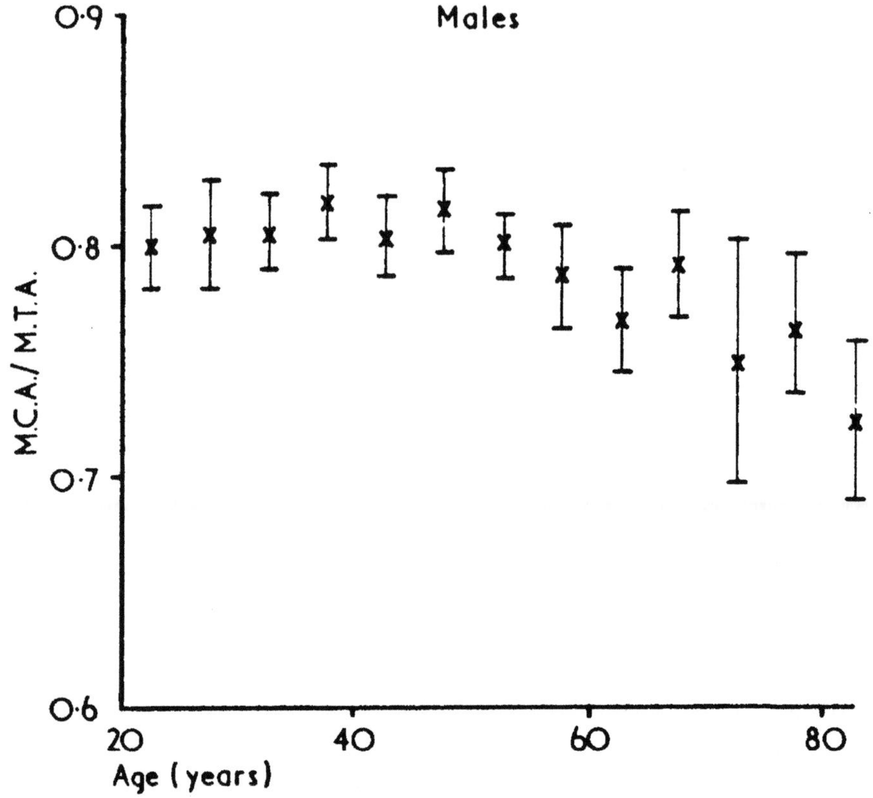

Figure 8. Metacarpal cortical/total area ratios for males (Courtesy: BEC Nordin)

1976). Cortical thickness data for other skeletal sites (figures 7, 8, 9) has been published (Meema and Meema, 1963; Bloom and Laws, 1970; Helela, 1969; Anton, 1969; Fisher and Hausser, 1970; Smith and Walker, 1964; Barnett and Nordin, 1960).

RADIOGRAPHIC PHOTODENSITOMETRY

Photodensitometry is a quantitative method that gives an indication of the bone mineral content determined from radiographic films of the skeleton. The method may be described as *radiographic absorptiometry*, in which the bone mineral content is determined by measurement of the optical density of the film. This is probably the oldest noninvasive method for assessing bone mineral. Variations in the thicknesses of tissues overlying the skeletal region of interest can affect the film density. Therefore, photodensitometry is not generally applicable to the axial skeleton and is usually restricted to the appendicular skeleton. The phalanges, radius, tibia, and other appendicular bones are selected for this technique.

Because routinely obtained radiographs may vary widely in radiographic

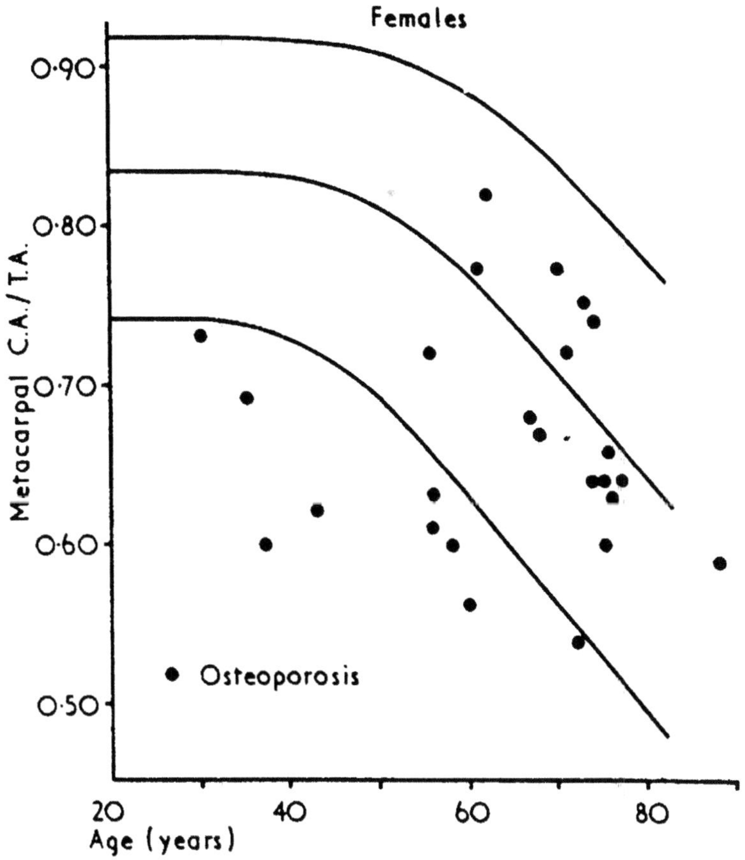

Figure 9. Metacarpal cortical/total area ratios in normal females and osteoporotic females (Courtesy: BEC Nordin)

film density, a standardization technique is used that compensates for small changes in the x-ray exposure factors (kVp, mA, exposure time, and film-processing). An aluminum wedge is simultaneously exposed and appears in the radiographic image; the wedge serves as a standard in which its measured optical density is compared with the optical densities for bone. Changes in the exposure factors or other factors are detected as changes in the optical density of the aluminum wedge; a correction based on this measured change is then applied to the optical density value for bone. A commercially available densitometer is used to determine the optical densities in the regions of interest of the radiograph. Densitometers may measure the optical density of a spot, line, or area. Radiographic methods in which a standard is not used, but which instead rely on a comparison between the optical densities of suspected bone and normal bone usually yield unacceptable results (Wahner et al., 1984).

The most acceptable photodensitometry methods incorporate a soft-tissue (water) phantom, in which the hand is immersed. The film is placed beneath

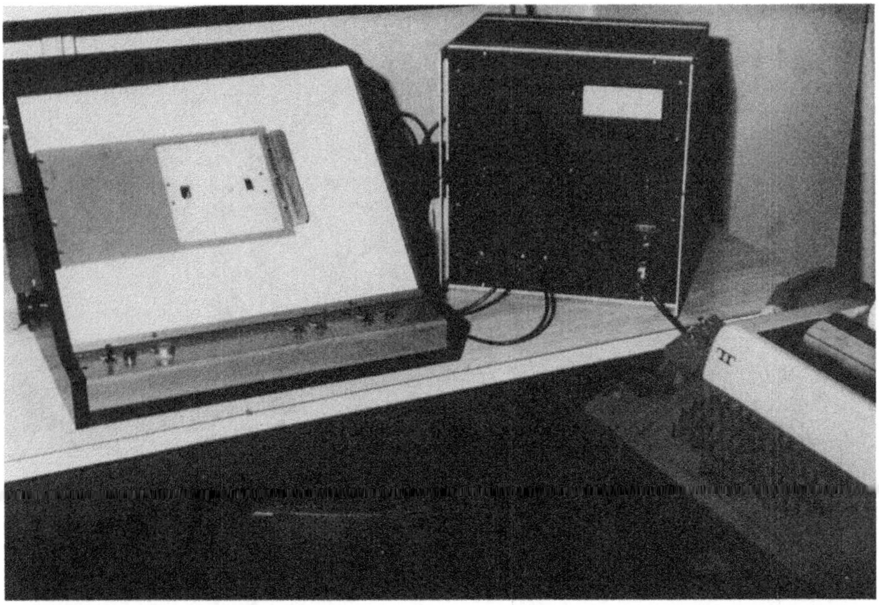

Figure 10. Semi-automated morphometer for cortical bone measurement (Courtesy: A Horsman)

the phantom for the exposure. A microdensitometer and computer system are used for the high resolution analysis of the radiographic film. This method has been used for assessing the bone mineral density of the metacarpals in studies of the response of bone to various treatment regimens for osteoporosis and other metabolic bone diseases. The results are expressed as areal densities (Colbert and Bachtell, 1981). Under the best conditions, however, the method does not provide the best precision and accuracy, as compared with other photon absorptiometry procedures (Colbert et al., 1970).

A computerized method was proposed for increasing the precision of the photodensitometry method. For clinical measurements, Horsman et al. (1977) developed a semi-automated computer-controlled morphometer (figure 10) for measuring changes in the mean width of cortices of the second, third, and fourth metacarpals in oophorectomized women. The film was clamped between a glass plate and an illuminated opaque Perspex screen engraved with a graticule. The morphometer was interfaced with a PDP-12 computer. A motor-driven vertical cursor and two horizontal markers attached to a precision linear potentiometer provided a computer signal that recorded the location of the densitometry measurement. The control panel of the morphometer allowed the operator to control the computer software. The measurements were made at the mid-points of the diaphyses of the metacarpals. The operator positioned the vertical cursor on the periosteal and endosteal boundaries, recording the position at the push of a button. The computer calculated the mean total width, mean medullary width, and mean cortical width for the six metacarpals measured for each patient. The errors associated with this automated method (<0.1 mm) were found to be comparable with those using calipers (Horsman and Simpson, 1975).

PRECISION AND ACCURACY (PHOTODENSITOMETRY)

Earlier evaluations of the radiographic photodensitometric methods were susceptible to large precision and accuracy errors (30%) in areas of heavy tissue cover (Mazess, 1982; Baker et al., 1959). Systematic inaccuracies and imprecision occur in radiographic photodensitometry because of inherent limitations in the use of x-ray tubes and generators. These limitations include: (1) nonuniformity of the radiation field, (2) unwanted scattered radiation, (3) polychromaticity of the x-ray spectrum, which contributes to beam hardening, and (4) variations in the x-ray spectrum and in the film response. In addition, the densitometric measurement is affected by the soft tissues on either side of the bone and within the marrow cavity.

The precision of routine photodensitometry is 5% to 10%. The accuracy for excised bones is 3% to 5%; for bones with a slight tissue cover, 5% to 10%; and for bones with large tissue cover, 10% to 30% (Mazess, 1979). The in vivo photodensitometry measurements demonstrated a good correlation ($r = 0.88$) with the in vitro bone ash per unit volume of the metacarpal. This level of accuracy is less than that obtainable with cortical thickness measurements and much less than that of photon absorptiometry. Aitken (1984) found a reproducibility of approximately 5%, which was better than that of radiogrammetry, but was inferior to that obtained with the use of six measurements (three middle metacarpals on each hand). The radiation dose associated with the radiographic photodensitometric method is about 40 mrem, the same as that of the radiogrammetry method. The major disadvantage of the photodensitometric method compared with radiogrammetry is the cost of a precision film densitometer (Aitken, 1984).

VIDEODENSITOMETRY

A scanning slit x-ray video absorptiometry method has been developed as an improvement of the photodensitometric method (Dobbins et al., 1981). Further developments of the method led to an in vivo system for the determination of the bone mineral content (BMC). Difficult measurements such as the femoral neck site were possible with this system (figure 11). A standard fluoroscopic machine with a 6-inch cesium-iodide image intensifier was used. A heavily filtered (0.2 mm brass filter) x-ray tube was used for the radiation source in conjunction with a single-phase generator operating in the fluoroscopic mode with tube voltages of 60 to 120 kVp. The x-ray tube (with 0.6 mm focal spot) was housed below the patient tabletop. The tabletop exposure rate was ap-

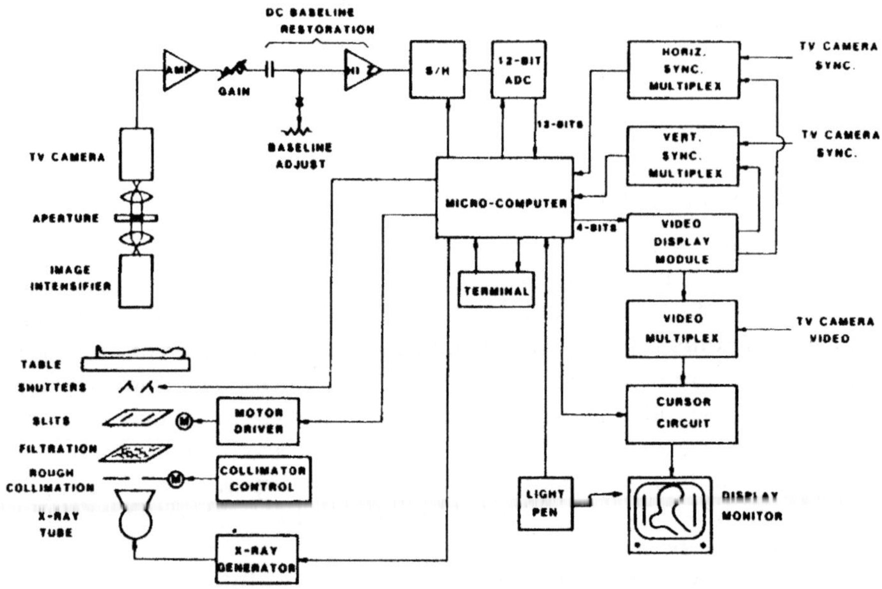

Figure 11. Scanning-slit videoaborptiometry system (Courtesy: JT Dobbins)

proximately 5 mR per mAs at 110 kVp, and the half-value layer was 8.4 mm Al at this kVp.

Two narrow (adjustable) scanning slits were used to reduce scattered radiation. The slits were scanned along the longitudinal axis of the patient using computer-controlled stepping motors. A 0.5-second pause at each location was used for visualizing the image on the TV monitor. The transmission data were digitized and stored on the computer, and a 256 × 256 × 4 bit video display was used for viewing the images. Completed images were stored on a hard disc and on floppy discs. The bone mineral content (BMC) was computed for a given area of pixel values as the difference of the logarithm of the intensity of bone plus tissue, minus the logarithm of the intensity for tissue alone. The bone mineral content per unit area (arbitrary units) was determined using bone phantoms of varying thicknesses. The linearity of BMC measurements for various kVp's and tissue thicknesses was very good. The coefficient of variation in the femoral neck BMC was 0.9%, which compares well with that of single-photon absorptiometry (1% to 2%), computed tomography (2%), and dual-photon absorptiometry of the femoral neck (2.2%).

The accuracy of the videodensitometric BMC measurement was affected by beam hardening and by different amounts of overlying tissue; a water bolus was used to minimize these effects. It was found that the excellent linearity and precision of the method allowed the monitoring of disease in individual patients over time. The radiation exposure to the skin, using the total patient scan time of 10 minutes, was about 185 mR (Dobbins et al., 1984).

3. SINGLE-PHOTON ABSORPTIOMETRY

Single-photon absorptiometry (SPA) was first described by Cameron and Sorenson (1963) in an effort to overcome the problems inherent in the use of film densitometry. The basic configuration for the single-photon systems commercially available today was introduced in 1972 (Mazess and Cameron, 1972). This device was designed to give a digital readout of bone mineral content and bone width. Several manufacturers now market the single photon absorptiometry system (Novo, Gammatec, Nuclear Data, Norland, Lunar).

The single-photon absorptiometry method does not distinquish between cortical and trabecular bone as the bone cross section is scanned. Like radiogrammetry, SPA is limited to the appendicular skeleton. With this method it is not possible to establish whether bone loss occurred in the cortex or in the marrow region of the bone. In addition, the porosity of the cortex is reflected by an increased transmission through the bone, although the method cannot differentiate between the presence of porosity and the loss of bone mineral.

Single-photon absorptiometry has been widely used in clinics around the world since the first systems were developed. As SPA was used in large populations of normals and patients, the limitations of the method became more apparent. The accuracy and sensitivity of SPA has been brought into question through this experience because of its limited application to individual patient diagnoses and because of its limited ability for discrimination between osteoporotics and normal subjects. Although SPA is still used in some clinics, this modality is being replaced by newer and better densitometric methods.

These limitations are discussed in this chapter, as well as the more recent improvements in the SPA systems.

PRINCIPLES OF MEASUREMENT

The units of bone mineral content (BMC) are grams per centimeter (g/cm) of ashed bone. This unit reflects the mass per unit length along the axial direction of the bone (figure 12).

In the single photon absorptiometry method, a linear scan of the radiation beam is performed at constant speed across the region of interest. The detector system measures the transmitted intensity of the radiation originating from the radionuclide source. The intensity is determined at each position for a preselected time interval (usually one second). The count rate (counts per minute) is determined over regions of soft tissue and bone.

The attenuation of the radiation beam is given by the following relationship:

$$I = I_o e^{-\mu/\varrho \cdot x},$$

where I and I_o are the measured (transmitted) and incident intensities (count rates), respectively; μ/ϱ is the mass attenuation coefficient of the medium; and x is the mass per unit area in the beam path.

The equation above is used to derive the bone mineral mass per unit area for a bone embedded in a uniform thickness of soft tissue, as follows:

$$x = \frac{\varrho \ln \left(\frac{I_o}{I}\right)}{\mu_b - \mu_s}$$

where ϱ is the density of bone mineral, μ_b, μ_s are the linear attenuation coefficients of bone mineral and soft tissue for the primary beam energy, I_o is the transmitted count rate for the soft tissue next to the bone, and I is the transmitted count rate for the path containing bone and soft tissue. I_o is the baseline count rate for regions of fixed soft tissue thickness; I is measured over the regions containing both bone and soft tissue in which the total tissue thickness is the same fixed thickness. The bone mineral mass per unit length of bone, i.e., the bone mineral content (g/cm), is determined by integrating "x" transversely across the bone width. Bone mineral mass per unit area multiplied by the cross-sectional area of bone equals the bone mineral content (BMC) (Cameron and Sorenson, 1963; Mazess et al., 1972).

For bone mineral measurements, the absorptiometer consists of a source and a detector, which move across the subject simultaneously viewing the same spatial position. The source and detector are mechanically coupled, and the source/detector arrangement is moved in a linear fashion over the region of interest using a stepping motor. The first digital readout SPA system utilized

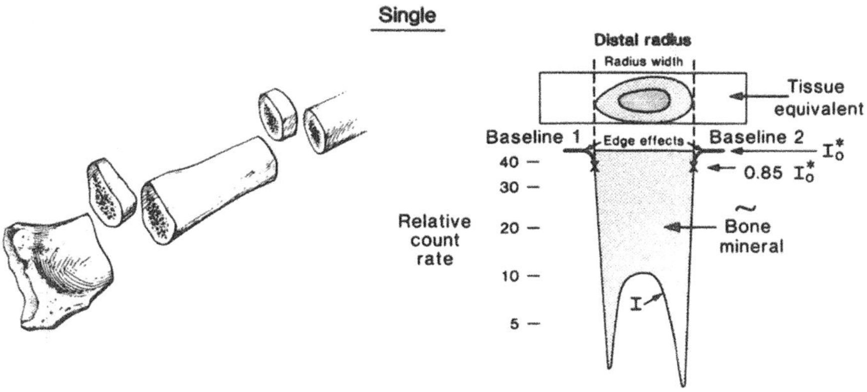

Figure 12. Bone mineral content, grams of ashed bone per 1 cm of axial length, proportional to area of the logarithmic plot (Courtesy: HW Wahner)

a scan speed of 2.0 mm/sec, a beam diameter of 2.0 mm, and integrated the accumulated counts for each 1.0 mm of source/detector movement. The counts for each interval were then recorded using digital data storage capabilities (Mazess et al., 1972).

The radioactive source (^{125}I, ^{241}Am, or ^{153}Gd) is selected on the basis of its primary gamma-ray energy, half-life, activity, and cost. Several studies of the optimal radionuclide source have been reported in the literature (Sandrick and Judy, 1973; Watt, 1975). The most common source is a sealed source (^{125}I) containing a tin filter. The source is enclosed in a lead source holder, to reduce the background count rate during measurement and to reduce the environmental exposure rate to the operator. The average energy of this source is 27.4 keV, which is sufficient for penetration of the human forearm. The source strength is appropriate for generating an attenuation curve (profile) from which an accurate determination of the bone mineral content of the forearm bones can be made.

The ^{241}Am (60 keV) source is more appropriate for larger appendicular bones with greater thicknesses of overlying tissues, such as the humerus, femur, and tibia (West and Reed, 1970). Although the ^{153}Gd source (41 and 100 keV) is useful in these regions, it is more suitable for bone mineral content measurements of the axial skeleton. ^{153}Gd is not the primary choice for the single-photon method. The activity of the ^{125}I source is generally in the range of 100 to 200 mCi. This radionuclide source must be replaced every 3 to 4 months in order to maintain an adequate intensity for good precision in the bone mineral content determination. An advantage of the ^{241}Am source is its long half-life, 458 years. The ^{153}Gd source has a long half-life, 242 days, as compared with that of ^{125}I, 60 days.

Other investigators have suggested the use of additional radionuclides as sources for SPA. Curium (^{244}Cm), primarily an alpha emitter with half-life 17.6 years, has a series of low-energy photons (14.3, 18.3, 21.4 keV), which require detection by a Si (Li) detector. The increased energy resolution of the Si (Li) detector and the use of lower energies provides good differentiation between soft tissue and bone for small bones. Promethium (^{145}Pm), with a half-life of 17.7 years, has a 44 keV K x-ray that is detected with a NaI(Tl) or CsI scintillation detector. Acceptable intensity profiles are provided by the ^{145}Pm source for the midshaft of the radius and ulna in humans (Friedman et al., 1974). These sources have not been used in commercial systems.

The detector system consists of a NaI(Tl) scintillation crystal attached to an electron photomultiplier tube, in which gamma-ray photons enter and create light pulses. These light pulses are amplified by the photomultiplier tube, and a voltage pulse is created that is proportional to the energy deposited in the crystal. These pulses are directed to an electronic pulse-height analysis circuit, which sorts the pulses according to their amplitude. An energy window including the primary ^{125}I energy peaks excludes pulses corresponding to other energies and counts the number of pulses entering the detector. The number of pulses per second is a measure of the transmitted count rate, which will vary as the source/detector mechanism scans across the skeletal region of interest. The count rates corresponding to different regions of interest are stored by the computer system or can be displayed as a count rate profile (plot of the count rate versus position). A source collimator limits the diameter of the beam at the skin entrance; a collimator on the detector limits the beam to 1/8 inch or 1/16 inch as desired by the clinical requirements.

The bone mineral content (BMC) determination by SPA is dependent upon the ability of the system to detect and define the bone edge. The edge is detected by observation of the transmitted count rate as the system scans across the interface between soft tissue and bone. This count rate will decrease as the beam encounters bone in addition to soft tissue. The bone edge is generally defined as the position for which the observed count rate (I) is 85% of the soft tissue count rate I_0. The first digital readout SPA utilized a 70% intensity threshold for defining the bone edge using the ^{125}I source (Mazess et al., 1972). Because the integrated area under the intensity profile is directly proportional to the calculated bone mineral content, the accuracy of the computer algorithm in defining the bone edge influences the boundaries over which the area integration is made. The bone width is also influenced by the choice of the bone edge. The bone width is determined along the direction of the linear scan path, and no information regarding the other dimensions of the bone cross section is available using the SPA method. Therefore, in repeated clinical BMC measurements, repositioning is very important since the slight rotation of the long bone will produce a difference in the bone width and thus a difference in the integrated area under the intensity profile.

A single-photon absorptiometric system that was used at the Mayo Clinic consisted of a 200-mCi ^{125}I radionuclide source that moved simultaneously

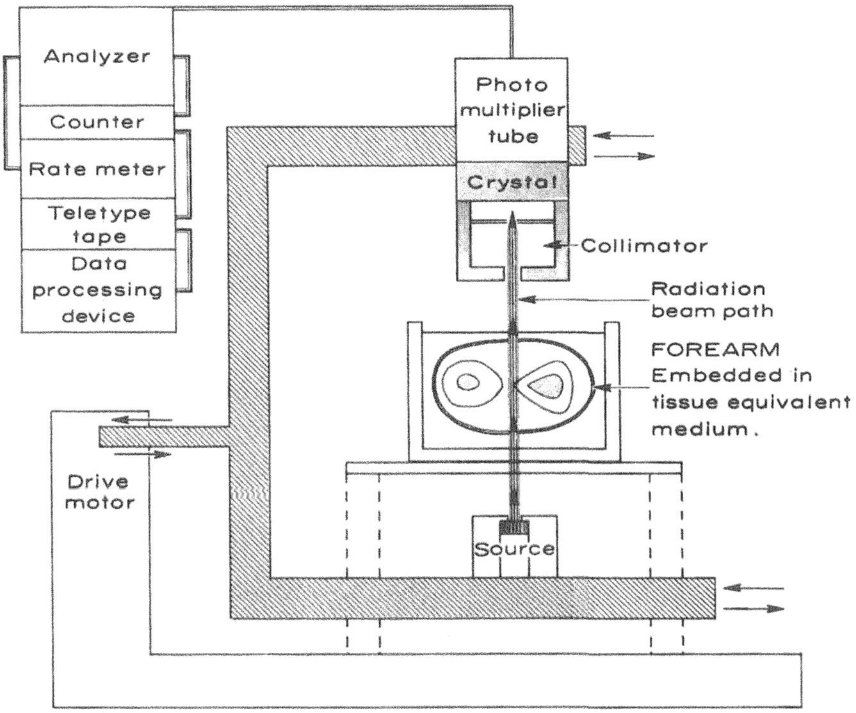

Figure 13. Single-photon absorptiometer for forearm measurement (Courtesy: HW Wahner)

(motor driven at 2.6 cm/min) with a NaI(Tl) detector placed in opposition (figure 13). The transmitted intensities were determined along the scan plane through the forearm, and an intensity profile or curve was plotted on graph paper. The integration of the intensity profile yielded a value which was proportional to the cross-sectional area of the radius and to the amount of bone mineral in the section of the radius scanned. Each bone edge was arbitrarily selected from the intensity profile as 85% of the baseline (soft-tissue) intensity prior to integration (Wahner, 1983). The source was collimated to provide a 2-mm diameter beam at the aperture, which diverged to a larger diameter at the level of the bone; a 3-mm diameter aperture was used at the face of the detector. The separation between the source and detector was 18.7 cm. Super Stuff (WHAM-O-Manufacturing Co., San Gabriel, CA) was used as bolus material and was placed around the forearm to provide the required constant tissue-equivalent thickness (about 4 cm).

A standard phantom consisting of an aluminum tube placed under 4 cm of water was scanned prior to the BMC measurements. The coefficient of variation of the bone mineral content of the standard was 1.8%. This standard served as a quality control evaluation on a daily basis. Other standards provided a regular assessment of the bone width and the bone-edge detection characteristics of the SPA device. The reproducibility for in vivo BMC measurements yielded coefficients of variation that were comparable to other SPA designs. The radiation dose to the skin was 1.6 millirad per procedure.

The calibration of the system was performed by determination of the bone mineral content at 1.0-cm intervals in dried defatted human radii at the midpoint of the radii scanned under 4.0 cm of water. After sectioning of the radii into 1.0 cm sections, the bone sections were weighed and ashed. The ash weight in grams per centimeter was plotted versus the bone mineral content value, providing a calibration curve. The width of each section was determined (along the direction of the scan) using calipers, and plotted versus the bone width (cm) provided by the bone mineral analyzer. Correlation equations were determined for bone mineral content and bone width, which were used to determine the ash weight (g/cm) from the bone mineral content value measured in vivo. The correlation coefficent between bone mineral content (g/cm) and ash weight (g/cm) was reported as $r = 0.92$; the correlation coefficient between the actual diameter (cm) and the calculated diameter (bone width) was $r = 0.93$ (Wahner et al., 1983).

Because the single photon method and the bone mineral content values are strongly dependent upon the bone volume and cross-sectional area, it is best to normalize the values to remove the dependence on skeletal size variations. Therefore, the bone mineral content divided by the bone width (g/cm^2), is the preferred unit of measurement.

Single-photon absorptiometry using ^{125}I has been used for bone mineral measurements of the forearm, jaws, tibia, and calcaneous; thicker bones such as the humerus or femur have been selected, provided the radiation source ^{241}Am was used for gaining penetration through these bones. The most commonly used measuring site is the distal third or the middle of the radius, which consists primarily of cortical bone. The predominant sites used at the Mayo Clinic for SPA have consisted of the distal site (10% of the radius length) and the midradius. The distal site consists of about 25% trabecular bone, and the midradius consists of about 10% trabecular bone (Wahner, 1983).

The effects of weightlessness on the resorption of bone mineral in astronauts has been investigated with the use of the single-photon absorptiometry method as well as other methods (Vogel and Wittale, 1976). These studies have indicated the need to find practical ways to prevent bone loss over extended periods in gravity-free space environments.

West (1973) performed measurements of the bone mineral content ("bone index", g/cm) of the femur using the source ^{241}Am (activity, 70 mCi) in a transmission arrangement. The photon beam was collimated to a cross section of 2 mm × 10 mm, with the 10 mm dimension parallel to the axis of the bone. A NaI(Tl) detector was used, and a computer analyzed the data and calculated the bone mineral content. The site of the measurement was one-fifth the distance from the lateral epicondyle to the greater trochanter. A skull x-ray stand was modified to support the photon source and scintillation detector. The source consisted of seven 2-mm diameter ceramic beads encased in a thin-walled stainless-steel cylinder, which provided a line source having the dimensions 2 mm × 14 mm (West and Reed, 1970).

The patient was seated on motorized chair, which was moved vertically, instead of moving the source/detector mechanism. The femur was supported in a horizontal position and moved downwards across the photon beam at a speed of 0.3 mm/sec. The femurs of 45 male skeletons were scanned, and a high correlation (r = 0.91) was found between the *bone index* and the femur mass. The bone index was also well correlated (r = 0.86) with the total skeletal mass in this study. A similar method has been described using ^{241}Am (Heron et al., 1978). The results obtained by West compared well with those of Mazess (1971), in which it was found that for ^{125}I SPA, the *scan integral* (analogous to the bone index) was well correlated with the femur mass (r = 0.94); the scan integral was also well correlated with the total skeletal mass (r = 0.92).

The major advantage to the use of a monochromatic source of radiation is the uniformity of the radiation field intensity and the reduction of scattered radiation and beam hardening (Aitken, 1984). The major disadvantage, as in photodenitometry, is the variability of the soft-tissue composition surrounding the bone being measured. The presence of adipose tissue significantly affects the transmitted intensities through soft tissues; changes in the volume and distribution of adipose tissue in a subject may lead to an apparent but false change in bone mass. An inherent problem in single-photon absorptiometry is the inability to accurately localize the scan path, which leads to errors when the measurements are repeated at a later date. Anatomical landmarks have been used for localization and have often reduced the errors associated with repositioning of the forearm.

X-RAY TUBE SOURCES FOR SPA

Archer-Hall et al. (1973) described a single-photon densitometer using a conventional x-ray tube source. The measurement apparatus was designed for interfacing with the collimator of the x-ray machine. The x-ray beam was intercepted by a lead plate containing two slots. A detector was attached below one of the slots and monitored the output of the x-ray tube. The second slot collimated the beam (2 × 10 mm) as it penetrated a water bath containing the patient's limb. The forearm, placed in a water tank, was moved at a speed of 1 cm/sec across the x-ray beam path by a motor drive. The transmitted beam passed through a slit (0.25 × 9.5 mm) to the second detector. The detectors consisted of small pieces of CsI(Tl) viewed by photocells, which produced a current rather than pulses. The variation of the detector output was considerable (up to 10% in amplitude) due to variations in the line voltage, and the monitor detector was needed to correct for this large variation. Changes in the x-ray spectrum produced by shifts in the line voltage were also compensated by the monitor detector.

As the forearm was moved perpendicular to the x-ray beam, the transmitted intensity was integrated at a rate of 100 times per second. An oscilloscope was used to display a plot of the intensity versus position, using a potentiometer attached to the moving carriage. The transmitted intensity was plotted for each 0.1 mm of movement and provided a profile of mineral of the ulna. Hard copies of these profiles were obtained from the oscilloscope display. An ivory step wedge was use to calibrate the system, although more suitable calibration materials were considered. An ivory slab (5-mm thick) and other absorbers, which approximated the Perspex base of the water tank and the water, were placed in the beam path of the monitor detector to provide a similar x-ray spectrum for detection. The patient's forearm was clamped in position in the water bath. It was found that the best discrimination between bone and water was obtained using the exposure factors: 90 kVp and 50 mA. The reproducibility error of the measurements was less than 2%, and the spatial resolution was estimated as 0.25 mm. In vivo measurements were performed on the ulnae of five subjects in which the reproducibility was found to be comparable to that achieved with cadaver bones. The marrow dose was estimated as 150 mrad per scan.

MULTIWIRE PROPORTIONAL COUNTERS

The use of multiwire proportional counters in absorptiometry has been reported by several investigators (Zimmerman et al., 1976; Horsman et al., 1976; Horsman and Currey, 1983). These systems produced transmission images of the appendicular skeletal sites. From these images the mass per unit area (g/cm^2) was derived at any selected point. Horsman described the multiwire proportional counter (MWPC) as a gas-filled chamber containing three planes of closely spaced wires. The MWPC was the detector system for determination of the transmitted radiation intensities, which emanated from a sealed radionuclide source placed above the detector. The appendicular bone chosen for the study was located between the radiation source and the MWPC detector system.

The cylindrical detector chamber was 5 cm deep and 57 cm in diameter, and contained three parallel planes of wires. The central plane of wires formed the anode, and the upper and lower planes formed the cathode. A uniform electric field existed between the anode and the cathode. The chamber was filled with a gaseous mixture consisting of 70% xenon and 30% isobutane at atmospheric pressure. The cathode plane of wires was equidistant (8 mm) from the anode plane, and the voltage applied across the anode and cathode was 5 kV. The anode wires were made of gold-plated tungsten, and the cathode wires were made of beryllium-copper. Any nonuniformities in the wire spacing resulted in changes in the efficiency of the proportional counter (Horsman et al., 1977).

The gadolinium (^{153}Gd) radionuclide source, with the half-life of 242 days, had an acitivity of approximately 50 mCi and an active diameter of 3 mm. The 42 keV europium x-rays emitted by the source coincided well with the maximum efficiency of the MWPC. The transmitted radiation entered the detector through a thin window (Melinex) 20 cm in diameter and interacted with the xenon gas atoms. At the 42 keV energy represented by the europium x-rays, ionization of the gas (removal of a K-shell electron) occurred. The removed electrons were attracted to the anode wires, and the position of a detected event was determined by the length of time required for a pulse of current produced by the event to be detected. Fluorescent K x-rays escaped the chamber undetected and did not interfere with the detected events. The spatial resolution of the MWPC system was about 1 mm.

The transmitted intensities and the corresponding locations were presented as an image on a color TV monitor. The image contained 128 × 128 picture elements (pixels), in which each element represented an active area of the chamber of 1.45 × 1.45 mm. The color of each pixel corresponded to the transmitted intensity detected by the MWPC. The logarithm of the ratio of the intensity (counts) in each pixel representing bone to the intensity in a pixel representing soft tissue only (baseline count rate), was found to be proportional to the thickness of bone mineral. A profile of these log ratios was generated along a line perpendicular to the long axis of the appendicular bone. Summation of the log-ratio values over the bone width provided a measure of the bone mass per unit length.

Also, by utilizing the second dimension of the image, it was possible to obtain the total mass of the bone represented in the image. A computer was used to perform these calculations and was connected to the MWPC for data collection and processing. Linear relationships were demonstrated between the mass of bone samples and aluminum samples and the total area (integrated counts) under the scan profile (figure 14). The precision of the measurement of bone mass in excised radii (immersed in a water bath) was given as approximately 2% (Horsman and Currey, 1983).

A later modification of the MWPC system included a rotating focused collimator placed between the appendicular skeleton and the entrance window of the MWPC. The collimator was focused on the radiation source, which produced a conical beam. Measurements in patients provided a precision of better than ±5% (Horsman et al., 1983). This method required an exposure time of 5 minutes, producing a radiation dose to the patient of less than 0.1 millisievert for examinations of the forearm.

Another interesting application is the multiwire gamma camera (MGC), which was developed for measurement of the bone mineral content of the os calcis in humans. This device used the nearly monochromatic radiation produced by ^{125}I. The main advantage of the multiwire system is its speed in providing an image. Bone mineral content determinations using the MGC have provided excellent agreement with the conventional single-photon absorptiometry methods using ^{125}I. The precision of the measurement by MGC was reported for the os calcis BMC as better than 1% RMS error, with an acquisition time of 100 seconds using a 500 millicurie ^{125}I source (Lacy, 1984).

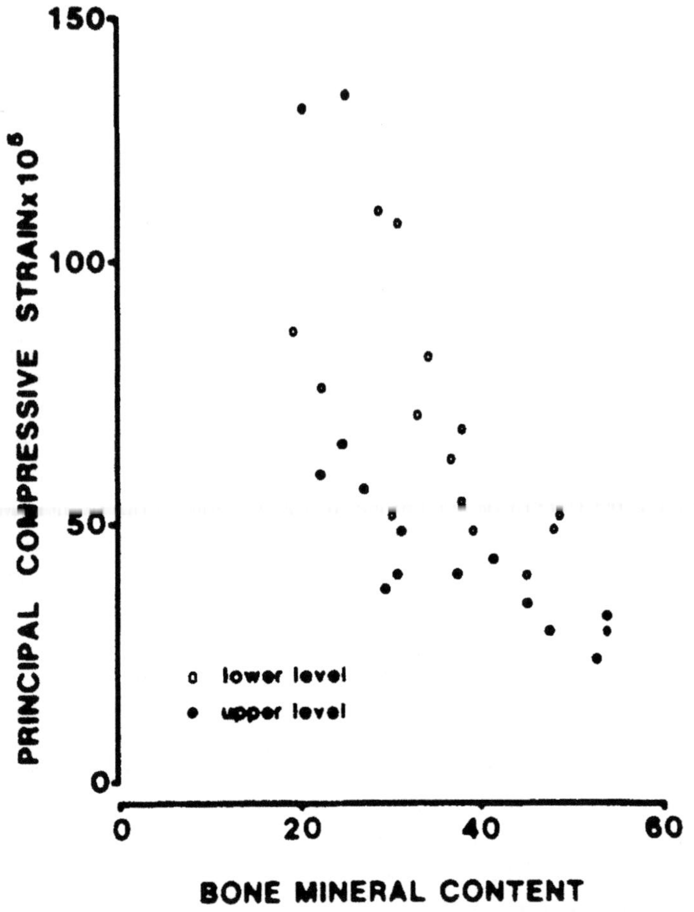

Figure 14. Relationship between compressive strain and bone mineral content of distal radius sites: 3 cm from styloid tip (lower level; r = −0.77), 6 cm from styloid tip (upper level; r = −0.86) (Courtesy: A Horsman)

TWO-DIMENSIONAL SPA

Single-photon absorptiometry of the appendicular skeleton using ^{125}I has been described in which a two-dimensional scan is performed. The main advantage of the method over the linear SPA scanning method is its ability to estimate total bone calcium in appendicular bones. The instrumentation required for these transmission measurements is the same as previously described for single-photon absorptiometry, except that the system is mechanically designed for rectilinear (two-dimensional) motion.

The scan plane (x-y) is parallel to the long axis of the bone. In the forearm, the transmitted intensities of the radius and ulna are simultaneously displayed. These intensity profiles allow the operator to identify and match the same scan sites in repeated measurements in vivo and to correct repositioning errors that

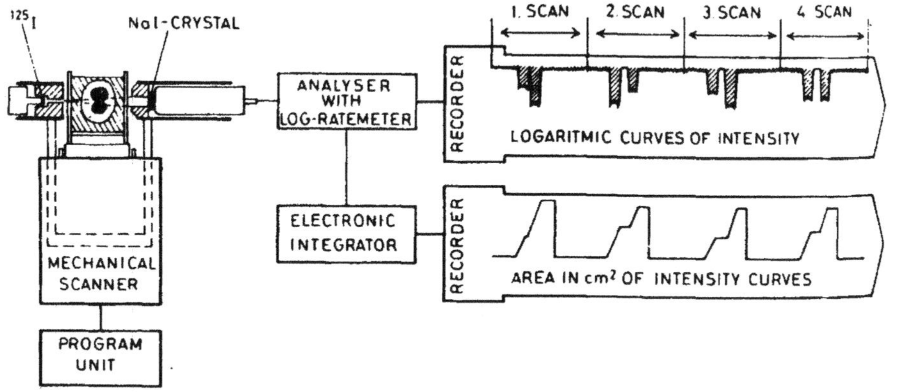

Figure 15. SPA Scanner, electronics, and intensity profiles (Courtesy: C Christiansen)

may occur due to rotation of the forearm. The forearm is positioned in a plastic container filled with distilled water to maintain the constant thickness required for SPA.

A commercial two-dimensional system is the GT 30, available from Gammatec (Stormly 16, 2890 Hareskov, Denmark). The radionuclide source (^{125}I) is supplied by Studsvik (Sweden) and is a point source with a diameter of 0.2 mm. The detector utilizes a 1.5-mm thick NaI(Tl) crystal and a 2.6-mm rectangular collimator. The scanning speed is 12 cm/min and the line spacing between linear scans is 4 mm. The system gives a measurement of the bone mineral mass per unit area or per unit length of bone, as in other single-photon absorptiometry techniques.

The system has been used for in vivo bone mineral measurements. The reproducibility of BMC measurements in normal subjects was found to be about 2%, while the variation in BMC in subjects with low values was on the order of 3% to 4%. The correlation coefficient between the measured calcium content and bone mineral content was found to be 0.964, indicating that the method provides a good indicator of total bone calcium for appendicular sites. The radiation dose to the patient, using the two-dimensional single-photon absorptiometry method, was reported as 3 to 4 millirad (Christiansen et al., 1975). A later study using the two-dimensional forearm scanner (figure 15) yielded a mean coefficient of variation in normal subjects of 1.4% (over a period of 1 year); it was estimated that the method is capable of a long-term reproducibility of 1.7% in BMC for osteopenic patients. This precision was found to be acceptable for the clinical determination of calcium balances (Christiansen and Rodbro, 1977).

PRECISION AND ACCURACY (SPA)

The primary errors associated with single-photon absorptiometry are as follows: (1) instability of the instrument over time, including radionuclide

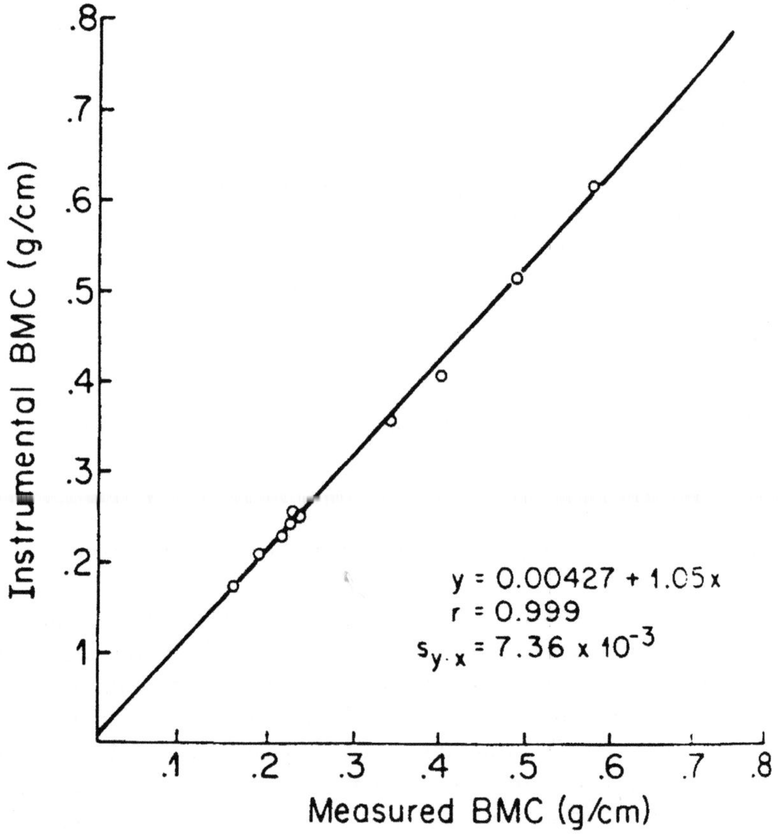

Figure 16. SPA data versus measured ash content (Courtesy: SN Rustgi)

source changes, malfunctions, and long-term drift; (2) beam hardening (2%), source composition (2%), beam spatial resolution and electronics (0.5%), scattered radiation (0.1%), repositioning (1% to 4%), and counting statistics (1% to 2%); (3) instrument differences between laboratories such as differing source-detector geometries and design differences; (4) source contamination with ^{131}I and spectral changes; and (5) forearm positioning and repositioning for repeated studies (Wahner, 1983).

The resultant value for bone mass is analogous to a value for cortical area (actually cortical volume) as measured by radiogrammetry. It is necessary to correct this value for bone size when comparing an individual's value to that of the normal population. However, in making this correction it should be noted that the bone width as measured by single-photon absorptiometry, is less accurate and less precise when compared to the radiographic measurement of total bone width. Some investigators feel that the accuracy of the single-photon absorptiometric method has not been adequately evaluated, i.e., through stringent comparisons between in vivo and in vitro measurements of human bone tissues, although very good correlations have been obtained for cadaver studies (Aitken, 1984).

Gupta has determined the accuracy of the single-photon technique as measured by the determination of the linear regression of ashed weight of bone versus the measured bone mineral content. For these experiments, the correlation coefficient was greater than 0.99 (Gupta, 1984; Chesney and Shore, 1981) and the reproducibility was represented by a coefficient of variation of 2.5% (Johnson et al., 1968; Smith et al., 1972).

The precision of single-photon absorptiometry in clinical studies is approximately 5% (Cameron et al., 1968; Wahner et al., 1977). The reproducibility is primarily affected by the repositioning errors associated with repeated measurements at the same bone site. This precision is inadequate for clinical and research applications (Wahner et al., 1984). The original design of the single-photon system has been modified over the years to increase the reproducibility of bone mineral content measurements. These modifications include the use of multiple scan paths separated by about 1.0 mm, data averaging, laser beams or light localizers for reducing repositioning errors, water baths instead of tissue-equivalent material for improving the ability of the operator to visualize the bone site during repositioning, and automated positioning algorithms such as the automatic determination of the distance between the ulna and the radius. With these modifications and improvements, the coefficient of variation can be reduced to 1% to 2% in population studies. The commercial instrumentation can usually be modified to reach this improved level of precision (figure 16).

The most critical factor that can affect the accuracy of the BMC measurement is the presence of fat in the soft tissue regions surrounding bone. Because the density of fat is less than that of soft tissue, this will result in an artificially low bone mineral content (Wahner et al., 1984).

EFFECTS OF ADIPOSE TISSUE

The presence of fat tissue within bone is also a problem in single-photon absorptiometry. During the SPA scanning procedure, the radiation beam may encounter regions of trabecular bone that contain fat. The penetration of the beam through these fatty regions is greater, and the transmitted intensities are therefore higher than expected. In this case the intensity profile describing the bone mineral rises above the baseline for soft tissue, and a low value for BMC is calculated. Since the theoretical basis for the SPA method assumes the presence of a two-component system, water-equivalent materials, and bone, the measurement is invalidated by the additional presence of intraosseous fat.

Karjalainen (1973) presented an empirical correction factor to the BMC for the presence of fat. Lahtinen et al. (1980) further investigated the correction coefficient K by which the measured bone mineral density (g/cc) must be multiplied to obtain the actual bone mineral density. In vitro measurements were performed on human distal radii removed from cadavers. The SPA device utilized an ^{241}Am source. The intraosseous fat was collected from cadaver radii, and the fat content was determined. It was shown that an error of 50% to 60% was possible in BMC measurements of very osteoporotic bones. However, this large error was not found in bones with higher bone mineral density. In fact, the correction factor was not needed for bones with a mineral density greater than 0.350 g/cc.

It was noted that the fat corrections for BMC measurements in which ^{125}I was used as the radiation source were smaller than those found using the ^{241}Am source. The authors concluded that the fat correction factor K was necessary for finding the BMC of bones containing significant amounts of trabecular bone tissue, such as the distal radius.

Rickers et al. (1981) investigated the effect of the additional fat in obese patients and concluded that neglect of this problem gives a systematic underestimation of BMC, leading to false conclusions in cross-sectional as well as longitudinal studies in human subjects. BMC was measured on the distal part of the forearm using an ^{125}I two-dimensional scanning photon absorptiometry device (Gammatec GT 30). The method had a long-term reproducibility in patients of better than 2%. The underestimate of BMC due to fat was found to be 30% in the most extreme cases. A study of six normal (non-obese) subjects was performed in which the BMC was measured. These subjects were again measured with increasing amounts of porcine fat added in 5 mm layers encircling the distal radius sites. The underestimate was found to be proportional to the thickness of the fat layer and was highly correlated ($r = 0.77$) with the percent overweight. In obese subjects, therefore, the correction for the fat layer on the forearm is mandatory for the interpretation of the BMC.

CLINICAL MEASUREMENTS

BMC measurements on the radius and ulna shafts are highly correlated ($r = 0.85$) with BMC of the femoral neck, but only moderately correlated ($r = 0.6 - 0.7$) with the BMC of the spine (Wilson, 1974). The precision of BMC measurements in clinical work is typically 2% to 4%. It is evident that a measurement of BMC in the appendicular skeleton provides a satisfactory indication of the strength of the femoral neck, but such appendicular measurements are not indicators of the strength of the spine.

Normal values of bone mineral content for different populations have been reported in the literature for the single-photon method. All measurement sites in the appendicular skeleton provide similar BMC values, which vary slightly as a result of the variation in trabecular bone content (Seeman et al., 1982). Normal BMC for the distal tenth of the human radius and at midradius, expressed in g/cm, and normalized g/cm^2, are given by Wahner et al. (1984). Normal BMC data is also presented for men. As measured by the SPA method, the bone mineral content (BMC) reaches a maximum at 30 to 35 years of age, with males having higher BMC than females. It has been demonstrated by

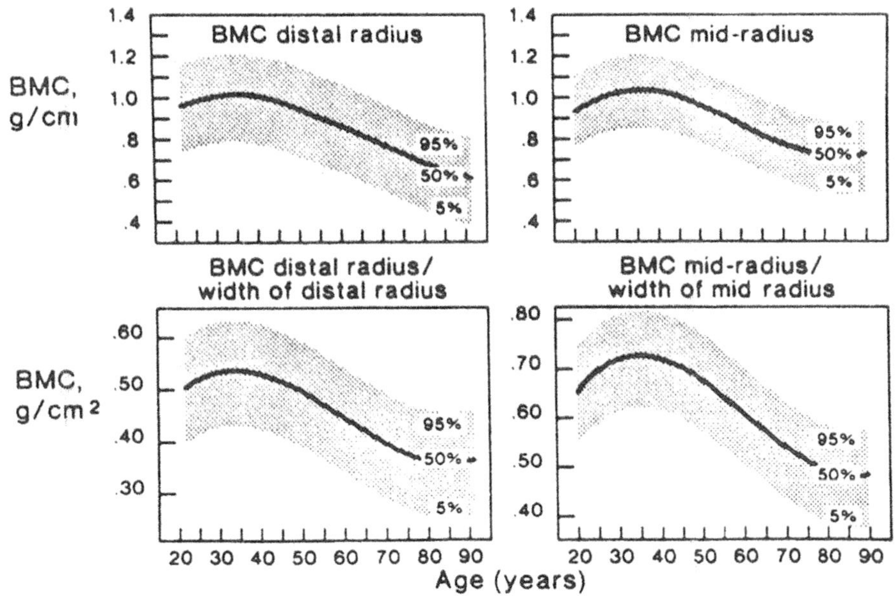

Figure 17. Normal female BMC at distal tenth of radius and at midradius versus age (Courtesy: HW Wahner)

single-photon absorptiometry that BMC decreases with age in both males and females, with females experiencing a more rapid decline in BMC with age.

In females, the highest rate of bone loss occurs near menopause; this rate lessens beyond age 65 (figure 17). Single-photon BMC at the distal radius site indicates slightly greater bone loss due to the presence of more trabecular bone. Between the age of 51 and 65 years, the rate of bone loss at the distal and midradius sites is 0.0118 and 0.0108 g/cm per year, respectively (Wahner et al., 1984). The normal decline of bone mineral content for elderly women is about 30% for the midradius and about 39% for the distal radius. In males (figure 18), the loss of bone mineral with age is linear and insignificant for the midradius; in the distal radius the rate of decline in BMC is 0.0032 g/cm per year (Riggs et al., 1981).

Normative data for various populations have been determined by single-photon absorptiometry. Bone mineral content of the radius was measured in an Ecuadorian population chosen for its infrequent occurrences of fractures. In that study, it was found that bone mass, adjusted for age, height, weight, and bone width, was 15% below values for the United States Caucasian population (Mazess, 1978). Trotter demonstrated that over their lifespan, American blacks have a larger skeletal mass than age- and sex-matched whites (Trotter et al., 1960). Greenspan has developed normative data in black males (Greenspan, 1978).

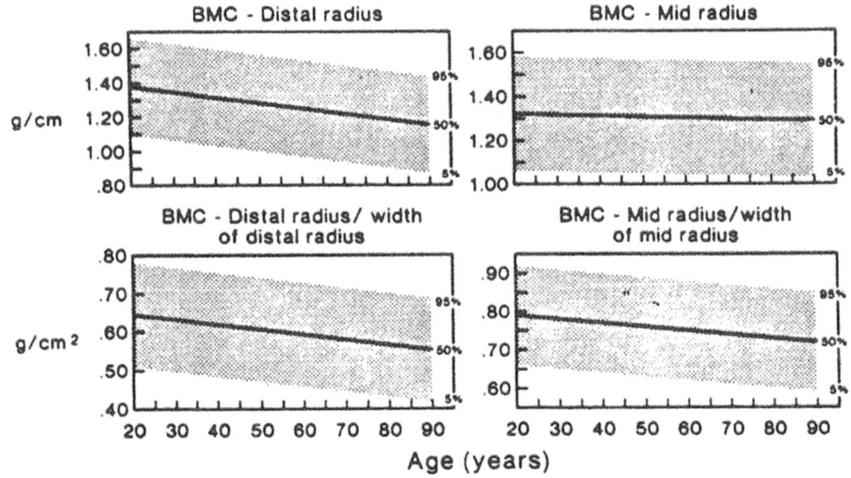

Figure 18. Normal male BMC at distal tenth of radius and at midradius versus age (Courtesy: HW Wahner)

The single-photon method has been used successfully to demonstrate the reduction of total skeletal calcium of patients on drug regimens. The method has also been used to demonstrate increased total skeletal calcium in patients receiving vitamin D. However, single-photon absorptiometry was found to overestimate the total skeletal calcium and the spinal bone mass in patients with osteoporosis, in which an appendicular skeletal site is selected (Wahner et al., 1984). Richelson et al. (1984) used SPA in a clinical study of the effects of estrogen deficiency on bone loss in postmenopausal females. The SPA method used in the study, a modification of the method by Cameron and Sorenson, was performed in the midradius, which contains an estimated 99% cortical bone. The system included a rectilinear scanning procedure. The measured BMC was determined as the mean value of eight scan passes made at 0.5-cm intervals over the radius. This method was reported to have a reproducibility error of 1%. This level of precision approaches the limit possible in clinical studies.

The single-photon method was found to underestimate the total-body calcium and spinal bone mass in patients undergoing steroid treatments for rheumatoid arthritis, in which cortical and trabecular bone loss is localized in the distal radius (Krolner et al., 1980). Single-photon absorptiometry of the radius has been recommended as a good method for monitoring bone mineral loss in patients with renal failure who are on maintenance dialysis. The SPA method is considered better than radiogrammetry, since a loss of 40% of bone mineral is required before the loss is measurable. SPA is preferred over bone biopsy because of the traumatic nature of repeated biopsies (Gupta et al., 1984; Griffiths et al., 1973; Gupta, 1983). BMC was found to decrease by 3.8% (mean decrease) in 77% of patients studied over a 26-week period (Catto et al., 1973) during dialysis. In this study it was found that SPA had greater sensitivity to BMC changes than did radiography of the hand.

It was demonstrated in another study that BMC, as measured by single-photon absorptiometry, was reduced by 12% in nondialyzed females and males with chronic renal failure; the study also showed that BMC (radius, ^{125}I) was normal in dialyzed patients with chronic renal failure (Andresen and Nielsen, 1982). This result is in conflict with those of other studies, which have demonstrated significant changes in BMC in patients with chronic renal failure (Andresen and Nielsen, 1982; Griffiths et al., 1973; Rickers et al., 1978).

The single-photon techniques allow detection of changes as low as 2% to 3% of bone mineral content (Lukert, 1984). The single-photon method used for screening may yield normal bone mineral content values, but these values do not exclude spinal osteoporosis. Single-photon absorptiometry may also be used as a low-cost mass screening method for elderly adults (Mazess and Cameron, 1985). Studies have indicated that bone mineral content of the radius may be more useful in predicting bone loss of the hip than of the spine. Wahner has concluded that the single-photon method is not reliable in the diagnosis and quantification of early bone loss in osteoporosis and other metabolic bone diseases.

Although it has been argued that the BMC of the radius is indicative of overall skeletal status and that BMC of the radius or the os calcis in patients with osteoporosis is on the average significantly below the BMC for normal controls, it has also been pointed out that the BMC reductions for these sites is less than that for the spinal sites (Mazess and Cameron, 1985; Wahner et al., 1983). It has further been stated that measurements of radius BMC and os calcis BMC cannot be used to accurately predict the mineral density of the critical fracture sites, such as the spine and the proximal femur (Mazess and Cameron, 1985; Mazess et al., 1984; Hangartner et al., 1983). Contrary to other opinions, Mazess has stated that single-photon absorptiometry is useful in metabolic bone disease, particularly in renal osteodystrophy and in many pediatric diseases.

Shimmins et al. (1972) investigated the use of both ^{125}I and ^{241}Am as sources for a single-photon absorptiometry system. The midshaft of the metacarpal, midshaft and distal radius, and midshaft of the femur were separately measured for bone mineral content in human subjects. The coefficient of variation in vivo was found as 2.3%. Studies were performed in which the BMC values using the ^{125}I and ^{241}Am methods were compared with the ash weight per centimeter in cadaver specimens. The ash weight per centimeter was well correlated ($r = 0.997$) with the BMC of the midshaft of the femur using ^{241}Am. The ash weight per centimeter was similarly well correlated ($r = 0.95$) with the BMC of the distal radius using ^{125}I. The ash weight per centimeter for the midshaft of the third metacarpal was also well correlated ($r = 0.98$) with the BMC using ^{125}I. This study demonstrated the superiority of the single-photon absorptiometry method over x-ray generator methods previously used by Shimmins et al. (1972), a significant finding for the evaluation of the metacarpals as well as for the radius and femur.

A large population study was performed on Japanese residents in Hawaii, in which SPA was used to measure the bone mineral status at five skeletal sites: distal radius and ulna, proximal radius and ulna, and os calcis (Yano et al., 1984). The single-photon absorptiometric technique used in the study was similar to that used in the study of bone loss during the Apollo and Skylab space missions (Vogel, 1975; Vogel et al., 1979). The rectilinear scanner (figures 19 and 20) had the capability of scanning in either the horizontal or vertical plane. The BMC of the forearm was determined by scanning in the horizontal plane, and for the os calcis, the vertical plane was scanned. Transmission measurements were counted at increments of 0.4 mm along a single traverse of the radius and ulna, and the separation between scan paths was 3 mm. The scan extended over a 2-cm interval beginning at the separation of the distal radius and ulna. The transmitted intensities were converted to a line image displayed on an oscilloscope for verification of the scan location.

For the proximal measurements, the scans were performed at the junction of the distal and middle one-third of the ulnar length. The os calcis scan included a 2.5-cm section through the central portion corresponding to the area of least mineral content as well as the area of greatest mineral loss during bed-rest studies. The recording of the bone profiles ensured the exact repositioning of the bones in repeated studies. Calibrations were performed twice daily using the Witt simulated three-bone standard (Witt et al., 1970) for the radius and ulna, and the Heuck step wedge (Heuck and Schmidt, 1960) for the os calcis.

This study (Yano et al., 1984) represents a comparison of the five measurement sites using SPA. Using multiple linear regression of the bone mineral content (BMC) on age, weight, height, strenuous exercise, and use of estrogen, it was concluded that the bone mineral content was predicted better in women than in men and that the predictability was best for the os calcis, intermediate for the radius, and least for the ulna in either sex. It was found that weight was the best predictor of bone mineral content of the os calcis for both sexes, a reasonable conclusion since the os calcis represents a weight-bearing bone. This study suggests that single-photon absorptiometry of the os calcis is a better predictor of bone mineral status than other appendicular sites.

Thomsen et al. (1986) used the single-photon absorptiometric method to study postmenopausal bone loss. The bone mineral content of the forearm was measured in healthy subjects, since this measurement was known to be well correlated with total body bone mineral. The densitometer (using ^{125}I) was scanned across the distal part of the forearm, and the BMC was calculated as the mean for six scans on each arm. The first scan site at the distal position was denoted by a separation of 8 mm between the ulna and radius; the remaining five scans were performed at intervals of 4 mm proximal to the first scan site. The long-term reproducibility in normal subjects was 1.2%. The BMC values were previously shown to be well correlated ($r = 0.98$) with the dry defatted

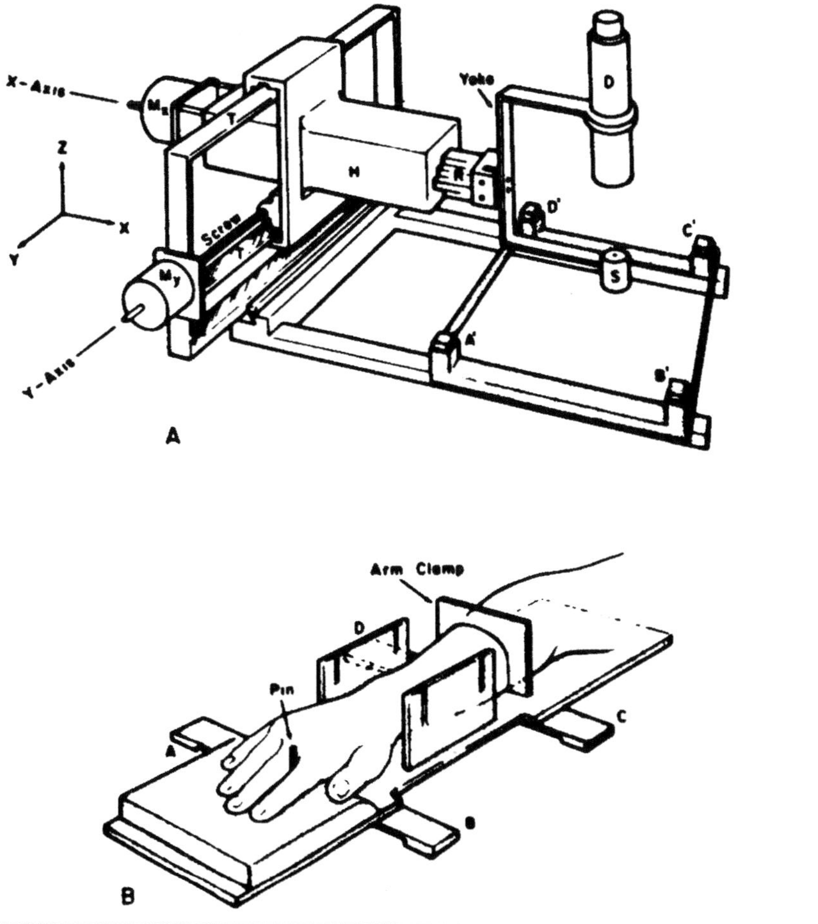

Figure 19. Forearm SPA scanner (Courtesy: K Yano)

bone weight of forearm bone slices (Nilas et al., in press). The BMC was corrected for fat in the subcutaneous tissue (Nilas et al., 1985).

Elias et al. (1985) utilized the ^{125}I SPA method in a recent study of postmenopausal osteoporosis. A linear distance of 1.5 cm of the radius and ulna were scanned at a point beginning about 2 cm proximal to the radial styloid process. The bone mineral content was expressed as the integral of the scanned area of the bone profile. Aluminum standards were scanned at each sitting to correct for machine drift. The precision of the technique was reported as 2.5%.

SPA IN CHILDREN

Several investigators have reported the use of single-photon absorptiometry in children (Mazess and Cameron, 1972; Stichen et al., 1976). Normative data for the radius were reported in these studies, in which ^{125}I was used as the radio-

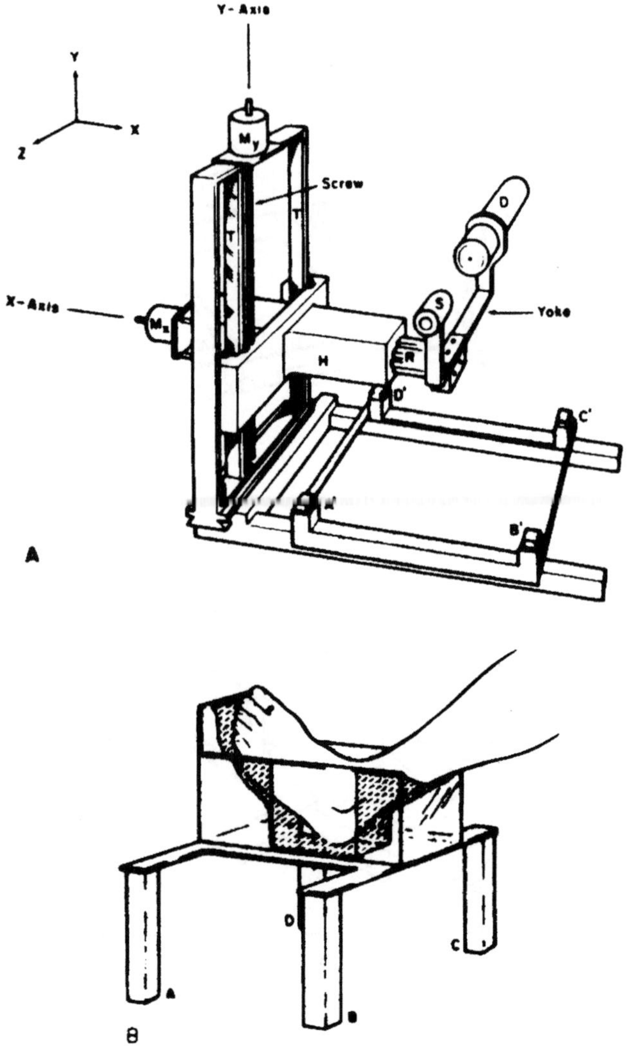

Figure 20. Heel SPA scanner (Courtesy: K Yano)

nuclide source. Normative data for the os calcis in children were also reported (Klemm et al., 1976). The use of ^{241}Am was reported for measurements of the BMC of the forearm in normal children in Sweden. It was stated that, although the ^{125}I method was advantageous compared to the ^{241}Am method, the latter method can be successfully used in small bones, such as the fingers of adults, and, in children, the radius and ulna; studies of the bone mineral accretion rate (figure 21) have also been performed in adolescents (Landin and Nilsson, 1981; Landin and Nilsson, 1983).

Data are available on the BMC of the midshaft of the radius in normal sub-

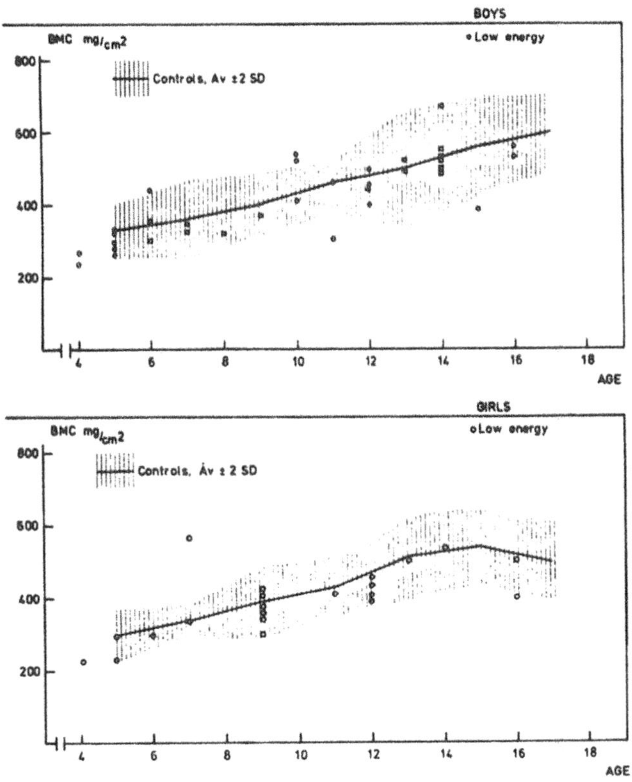

Figure 21. Bone mineral content in boys and girls with low-energy fractures as compared with normals (Courtesy: L Landin)

jects between the ages of 5 and 20 years (Chesney et al., 1977; Mazess and Cameron, 1974). Minton et al. (1979) and Roberts et al. (1981) have used SPA in studies of the mineral accretion rate in premature and term infants and to assess the effects of various infant formulas on bone mineralization. Greer et al. (in press) have defined the accuracy and precision of the SPA method in neonates and have extrapolated a range for the intrauterine bone mineral content.

However, no data have been collected on normal preschool children between the ages of 1 and 5 years; this fact prevents the SPA method from being used in the diagnosis of demineralization in children with metabolic bone diseases in this age group. The problem of repositioning for SPA forearm measurements in serial studies of children is compounded by the growth of bone during the earlier years. There is a need for assessing total-body bone mineral status, particularly in disorders such as childhood leukemia and immobilization, in which specific appendicular sites may not reflect overall bone demineralization. Despite these problems, the single-photon absorptiometry method has proven to be an accurate and reproducible method for determining bone mineral content in children (Chesney and Shore, 1982).

FRACTURE RISK

Single-photon absorptiometry has been used to establish a bone mineral content value that represents the threshold for high risk of skeletal fractures. A study was conducted in which the value 325 mg/cm^2 was selected as the "at risk" value, which is used for screening women with suspected metabolic bone disease. The study included measurements of spinal BMC using dual-photon absorptiometry (DPA). The "at risk" value was derived on the basis of the correlation between the spinal BMC and the BMC at the distal radius site (the point at which the radius and ulna are separated by 5 mm.). Because the SPA instrumentation was easily transported to screening clinics and other locations, as compared with the spinal DPA system, the SPA method was the preferred screening method. It was shown that, with the use of this distal radius site, the "at risk" value useful in screening included 95% of all BMC values reflected by patients having fractures. It was concluded that the "at risk" BMC value (figure 22) could be used (in conjunction with the midradius BMC value) as a preliminary test for both generalized and trabecular bone mass loss in women (Grubb et al., 1984). Women with distal (5 mm) radius BMC values less than 325 mg/cm^2, should be considered for further evaluation.

Another recent study, however, has concluded that single-photon absorptiometry is of limited usefulness in distinguishing patients who are at high or low risk for fracture on an individual basis. Significant individual variations in bone geometry limit the usefulness of the fracture risk index. Cross-sectional variations in the bone at the scan site are not represented in the measurement of bone width. A study of the femur, tibia, and femoral neck indicated that the assumption of a cylindrical cross section is not justified and that the cross-sectional geometries from one individual to the next are significantly different. The BMC determination, if normalized to the individual's bone width, is an inaccurate normalization because of the undetected differences in geometrical area in the case of these skeletal sites (Ruff and Hayes, 1984).

RADIATION DOSE TO PATIENTS

The radiation dose to the patient undergoing single-photon absorptiometry has been reported in the literature. For purposes of comparison, the radiation dose is generally less than that of a standard chest radiograph. The SPA method utilizes a highly collimated beam of approximately 2 mm diameter. Only a small linear path across the appendicular skeleton is irradiated during the scan. The radionuclide source ^{125}I, with energy near 27 keV and a half-life of 60 days, produces a radiation beam that is readily absorbed at this low energy by soft tissue and bone. Only a small percentage of the intensity is transmitted through the limb. The radiaton beam scans at a constant rate across the limb,

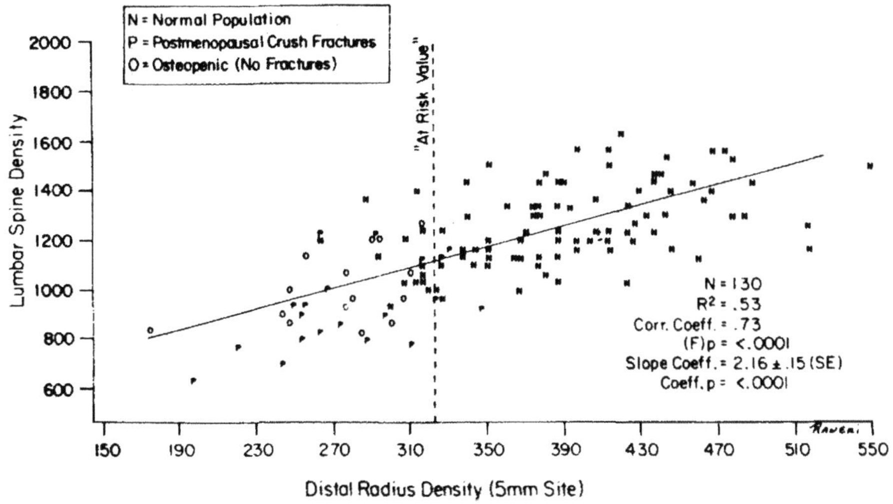

Figure 22. Lumbar density versus distal radial density for normal subjects and patients (Courtesy: SA Grubb)

and the time for a complete linear traverse is less than 1 minute. Wahner has reported the peak skin dose as 13 millirad (Wahner, 1984). Aitken (1984) has noted that although the SPA measurement yields a low radiation dose (5 to 10 mrem per scan), the customary use of four scans on each occasion raises the total radiation dose to about 40 mrem, a dose comparable with radiogrammetry.

4. DUAL-PHOTON ABSORPTIOMETRY

The potential of dual-photon absorptiometry (DPA) for noninvasive bone measurements was originally reported by Reed (1960) and by Cameron and Sorenson (1963). The first equipment utilizing this technique was constructed by Reed and Atkinson (1965; Reed, 1966), and methods for measurement of the BMC of the lumbar vertebrae in vivo were subsequently elaborated (Roos et al., 1970; Roos, 1974; Roos and Skoldborn, 1974; Roos, 1975; Roos et al., 1980; Hansson et al., 1980; Mazess et al., 1970; Wilson and Madsen, 1977; Krolner, 1985). Krolner described in detail the methodology of lumbar spine DPA, noting that forearm BMC measurements are not very useful in predicting BMC in the axial skeleton (Dalen and Jacobsen, 1974; Madsen, 1977) especially in diseased states (Krolner et al., 1980; Krolner et al., 1982c). Dunn et al. (1980) developed the dual-photon method for measuring the bone mineral content in the hip.

PRINICIPLES OF MEASUREMENT

Dual-photon absorptiometry is based upon measurement of the transmitted intensities at two photon energies through a medium containing bone and soft tissues. Although two separate radionuclide sources having different energies could be used, the radionuclide source ^{153}Gd is well suited for the method since the photopeaks of approximately 44 and 100 keV (europium K x-rays, 42 and 48 keV; gamma rays, 97 and 103 keV) are provided by a single source.

The following two equations, describing the transmission of photons of different energies through bone and soft tissue, are used to derive the bone mineral content, M_{bm}:

$$I_{44}(x, y) = I_{44}(o)e[-(\mu/\varrho)_{44,st} \cdot M_{st} - (\mu/\varrho)_{44,bm} \cdot M_{bm}]$$

$$I_{100}(x, y) = I_{100}(o)e[-(\mu/\varrho)_{100,st} \cdot M_{st} - (\mu/\varrho)_{100,bm} \cdot M_{bm}]$$

$I_{44}(x, y)$ and $I_{100}(x, y)$ are the transmitted radiation intensities at a point (x, y), which corresponds to the two photon energies, 44 and 100 keV, respectively. $I_{o\,44}$ and $I_{o\,100}$ are the incident intensities at the entrance surface of the radiation beams. (μ/ϱ_{44} and μ/ϱ_{100}) are the mass attenuation coefficients for soft tissue (st) and bone mineral (bm) for each of the two photon energies (Wahner, 1984).

Solving these two equations simultaneously for the bone mineral mass M_{bm} is easily performed, since the incident intensities and the transmitted intensities are obtained from measurements, and the mass attenuation coefficients are known for the two energies used; the unknowns of the two equations are M_{st} and M_{bm}, which are found upon solving these equations with the appropriate values inserted (Peppler and Mazess, 1981).

$$M_{bm} = \frac{\dfrac{(\mu/\varrho)_{44,st}}{(\mu/\varrho)_{100,st}}\left[\ln\dfrac{I_{100}}{I_{100}(o)} - \ln\dfrac{I_{44}}{I_{44}(o)}\right]}{\dfrac{(\mu/\varrho)_{44,st}}{(\mu/\varrho)_{100,st}}\left[(\mu/p)_{44,bm} - (\mu/\varrho)_{100,bm}\right]}$$

The principal advantage of the dual-photon method over the single-photon absorptiometry and radiographic film methods is the elimination of the effects of soft tissue in the transmission measurement. The two criteria for accurate measurements of BMC by the technique of DPA are: (1) the BMC must be independent of the thickness of soft tissue and (2) the measured BMC must be proportional to the actual BMC (Smith and Tothill, 1982).

Monochromatic attenuation techniques have been found to be unsuitable because the presence of adipose tissue and intestinal gas in the path of the radiation gives uncontrollable variations in transmission (Roos and Skoldborn, 1974). These artificially high transmission values give misleading bone mineral content values. With the elimination of the dependence upon the overlying thickness of soft tissues throughout the body, the dual-photon method is applicable to the measurement of bone mineral content of the axial skeleton (figure 23) as well as the appendicular skeleton.

The first usable method (Roos and Skoldborn, 1974) for measuring bone mineral in the axial skeleton involved the use of dual-photon absorptiometry with the monoenergetic radionuclides ^{241}Am (100 mCi) and ^{137}Cs (5 mCi). The two sources were configured such that a single beam emerged which contained photons with primary energy peaks of 59.6 keV and 662 keV, respec-

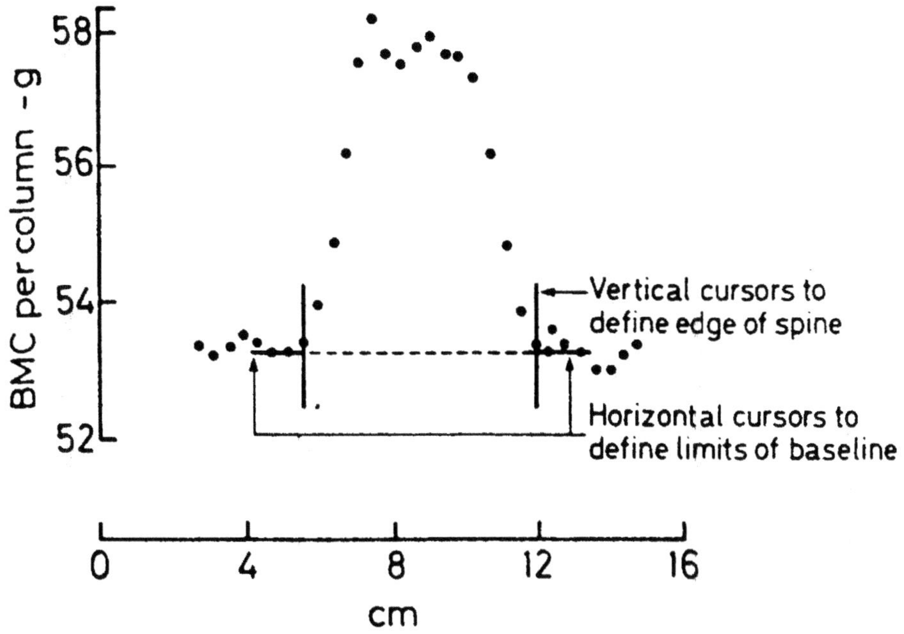

Figure 23. Profile of vertebral bone mineral content (Courtesy: P Tothill)

tively (figure 24). The ability to separate bone mineral from soft tissue when measuring two transmitted photon energies depends on the values of the corresponding attenuation coefficients and the thicknesses of the attenuating substances. The most common x-ray photon interactions in this energy range are: (1) the photo-electric effect and (2) Compton scattering.

Photoelectric absorption interactions contribute to the increased attenuation at low photon energies (below about 100 keV) in high Z substances such as bone mineral, while Compton interactions provide attenuation that is purely proportional to density above about 140 keV. It is the ratio of the attenuation coefficients for bone and for soft tissue that determine the ability of the system for detecting small differences in bone mineral density. The ratio between the mass attenuation coefficients for bone mineral and soft tissue increases when the photon energy decreases. Thus, at low photon energies, the ability to distinguish between bone and soft tissue is increased. The ratio is higher for the two primary photon energies of the ^{153}Gd source than for the photon energies represented by the source combination ^{241}Am and ^{137}Cs. The advantage gained by selection of the lower energy source may, however, be counteracted by the fact that the lower energy photons are more easily absorbed in tissues. This fact may result in a reduced transmitted intensity and reduced statistical precision.

Wooten (1971) suggested that the theoretical optimum for the lower energy

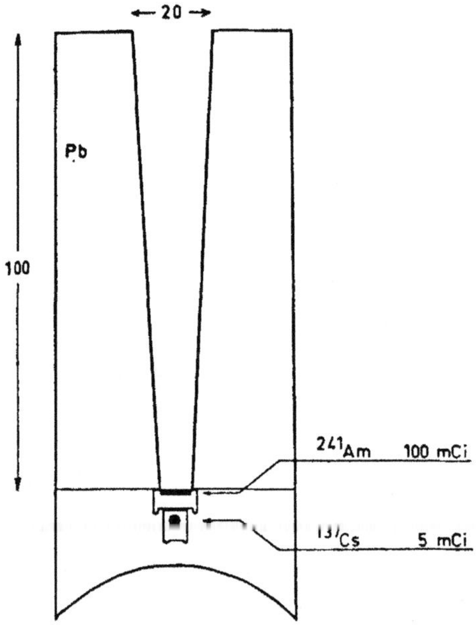

Figure 24. Dual source configuration (distances in mm) (Courtesy: BO Roos)

was on the order of 35 to 45 keV and for the higher energy was on the order of 200 to 800 keV. Other studies of the optimal energies of the dual photon source indicate that gadolinium (^{153}Gd) is near the optimum (Watt, 1975; Hanson, 1974). The half-life of ^{153}Gd is 242 days; this allows the source to be used for a period exceeding 1 year in clinical applications (Peppler and Mazess, 1981).

INSTRUMENTATION AND SYSTEM DESIGN

The typical dual-photon absorptiometry system consists of the following components:

1. Sodium iodide (NaI/Tl) scintillation detector
2. Radionuclide source — ^{153}Gd, having an activity of 1.5 curies (or other sources)
3. Pulse height analyzer and amplifier electronics
4. Source and detector collimation
5. Rigid source/detector support system with stepping motor
6. Data storage, printout, and digital display device

Commercial DPA systems often include a computer terminal with digital image display capability. The final data output for dual photon absorptiometry systems is often displayed in the form of a numerical printout of the intensity at each point in the rectilinear scan or as an image in which the transmitted beam intensity at each location corresponds to the brightness of a point in the displayed image.

The transmitted gamma-ray photons are absorbed in the scintillation crystal and produce light pulses, which are also absorbed and amplified by the photomultiplier tube. The sodium iodide crystal absorbs virtually all of the incident photons that reach the detector. The amplified signals are separated according to their voltage pulse amplitudes; this is the process of energy discrimination. Through energy discrimination, the primary gamma-ray energies, 44 and 100 keV, are individually counted as peaks in the spectrum. A digital counter accumulates transmitted counts for a period of 1 second in each energy channel, as the photon beam and the detector move simultaneously across a linear scan path. The count rate, corresponding to each position along the scan path, is recorded and stored in the computer. The bone mineral content can, therefore, be computed at each of these locations as the system scans the entire skeleton. Since the detector is incapable of counting all of the interactions that occur in the crystal, a correction is made for these losses. This dead-time correction is automatically performed by the pulse height analyzer.

Roos and Skoldborn selected the sources ^{241}Am and ^{137}Cs because of the absence of interference from any nearby photon energies and because both radionuclides have long half-lives and stable output. The compound radiation source was configured so that the 7.2-mm diameter ^{241}Am source was above the 3-mm diameter ^{137}Cs source, and the higher energy photons passed through the ^{241}Am source. Therefore, a single collimator was used, providing a single rectangular beam of 18-mm transverse dimension. In the measurement of the two transmitted intensities, the energy windows were maintained at 50 to 70 keV and 550 to 800 keV, respectively. Roos and Skoldborn presented the theoretical equations describing the calculation of the mass of bone mineral. The bone mineral content was given in terms of g/cm, based upon calibration measurements of phantoms of known equivalent mineral content. A correction was made for the interference produced by a certain fraction of the Compton-scattered photons of the ^{137}Cs source that were counted in the low-energy window.

Wahner et al. (1984) described a dual-photon absorptiometer designed for clinical usage (figure 25). The radionuclide source (^{153}Gd) was mounted in a lead-shielded assembly beneath the scanning table. The source holder included the collimator and the beam shutter mechanism, which was activated manually or by the computer. The detector assembly was mounted on a C-arm arrangement above the scanning table and patient. The sodium iodide detector crystal was 2.5 cm in diameter and 1.0-mm thick. The source-detector separation was 40 cm. The collimator diameter for the source and the detector was 6.0 mm. Stepping motors were used to control both the X and Y directions of the source/detector assembly during rectilinear scanning. Both motors were controlled by computer-generated signals. Potentiometers attached to each motor indicated the exact X, Y coordinates of the beam position at any given time.

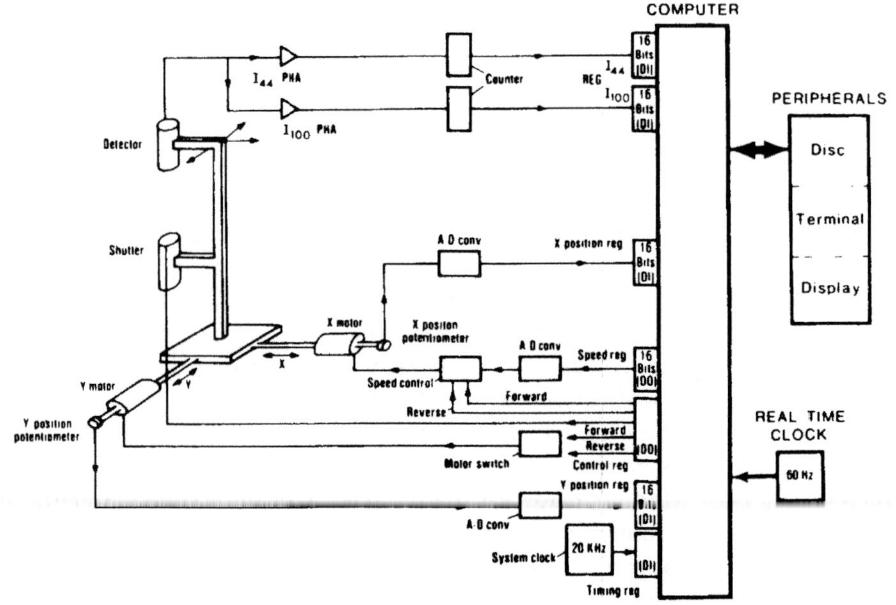

Figure 25. DPA scanner mechanism (Courtesy: WL Dunn)

Krolner and Pors Nielson (1980) modified the two-dimensional design of the DPA scanner described by Wilson and Madsen (1977). The exit collimator of the source had a diameter of 4.0 mm. The mean diameter of the radiation beam in the vertebral body was about 6 mm. The detector contained a 1.0×1.5-inch NaI(Tl) crystal with a circular lead-cadmium collimator (13-mm diameter). The energy windows of the two-channel analyzer were set at 30%. The distance from the radioactive source to the detector was 30 cm. A logarithmic attenuation curve was generated for each of the two energy peaks. The analog computer automatically corrected for the influence of the Compton crosstalk present in the 44-keV energy window. The signal (transmitted intensity) was considered to be proportional to the amounts of bone mineral in the path of the radiation beam. A greater signal was encountered when the path included fat tissue. The singal is given by the equation:

$$M = \frac{\ln \dfrac{I_{44}(o)}{I_{44}} - \dfrac{\mu_{s,44}}{\mu_{s,100}} \ln \dfrac{I_{100}(o)}{I_{100}}}{\mu_{b,44} - \mu_{s,44} \dfrac{\mu_{b,100}}{\mu_{s,100}}}$$

where I_{44} (o) and I_{100} (o) represent the incident intensities for the two energies 44 and 100 keV, I_{44} and I_{100} are the transmitted intensities at these two energies, $\mu_{s,44}$ and $\mu_{s,100}$ are the mass absorption coefficients for soft tissue at the two energies, and $\mu_{b,44}$ and $\mu_{b,100}$ are the mass absorption coefficients for bone at the two energies.

When fat was also measured, the following equation is valid:

$$M = m_b - \frac{\mu_{s,100}\,\mu_{f,44} - \mu_{s,44}\,\mu_{f,100}}{\mu_{s,100}\,\mu_{b,44} - \mu_{s,44}\,\mu_{b,100}} (m_{f,o} - m_f)$$

where m_b and m_f are the amounts of bone and fat, respectively, in the path of the radiation beam, and $m_{f,o}$ is the amount of fat at a point of calibration lateral to the vertebrae; $\mu_{f,44}$ and $\mu_{f,100}$ are the mass absorption coefficients for fat at the energies 44 and 100 keV.

It is noted that the influence of fat was eliminated if the thickness of fat was constant during the scanning movement. However, an erroneous result was obtained if the distribution of adipose tissue was nonuniform. The integration of the equation above for one scan yields the bone mineral content (mass per unit length, BMC). The zero-setting was determined during one longitudinal scan parallel with the lumbar spine and to the right of the transverse processes of the vertebrae. The mean value of this scan was used as the zero value. The scanning speed of the source/detector assembly was 4.0 mm/sec. The length of one scan across the spine was 12.0 cm. The scanning time required to perform a continuous rectilinear scan of all five lumbar vertebrae was 25 minutes. The BMC value was determined directly from the height of the integrated attenuation curve. Krolner has expressed the lumbar spine BMC in arbitrary units as the sum of the scan integrals (integrated over the attenuation curve) of L(2), L(3), and L(4) having the dimension of mass. The number of scans across these segments were in the range of 20 to 29 in normal subjects.

Krolner and Pors Nielson modified the examiner-defined baseline setting procedure described by Roos (1974). In addition, narrow-beam geometry was used in the determination of BMC; this improvement made it possible to select a well-defined spinal segment and to determine the BMC with the dimension of mass (Krolner and Pors Nielsen, 1978; Krolner et al., 1982a). The prototype device described by Krolner was designated the Gammatec BMC analyzer (Novo Diagnostic Systems, Wilton, Conn.). The patient couch was made of transparent Perspex. The patient was positioned with bent hips in a supine position to minimize the lumbar lordosis (curvature). The correct positioning of the spine was ensured by skin marks outlining the spinous processes of the vertebrae.

A highly collimated beam of photons from a ^{153}Gd (activity: 1.2 to 0.4 Ci) source was transmitted through the body using the rectilinear scanning mode. The scintillation detector NaI(Tl) opposite the source recorded the transmitted count rates in a two-channel pulse-height analyzer (44 and 100 keV windows). The scan steps were 4.0 mm, providing six to nine scans across each vertebrae. The position of the detector was adjustable at either 28 cm or 33.4 cm above the couch, the latter position being chosen for obese patients. It was found that the calculated BMC values obtained for the 33.4-cm distance were reduced by a factor 0.963 over those values obtained at the shorter distance. The transmitted count rates in the regions lateral to the vertebrae were 38,000 cps in the 100 keV channel and 11,000 cps in the 44 keV channel for a 1.0-Ci source activity. The dead time was 1.6 microseconds, and the background count rate was about 6 cps in the 44 keV channel and 12 cps in the 100 keV channel. The spillover of the 100 keV scattered photons into the 44 keV channel varied with the patient thickness. Experiments showed the spillover was 0.7% for an absorber thickness of 13 cm water, 1.0% at 19 cm, 1.5% at 25 cm, and 2.1% at 31 cm. The dead time and background count rate were neglected in the calculations, while a correction for a spillover of 1.0% was included. The attenuation curve (bone density profile) for each vertebra provided a method for identifying the location of the scans relative to the anatomy, increasing the reproducibility of positioning. The operator selected the baseline transmission count rate, which defined the width of the bone and the boundaries of the integration of the attenuation curve.

Madsen (1977) reported on a study of the bone mineral content in human subjects in which the DPA method incorporated the Ohio Nuclear whole-body scanner. The radioactive source was a 4-mm bead of ^{153}Gd with an activity of approximately 1 Ci. The source was mounted 25 cm below the scanner table top and a NaI(Tl) scintillation detector was mounted 30 cm above the table directly opposite the source. The detector was collimated with a slit collimator 1.25 × 3.75 cm. The source was collimated with a 1-cm diameter circular collimator located 20 cm above the source. The source and detector moved simultaneously in a rectilinear raster pattern at a rate of 0.25 cm/sec at intervals of 1.25 cm. Transmission counts were sampled every 2 seconds and were recorded on magnetic tape.

The subjects were placed in the supine position on the scanner table, and the scans were started along a line joining the tops of the iliac crests. The width of the completed scan was approximately 30 cm, with the spine positioned in the center of the scan. A measurement consisted of eight rectilinear passes so that a section of lumbar spine 10 cm in length was examined. The mean value of eight passes was taken to represent the mineral content of the region of interest. The standard error of the measurement was approximately 6%; the radiation dose was found to be less than 2 mrad.

The precision of the vertebral BMC in vivo was determined in four subjects over a 1-month period; the coefficient of variation of the BMC was found to range from 0.7% to 3.8% (average 2.3%). Measurements of a phantom were found to have a coefficient of variation of 1.7% over a 6-week period. The accuracy of the method was evaluated in a phantom and resulted in a standard error of the estimate of 1.2% in predicting mineral content. Madsen concluded that the bone mineral of the spine must be evaluated directly and not inferred from appendicular bone. He also found that the average lumbar spine BMC (g/cm) was moderately correlated with the ulnar BMC (g/cm) ($r = 0.642$) and

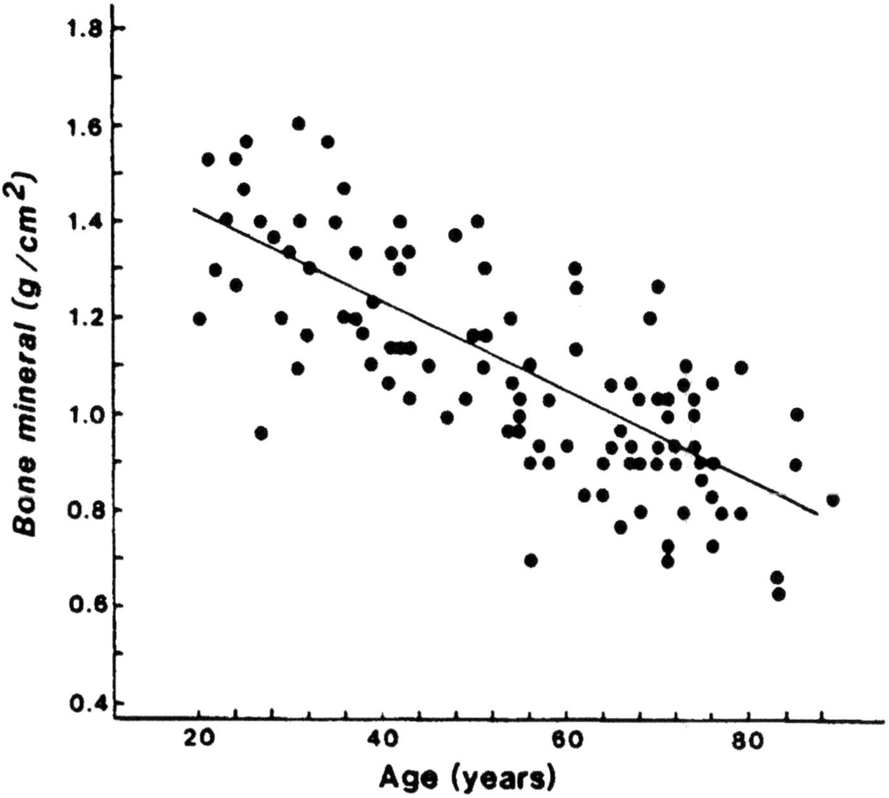

Figure 26. Bone mineral density of the lumbar spine in 76 osteoporotic females (dots) including one or more vertebral compression fractures and the mean normal values and normal ranges by DPA (Courtesy: BL Riggs)

the radius BMC (g/cm) (r = 0.675). In addition, Madsen reported that the rate of bone loss with age was greater in the peripheral bones than in the spine and suggested that measurement sites on the appendicular skeleton may provide a more sensitive indication of age changes in bone mineral content throughout the skeleton than sites on the axial skeleton.

Another dual-photon system was developed using a commercial Ohio-Nuclear (subsidiary of Technicare Corp., Solon, Ohio) dual-probe rectilinear scanner (Riggs et al., 1981). The radiation source was ^{153}Gd (1.5 Ci), and the detector consisted of a NaI(Tl) scintillation crystal and photomultiplier tube. The photon beam was collimated to a diameter of 6.0 mm and scanned a 20-cm path across the spine. Each intensity measurement was accumulated over a 1.2-mm distance, and the distance between scanning paths was 5 mm. The high-precision scanning mechanism of the Ohio-Nuclear device provided excellent localization of the transmitted beam. The size of the beam was made smaller compared to previous techniques; and an edge-detection algorithm

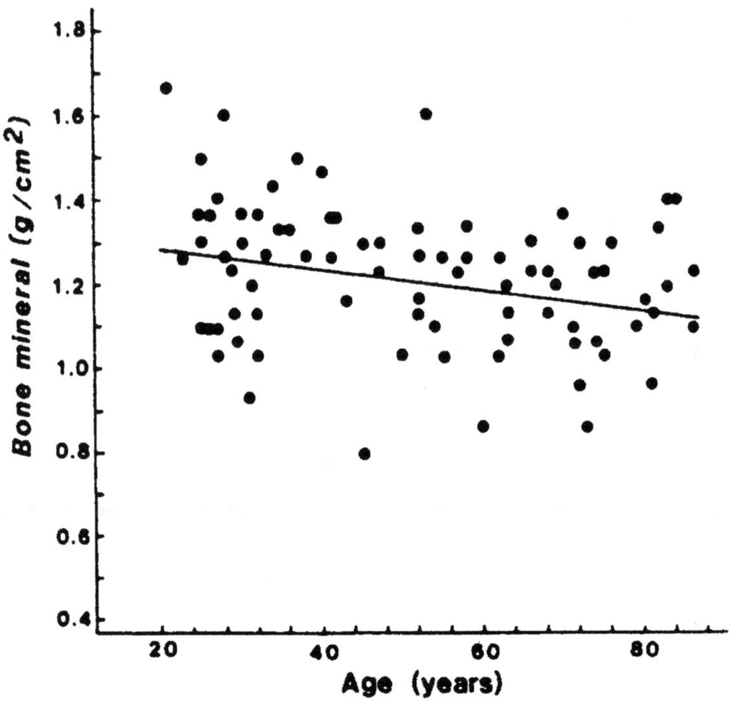

Figure 27. Bone mineral density of lumbar spine in 105 normal women by DPA (Courtesy: BL Riggs)

was found to improve the overall precision and resolution of the measured data. The scanning pattern, as well as the data acquisition, was controlled by a PDP-11/VO3 computer system. The computer algorithm performed point-by-point determinations of the density of bone mineral. The edge-detection program provided recognition of bone edges by evaluating the relative change in mineral density values between points.

Corrections were made for crossover of the energy spectra from the 100-keV to the 44-keV channel (4% to 6%) and for dead time of the counting system. A second computer was used for image display; intensity-modulated images of the spine were displayed on a 64 × 64 matrix with 16 levels of gray. Regions of interest were selectable on the screen, using a light pen, in which the BMC distribution was displayed. The BMD, bone mineral density, expressed in grams per square centimeter, was derived by dividing the BMC by the projected area of the spine (figures 26, 27, and 28). In the L(1) to L(4) region of the spine, this value included the vertebral bodies and the disk interspaces. The average coefficient of variation in five volunteers was 2.3%, demonstrating the in vivo reproducibility of the lumbar spine measurements. Riggs et al. (1982) have published bone mineral density (BMD) values for the proximal femur in normal men and women.

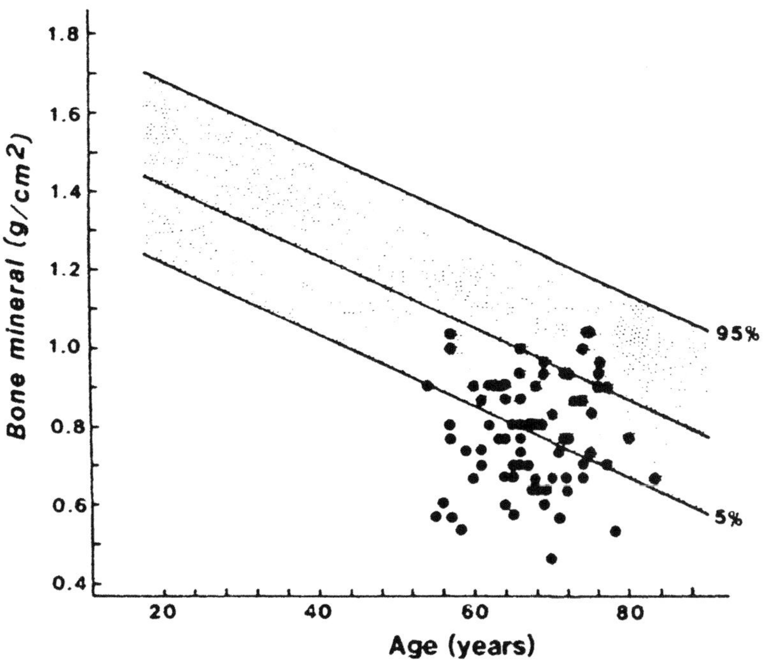

Figure 28. Bone mineral density of lumbar spine in 82 normal men by DPA (Courtesy: BL Riggs)

Richelson et al. (1984) used the dual-photon method (previously described by Wahner) for determinations of the bone mineral densities of the proximal femur (neck and intertrochanteric areas) and the lumbar spine in a study of estrogen deficiency and its relation to bone loss in postmenopausal females. The reproducibilities of the method were found as 2.2% and 1.5%, respectively. The femoral neck site was estimated to contain 75% cortical bone and 25% trabecular bone. The femoral intertrochanteric area was estimated to contain 50% cortical and 50% trabecular bone; the lumbar spine composition was estimated as 40% cortical bone and 60% trabecular bone in these studies.

The dual-photon method has been used in conjunction with a gamma scintillation camera (Mirell et al., 1985). The system was designed for measurement of the bone mineral content of the spine. The irradiator used a 10-mCi ^{133}Xe source and a 2-mCi ^{99m}Tc source, which were simultaneously exposed for 5-minute intervals. The sources were positioned at the focal point of the converging collimator, and conical beams were projected toward the camera face. The subject was in a supine position between the scintillation camera and the sources. Phantom measurements were performed to correct for the non-uniformity inherent in the image and for the beam angulation.

A set of calibrated bone mineral phantoms ranging in BMD from 0.5 to 2.0

g/cm^2 were used to calibrate the system. The accuracy error of the BMD measurement in phantoms was 2%. The use of two separate radiation sources eliminated the problem of crossover from the high-energy peaks, as is found with dual-energy radionuclide methods using ^{153}Gd. The use of a combination of long-lived radionuclide sources such as ^{241}Am (60 keV) and ^{57}Co (122 keV) was suggested by the authors.

BEAM HARDENING AND CROSSOVER CORRECTIONS

A necessary procedure in the use of DPA is the correction for overlap of the two primary energy peaks in the accumulated gamma-ray spectra. Approximately 5% of the count rate detected in the 44-keV energy channels is a result of spillover (overlap) from the 100-keV energy channels. This correction can be automatically performed by the computer system after the count rate data is accumulated. The effect of beam hardening has been described by Krolner as the increased contribution of scattered radiation, background radiation, and Compton crosstalk to the total count rate in the 44-keV channel for higher absorber thicknesses (patient thicknesses) and for higher BMC levels. The 44-keV radiation is not completely monoenergetic (Roos, 1974; Wilson and Madsen, 1977; Krolner and Pors Nielsen, 1980).

Smith and Tothill (1982) investigated the crossover correction in DPA using ^{153}Gd (figure 29). The crossover of the Compton-scatter spectrum of the 100-keV photons into the 44-keV window was believed to affect the absolute determination of the BMC. Compton events are produced within the crystal of the detector and may also arise from photons scattered within the patient. The *crossover correction* was expressed as a percentage of the 100-keV photopeak.

The gamma rays associated with the ^{153}Gd source are characterized by the following energies (and approximate abundance): 103 keV (23%), 97 keV (31%), and 70 keV (2.6%); and europium K x-rays with energies 41 keV (86%) and 47 keV (23%). The peak at 103 keV cannot be resolved from the 97 keV peak using a NaI(Tl) detector. Similarly, the 41-keV and 47-keV peaks cannot be resolved. The primary peaks are therefore considered to be at 44 keV and 100 keV, respectively. Smith and Tothill determined the ratio of counts in the 44-keV window to the counts in the 100-keV window as approximately 2:1. This ratio was decreased to 1.1:1 using an encapsulated sealed source with a stainless steel window (0.2 to 0.25-mm thick) and a 10-cm diameter, 5-cm thick NaI(Tl) detector.

A formula for the determination of the beam-hardening correction for a fixed absorber thickness was developed (Krolner and Pors Nielsen, 1980). The lumbar BMC was shown to decrease with increasing absorber thickness; this decrease was enhanced by the use of a lower source activity. The relative BMC change following a shift in absorber thickness of 1 cm is 0.5% at the 17-cm level, 1.0% at the 20-cm level, and 2.0% at the 27-cm level. The results of measurements on human lumbar spine sections in vitro confirmed the absor-

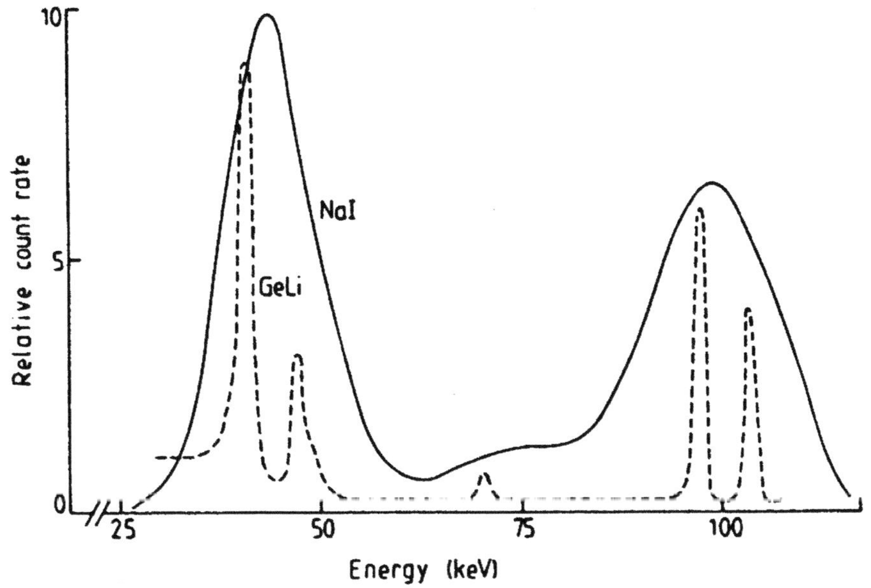

Figure 29. Spectra for ^{153}Gd as determined with two different detectors (Courtesy: MA Smith)

ber thickness correction suggested by Krolner. The accuracy of BMC measurements using spine standards is high, provided beam-hardening corrections are used (Krolner and Pors Nielsen, 1980).

Mazess et al. (1974) reported a crossover correction of 1.9%. Wilson and Madsen (1977) found a crossover correction of 3.0%. Wahner and Dunn (1980) and Riggs et al. (1981) found crossover corrections of 6.0% and 4% to 6%, respectively. Krolner and Pors Nielsen (1980) reported a crossover correction of about 1%. Peppler and Mazess (1981) demonstrated a variation in the crossover correction as a function of soft-tissue thickness. However, Wilson and Madsen (1976) specifically stated that the crossover correction did not change with changes in the soft-tissue thickness.

Gotfredsen et al. (1984) determined the spillover for ^{153}Gd for their TBBM system by placing layers of aluminum between the source and detector until all 44-keV photons were preferentially absorbed, leaving only the Compton-scatter events from the 100-keV photons. The correction for Compton events in the lower energy channel was 2.4%, expressed as a fraction of the count rate in the 100-keV channel.

The standard method for calculating the crossover correction had been to use copper to filter out the 44-keV peak at the source collimator. Smith and Tothill (1982) found that the filtered ^{153}Gd spectrum underestimated the contribution to the 44 keV channel. They found that the magnitude of the crossover correction varied with the thickness of soft tissue, using the larger collimation geometry. It was suggested that the low abundance 70-keV peak in the ^{153}Gd

spectrum contributed appreciably to the lower energy channel. These investigators used monoenergetic (Hg and U) x-rays to simulate the upper portion of the ^{153}Gd spectrum and introduced a new crossover correction. It was suggested that the contribution from the 70-keV peak was perhaps 30% of the total crossover correction. It was also found that the error due to background was significant when calculating the crossover correction; Compton-scattered photons from a contaminant ^{152}Eu in the ^{153}Gd source were significant.

Smith and Tothill found that a crossover value of only 3% would reduce the counts in the 44-keV window by 19% in a subject of thickness 22 cm with average bone density; and by 25% in a subject of thickness 27 cm and high bone density. It was shown that for a 22-cm thick subject the crossover correction was 2.8% using the standard Cu filter technique, whereas the true crossover correction was 4.4%; this difference in the crossover correction values produced an error of 15% in the BMC measurement of a normal subject (Smith and Tothill, 1982). Smith and Tothill, therefore, found the previous standard method (using Cu filters) for measuring the crossover correction to be inadequate.

CORRECTION FOR FAT

For in vivo spine BMC measurements, the most important source of error is the inhomogeneously distributed fat, including intervertebral fat. The presence of fat influences the choice of the baseline for integration, and this corrected zero-level must be chosen for each individual vertebra. A *fat inhomogeneity index* (FII) has been used to define the amount of inhomogeneously distributed fat in which the FII is dependent upon the number of accepted scans and the mean transmission value lateral to the vertebrae (Krolner, 1985). It has been shown that an increase in the fat thickness over (or within) the vertebrae of 1.0 g/cm^2, compared to the fat thickness lateral to the spine, will reduce the measured BMC by 0.046 units/cm^2 or approximately 7% in a healthy young woman (Krolner and Pors Nielsen, 1980). It was also found that the accuracy error of inhomogeneously distributed fat over the vertebrae was small compared with that of intravertebral fat, at least when several vertebrae were studied. The precision of lumbar BMC in vivo was found to be significantly reduced at high values of the fat inhomogeneity index.

The accuracy of lumbar BMC measurements was determined on seven excised human lumbar spines placed in toto in a water bath; the vertebrae were subsequently ashed. The dry-ash weights of the L(2), L(3), and L(4) vertebrae were well correlated ($r = 0.986$) with the lumbar bone mineral content using DPA. It was also shown that the lumbar spine BMC was underestimated by an average of 10% if intravertebral fat was not considered. It was concluded that changes in intravertebral fat content may account for nearly one-tenth of the apparent diminution of lumbar BMC with advancing age (Krolner and Pors Nielsen, 1980; Krolner and Pors Nielsen, 1982a).

Further experiments included DPA measurements on progressively defatted vertebrae; it was found that the accuracy was not significantly affected by the presence of marrow fat. A 0.3% change of bone mineral density (BMD) resulted from a 5% change of marrow fat (Wahner et al., 1985).

PRECISION AND ACCURACY (DPA)

During the early development of dual-photon absorptiometry (DPA), the method was found to be inherently less precise than the single-photon technique (SPA) (Watt, 1975). The precision, determined in a bone phantom of known mineral content encased in lucite and scanned at least once per day, was represented by a coefficient of variation (including machine and positioning errors) of 1.8% (Dunn et al., 1980). By improving the counting statistics, bone mineral measurements have been made on the spine with high precision (coefficient of variation 3%) and with errors in accuracy of 1% to 5%, depending upon the source configuration and beam intensity (Peppler and Mazess, 1981). The linearity and accuracy of the BMC measurement in vitro was studied using a Perspex box-shaped standard containing a cylinder of 4.0-cm diameter positioned at 7.5 cm above the couch and having a total absorber thickness of 17 cm (Krolner and Pors Nielsen, 1980). The cylinder was filled with bone mineral in various concentrations, and scanned 10 times at each bone mineral equivalent value.

The estimated BMC (using DPA) was linear, with an excellent correlation ($r = 1.00$) with the true BMC of the standards. The average error (SEE) made by estimating the correct BMC from the sum of the scan integrals was 1.3%; this was given as the in vitro accuracy of the method. The BMC was underestimated by 3.6% to 5.7% without the "beam-hardening corrections." The accuracy error using ashed human vertebrae was higher than for spine standards, that is 3.5% versus 1.3%. This difference resulted from errors of bone-edge detection and unevenly distributed bone mineral within the vertebrae. The overall accuracy error of this DPA method in vitro was reported as less than 6%, while the precision error in vivo was less than 3%. In other experiments, it was demonstrated that the bone mineral densities measured in excised vertebrae in 20 cm of water were well correlated ($r = 0.995$) with in situ cadaver measurements using DPA (Wahner et al., 1985). In a clinical study of five human volunteers over a 4-week period, the coefficient of variation was 1.3% for the lumbar spine (L1-L4) BMC measurements and 2.2% for the neck of the femur. It was stated that this precision was within the limits necessary to observe changes of clinical importance (Dunn et al., 1980).

The reproducibility (precision) of lumbar BMC in healthy women suggested a precision error of 0.7 units within weeks (Krolner and Pors Nielsen, 1980), 1.0 units within months (Krolner and Pors Nielsen, 1982a), and 1.6 units within years (Krolner, 1983) if the data from one single individual were analyzed by the same examiner. However, measurements in vitro may give a better estimate of the precision error of lumbar BMC than measurements in vivo (Krolner and Pors Nielsen, 1982b). Repeated measurements on standard phantoms using dual-photon absorptiometry have indicated the long-term stability of these measurements. Wahner has stated the coefficient of variation as 1.8% for repeated measurements over a 9-month period. The precision of dual-photon measurements in patients and volunteers was represented by the coefficient of variation of 2% to 3% for spine and hip studies (Wahner et al., 1984). Krolner has suggested that the long-term reproducibility of the measurement of lumbar BMC in vivo, for an individual with a 19-cm absorber thickness and a FII of 1.5-cm fat, is 1.4% to 2.5% for the BMC range of normal premenopausal women, and 2.0% to 7.9% for the BMC range of women suffering from spinal osteoporosis (Krolner, 1982; Krolner and Pors Nielsen, 1982b).

It is possible to monitor the count rate in each of the two energy channels for the purpose of maximizing the count rate, while locating bone edges and identifying artifacts or anatomical variations. This technique is often useful for improving the reproducibility. The accuracy and reproducibility of the bone mineral measurements are also strongly dependent upon the constant speed maintained by the stepping motors of the scanner. Slowing of the stepping motors creates erroneously increased count rates and vice versa. The inhomogeneous distribution of fat within and around the vertebrae has been found to be the major source of variation in lumbar DPA, with other sources being the irregular structure of the vertebrae (unfavorable geometry), variations in patient thicknesses, the uncertainty of localization and repositioning of the bone areas of interest, and the activity and randomness of the radioactive decay of the source. In addition, according to Krolner and Pors Nielsen, the reading of the attenuation curves (bone profiles) is the single most critical step of the measurement procedure that affects the reproducibility more than patient factors and physical factors. Krolner concluded that the precision of the lumbar BMC methods now available is not sufficiently high to allow short-term studies of the rate of bone mineral loss in single individuals; however, the DPA method is extremely well suited for clinical investigations (group or population studies).

Wahner et al. (1985) recently assessed the accuracy of DPA using ^{153}Gd. Although limited to cadaver and phantom studies, it was found that DPA accurately indicates bone mass and bone density. Lumbar spine segments (L2-L4) removed from cadavers were measured with DPA (Lunar Radiation Corp., Madison, Wisconsin) while immersed in a 10-cm depth of 70% ethanol solution. The L3 vertebrae were ashed at 600°C for 24 hours to obtain the "area densities" (ash weight per unit area in grams per square centimeter). The vertebral area densities were compared with the *bone mineral densities* BMD (bone mineral content BMC divided by the projected anterior vertebral area, number of pixels times pixel size) obtained by DPA. A very good correlation ($r = 0.94$) was found and the relative accuracy to be found in normal subjects was estimated as 5% to 6%. Measurements were also performed on the femoral neck specimens with better accuracy (3% to 4%).

DaCosta et al. (1985) evaluated the reproducibility of DPA measurements using a phantom constructed of a section of human bony pelvis and lumbosacral spine. The reproducibility within a single day for the measurement of the bone mineral density (BMD, gm/cm^2) of the lumbar vertebrae (L2-L4) was demonstrated by a coefficient of variation (1 SD) of 0.97%. In repeated evaluations over a period of 4 months, the coefficient of variation did not exceed 1.9%. The reproducibility over a 7-month period (including a ^{153}Gd source change) was reflected by the coefficient of variation of 2.1%. It was found that BMD measurements using DPA were reproducible to within 2%.

The accuracy of dual-photon absorptiometry for assessing total-body calcium was determined by comparing the results of DPA with those obtained by total-body neutron activation analysis; the coefficient of variation was 0.99% (Dunn et al., 1980). In comparing DPA measurements for excised lumbar spine vertebrae with the measured ash weight of the vertebrae, a standard error of 3.0% has been reported (Wilson and Madsen, 1977).

TOTAL-BODY BONE MINERAL MEASUREMENTS

Dual-photon absorptiometry can be used for measurements of fat content in body areas not containing bone mineral (Jacobson, 1964; Witt and Mazess, 1978). A dual-photon absorptiometry system for the determination of total-body bone mineral (TBBM) was described early in the development of DPA. The device used a ^{153}Gd source with an activity in the range of 0.5 to 1.5 Ci. The source consisted of a 3.0-mm diameter bead in a stainless-steel capsule, yielding the nearly equal photon intensities represented by the 44-keV europium K fluorescence peak and the 100-keV (97- and 103-keV) peak. The ratio of the transmitted intensities of the two primary energy peaks was 1:10 for thick body areas such as the trunk (Watt, 1975).

In addition, methods have been developed for determining total-body bone mineral (TBBM) and lean body mass (LBM). Peppler and Mazess (1981) described a nuclear medicine rectilinear scanner that was adapted for dual-photon absorptiometry. The radioactive source used in the instrument was ^{153}Gd. The activity of the source was 1.0 Ci, providing a scan time of 70 minutes and a radiation dose to the patient of less than 1 mrem during the total body scan. The measurement of total-body bone mineral assumes a two-component system of bone mineral and soft tissue, respectively. It is assumed that the composition of bone mineral does not vary; however, soft tissue contains variable amounts of fat and lean. The variations of fat/lean composition will introduce differences in the effective attenuation coefficients for soft tissue at both energies. It is necessary to estimate the soft tissue composition in order to obtain accurate bone mineral and soft tissue masses (Peppler and Mazess,

1981). The lean body mass was determined from the relationship between the attenuation coefficients:

$$R_{st} = \frac{\mu_{44,st}}{\mu_{100,st}} = \frac{\ln \dfrac{I_{44}(o)}{I_{44}}}{\ln \dfrac{I_{100}(o)}{I_{100}}}$$

R_{st} is the ratio of attenuation coefficients of soft tissue at the lower and upper energies. R_{st} varies linearly from 1.288, representing 100% fat, to 1.451, representing 100% lean. The masses of soft tissue, M_{st}, and bone mineral, M_{bm}, were calculated and summed up over the entire body (Mazess et al., 1981).

The short-term precision (months) for the total-body bone mineral measurements was approximately 1.5% for cadaver skeletons. The short-term precision for normal human subjects was approximately 2%. The long-term (years) precision on cadaver skeletons was better than 3%. The precision for the determination of percent fat was 0.9%, which lead to an error of less than 1% in the total-body bone mineral. The accuracy, given as one standard error of the estimate, of total-body bone mineral (TBBM) in five cadaver skeletons was reported as 36 g (equivalent to about 13 g of calcium) with a correlation coefficient of 0.99. This represented an error of approximately 1% to 1.5% in normal subjects (adults), 2% in older women, and 2.5% in osteoporotic females (Peppler and Mazess, 1981).

Mazess et al. (1984) measured total-body bone mineral (TBBM) in grams, using a rectilinear transmission scanner. The dual-photon ^{153}Gd device was designed to scan over the entire body area (120 × 180 cm). The scanner used a transverse scan speed of 1 cm/sec with data collected at 0.5-second (5-mm) intervals. The approximately 70 transverse scan paths across the body were separated by a distance of 2.5 cm. The radiation beam was approximately 1 cm × 2 cm at the level of the body; a slit collimator (8 mm × 25 mm) was used on the detector. The transmitted intensities at the 44-keV and 100-keV peaks of the spectrum were corrected for count loss due to dead time, beam hardening, spillover from the 100 keV channel into the 44 keV channel, scattered radiation from the patient, and background.

The complete TBBM scan consisted of approximately 8000 pixels, in which about 3000 pixels contained bone tissue, 2000 pixels contained soft tissue alone, and 3000 pixels contained only air transmission intensities. The bone-mineral and soft-tissue content were calculated for each pixel (5 mm × 25 mm). The computer system contained algorithms for separating the skeleton into major anatomical segments (head, arms, legs, and trunk; and within the trunk, ribs, pelvis, and spine). In these segments the spine also included the sternum, the ribs contained the clavicles, and the pelvis included the sacrum and the femoral heads. The areal density, BMD (bone mineral content per unit area), was calculated for each area. Similarly, the TBBM/area was calculated for the total skeleton. It was stated that the use of the area density minimizes the influence of anatomical positioning and normalizes the measurement for skeletal size. The TBBM/area was determined with a precision of 1.4% for cadaver skeletons and 2.4% for in vivo measurements of one adult male subject.

The reproducibility in limb segments and the trunk was 2% for cadaver skeletons and 4% in vivo, while the reproducibility of the smaller subsegments of the trunk was 4% for cadaver skeletons and 6% in vivo (Mazess et al., 1984). This system was used to investigate the correlation between single-photon absorptiometry of the radius and dual-photon absorptiometry of the spine in predicting skeletal status. The TBBM was previously shown to be moderately correlated ($r = 0.8$) with spinal density.

Gotfredsen et al. (1984) reported on a dual-photon absorptiometry system for measuring total-body bone mineral (TBBM). The system consisted of a scanning table, a 1-Ci ^{153}Gd source, a NaI(Tl) detector, the counting electronics, a computer and data storage unit, and a printer. The source and detector were mounted opposite each other, the source below and the detector above the table. A cylindrical collimator was used to provide a beam of 250-mm diameter at the top of the scanning table. The detector collimation consisted of four openings (each 6 mm) in diameter and 5-mm thick separated by 1.5 mm), forming a slit collimator (6 × 28.5 mm). The detector crystal thickness was 50 × 7 mm. Two single channel analyzers were used for discrimination of the two energy peaks. The rectilinear scanning procedure required 90 minutes at a transverse speed of 1 cm/sec and longitudinal steps of 2.5 cm. Transmitter intensities were recorded at 0.5-second intervals (0.5-cm intervals), yielding 150 points per line and a total of about 11,000 pixels of data. The skeleton was divided into four regions consisting of 20 scan lines each (figure 30). The bone mineral mass m_b was determined from the following equations:

$$M_b = \frac{R_{st} \ln \frac{I_{100}}{I_{100}(o)} - \ln \frac{I_{44}}{I_{44}(o)}}{(\mu_{b,44} - \mu_{b,100})\, R_{st}}$$

where I_{44} and I_{100} are the transmitted intensities, $I_{44}(o)$and $I_{100}(o)$ are the incident intensities, and $\mu_{b,44}$ and $\mu_{b,100}$ are the mass attenuation coefficients at the energies 44 and 100 keV. R_{st} is defined as the ratio of the mass attenuation coefficients for soft tissue: $\mu_{st,44}/\mu_{st,100}$, where st refers to soft tissue. Similarly, the soft tissue mass m_{st} was determined as follows:

$$M_{st} = \frac{\ln \frac{I_{44}}{I_{100}(o)} - R_b \ln \frac{I_{000}}{I_{100}(o)}}{R_b\, (\mu_s t_{,100} - \mu_s t_{,44})}$$

where R_b is defined as the ratio of the mass attenuation coefficients for bone: $\mu_{b,44}/\mu_{b,100}$, where b refers to bone.

The amount of bone mineral in all measuring sites was summed to yield the TBBM. The mass attenuation coefficients required for calculation of the bone mineral mass were determined at 44 and 100 keV by measuring aluminum, water, and ethanol phantoms. Corrections for dead time losses, beam hardening, and spillover from the 100-keV to the 44-keV energy window were made. These three corrections changed the calculated TBBM by approximately 20% and appear to be necessary corrections. In addition, as the source decayed, the dead time correction required adjustment. The day-to-day precision error of the method using phantoms was 2.6%. The linearity of the system was demonstrated by a correlation coefficient r = 0.999 between the TBBM and the weight of aluminum samples. The short-term precision error determined in healthy subjects scanned at the beginning and at the end of a 2-month interval was 2.4% (CV). The precision of the R_{st} determination in healthy subjects was 0.4%. The long-term precision error in healthy subjects was 2% to 3%. The radiation dose per unit body area was estimated (film methods) as 50 mGy (5 mrad). The importance of the accurate determination of the correction factors, especially the correction for Compton scattering in the patient, was emphasized. Finally, the patient was required to lie still for 90 minutes during the scan; this requirement could be reduced with the use of faster scan speeds.

Gotfredsen et al. (1984) further published the results of TBBM measurements on whole cadavers and on the same healthy subjects scanned at two different institutions. The TBBM measurements were well correlated (r = 0.991) with the weight of the cadaver skeletons. The dry defatted weight of skeletal specimens was also well correlated (r = 0.996) with the actual calcium content (ashing). The correlation between the TBBM values obtained at the two institutions (University of Wisconsin, Madison and Glostrup Hospital, Denmark) was high (r = 0.99). It was concluded that the precision and accuracy of the TBBM method is better than that of other methods used to evaluate the total or local bone mineral content. The only other method for measuring TBCa, neutron-activation analysis (having a precision error of about 2% and an accuracy of 5% to 7%), requires much higher radiation doses. Both institutions participating in the TBBM study found comparable precision errors of 2% to 3% and accuracy errors of 1% to 1.5% in normal adults. These errors may be acceptable for the longitudinal evaluation of osteoporosis treatment in groups of patients as opposed to the diagnosis of individual patients.

In addition to the determination of total body bone mineral (TBBM), the ratio R of attenuation at 44 keV to that at 100 keV is a direct indication of the fat content of soft tissue (Mazess et al., 1970; Witt and Mazess, 1978, Preuss and Schmonsees, 1972). It was found that the value of R ranges from 1.32 at 100% fat tissue to 1.47 at 100% lean tissue; each change of 0.01 in the R value corresponds to a change of 4% in body fat. The percentage body fat %FAT, derived from the R value was used to calculate the mass of fat and the lean body mass LBM. The typical precision of an R value determination was about 0.005 (or about 2% body fat). The accuracy of the R value as determined in

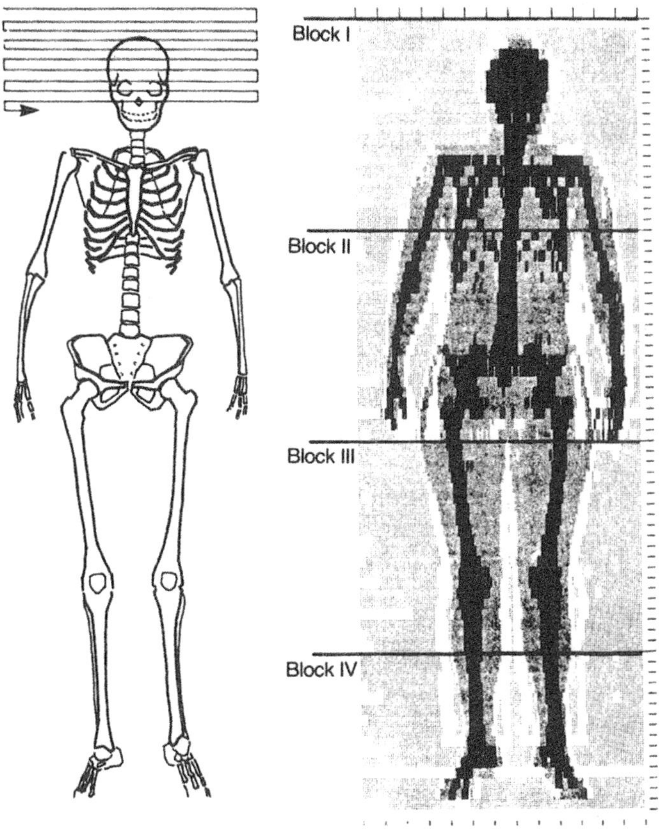

Figure 30. Rectilinear scan path and image display of total-body bone mineral (Courtesy: A Gotfredsen)

phantoms containing alcohol and water, which simulate fat and muscle, respectively, was very good (predictive error, defined as 1 SEE, was 1%).

It was found that the TBBM was not a constant fraction of the lean body mass LBM, as is often assumed; the TBBM as a percentage (5%) was low compared to previous assumptions. The percentage fat using dual-photon absorptiometry was moderately correlated ($r = 0.87$) with the underwater density determination of fat. The DPA method was, therefore, found to be useful in assessing these factors as they relate to the nutritional aspects of health (figure 31).

Als et al. (1985) developed a whole-body scanner for the measurement of total-body bone mineral (TBBM, g/cm^2). The device used a 1-Ci ^{153}Gd radiation source, and the scanning procedure required 90 minutes scanning time with the patient in a supine position on the scan table. The radiation source

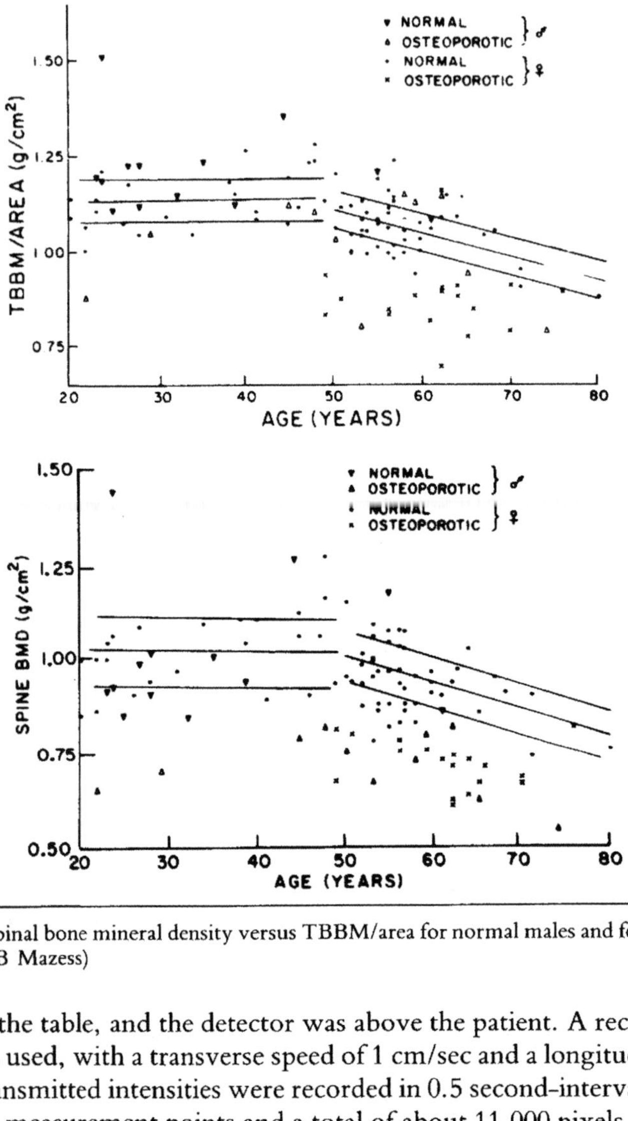

Figure 31. Spinal bone mineral density versus TBBM/area for normal males and females by DPA (Courtesy: RB Mazess)

was below the table, and the detector was above the patient. A rectilinear scan pattern was used, with a transverse speed of 1 cm/sec and a longitudinal step of 2.5 cm. Transmitted intensities were recorded in 0.5 second-intervals, yielding lines of 150 measurement points and a total of about 11,000 pixels. The reproducibility of the TBBM measurement was 2.4%, and the accuracy was 1.5%. The radiation dose in one scan procedure was 50 μGy (5 millirad) per unit of body area. In a study of 61 patients with rheumatoid arthritis, the TBBM was correlated (r = 0.89, SEE = 9.6%) with the distal forearm BMC measured also by ^{125}I SPA in the patient group.

The total-body mineral in vivo can be directly related to the total-body calcium as measured by neutron activation analysis (figure 32). Total-body neutron activation analysis (TBNAA) gives an approximate indication of total-body mineral, since calcium is a relatively constant fraction of mineral in the

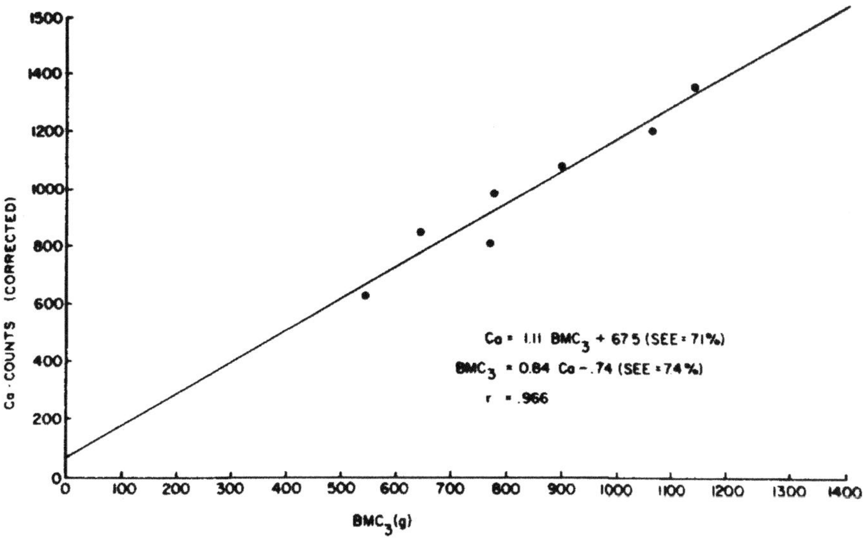

Figure 32. Spinal BMD and total-body bone mineral in normal and osteoporotic males and females (Courtesy: RB Mazess)

skeleton. Calcium represents approximately 38% to 39% of the mineral (ash) weight for mature compact bone (Woodward, 1964; Blitz and Pelligrano, 1969; Armstrong and Singer, 1965; Dyson and Whitehouse, 1970). The relatively high radiation dose received by the patient during TBNAA (0.3 to 5.0 rem) prohibits some applications of the method and limits the feasibility of repeated studies of the same patient (Peppler and Mazess, 1981).

CLINICAL MEASUREMENTS

DPA can be easily applied to the lumbar vertebrae as a noninvasive procedure. It provides a fairly accurate measurement of BMC in the vertebrae and an estimate of vertebral strength. The radiation dose is low compared to conventional spinal radiography. It is questionable, however, if knowledge of the lumbar BMC is of any use in clinical practice, i.e., whether it can be used for the guidance of a certain treatment in one individual patient. It remains, in fact, to be established that postmenopausal women having a low BMC are more prone to develop fractures than other postmenopausal women (Krolner, 1985).

Riggs et al. (1982) investigated the bone mineral density using DPA in subjects with postmenopausal and senile osteoporosis. The BMC (g/cm) was also assessed by ^{125}I SPA of the midradius and distal radius. The BMD (g/cm^2) was assessed in the lumbar spine and in the proximal femur (cervical and intertrochanteric regions) in 205 normal males and females. The DPA method consisted of the modified device (Dunn et al., 1980; Riggs et al., 1981) of the method of Mazess et al. (1974). Two distinct syndromes were described on the basis of the data obtained: (1) *postmenopausal osteoporosis,* which is characterized by the excessive and disproportionate trabecular bone loss involving a small subset of women in the early postmenopausal period, and (2) *senile osteoporosis,* which is characterized by the proportionate loss of both cortical and trabecular bone involving essentially the entire population of aging women and, to a lesser extent, aging men.

The validity of DPA measurements has been evaluated in clinical studies. The DPA method has been used in a longitudinal study of aging in postmenopausal women and its relation to the mineral content of the lumbar spine, in which the bone mineral content (g/cm) and bone mineral area (BMA) were determined (Lindquist et al., 1983).

In another clinical investigation, the center of the vertebral body (usually L3) was marked on the abdomen during fluoroscopy, with the patient lying on his or her back with legs bent. The transmission measurements were performed with the patient in the same position; positioning lights mounted on the detector allowed for the alignment of the radiation beam with the mark on the abdomen. Side supports for the knees made it easier for the patient to lie still during the procedure; no other restraints were used. The measurement path length was 160 mm, giving 41 measurement points at intervals of 4 mm. The measurement time for each point was 0.25 minutes, and the total time for the measurement was about 10 minutes. Three measurement paths were included, one on each side of the center of the vertebra at a distance of 5 mm, in which 15 minutes per path was required for an exam. The standard deviations for repeated measurements in phantoms and in patients were 3% and 3% to 8%, respectively (Roos and Skoldborn, 1974).

In a later evaluation of the device, the reproducibility for patient measurements ranged from 3.4% to 5.7%. The long-term stability of the device was better than 1% over a 5-month period as tested by phantom measurements (Ross, 1975). Hanson and Roos (1980) studied the relationships between age, height, weight, and the bone mineral content of the lumbar vertebrae. They measured the BMC using dual-photon absorptiometry (Roos and Skoldborn, 1974) in 109 excised lumbar vertebrae from 36 subjects, placing the vertebrae in a water phantom; the ashed weights of the vertebrae were determined. The investigators also determined the lumbar spine score (Barnett and Nordin, 1960) from lateral radiographs of the vertebrae and found no correlation between the BMC and this score. The BMC (using DPA) was, however, correlated with the age, height, and weight of the subjects and with the body weight above each vertebra. The decreasing BMC with age was demonstrated in male and female subjects.

Hansson and Roos (1986) investigated the bone loss due to aging in females in Sweden. The DPA method utilized the two radionuclides ^{241}Am and ^{137}Cs. Localization of the radiation beam was facilitated by the use of an x-ray tube and an image intensifier. Transmissions measurements were performed at 4-mm steps using a motorized couch upon which the patient was supine. The

BMC values were divided by the width to correct for vertebral size; this bone mineral areal content (BMAC, g/cm^2) reflected the *areal density* in other studies. It was noted that the BMC is more closely related to the compressive strength of vertebral bodies than is BMAC (Hansson and Roos, 1986, in press). The precision errors of the BMC and BMAC measurements were about 4%.

Bohr and Schaadt (1985) investigated the relationship between cortical and trabecular bone sites for measurement of bone mineral content using dual-photon absorptiometry. The DPA method (Schaadt and Bohr, 1982) incorporated a l-Ci ^{153}Gd source. Scanning was performed on healthy women at the femoral neck and shaft sites. The scan speed was 2 mm/sec; linear scans at intervals of 2 mm were performed. The femoral neck scan was done at an angle of 53° with the transverse direction, that is, approximately perpendicular to the axis of the femoral neck. In order to compensate for the normal anteversion of the femoral neck, the legs were rotated 15° inwardly. The average of five single scan integrals around the lowest value was chosen to represent BMC of the femoral neck (g/cm). For the femoral shaft, scanning was performed transversely across the middle of the bone and the results given as the average of five single-scan integrals (g/cm).

Autopsy specimens were also measured in a water bath using DPA. Following the DPA measurements, the specimens were sectioned and ashed, and the cortical and trabecular bone was separated. The calcium content was determined by atomic absorption analysis, and the amount of hydroxyapatite (HA) was calculated as 2.5 times the calcium content. HA of the femoral neck was well correlated ($r = 0.991$) with the BMC by DPA. Similarly, HA of the femoral shaft was well correlated ($r = 0.996$) with the BMC. The coefficient of variation for repeated in vivo BMC measurements was 1.4 ±0.7% for the femoral neck and 1.3 ±1.3% for the femoral shaft. This precision is comparable to those of other investigations. It was concluded that structures of the femoral neck containing mostly trabecular bone show a more rapid loss of bone with age than the average femoral neck, while structures consisting mainly of cortical bone lose bone at a slower rate, corresponding to the femoral shaft.

DPA was used for the determination of the relationship between lumbar spine bone mineral density (g/cm^2) and strength of the back extensor muscles (Sinaki et al., 1986). A population of 68 healthy postmenopausal Caucasian women was selected for the study. A strain-gauge dynamometer was attached to the back muscles with the subject in a prone position, and it measured the isometric strength (lbs) of the back extensor muscles. The reproducibility of the dynamometer measurements was 8.7%, and the reproducibility of the BMD measurements was 2.3% (Seeman et al., 1982). The bone mineral density (g/cm^2) was slightly correlated ($r = 0.32$) with the measured arm span, slightly correlated with height ($r = 0.38$) and weight ($r = 0.35$), and slightly correlated with back extensor strength ($r = 0.34$). It was concluded that the data suggest that the strength of back muscles may contribute to the bone mineral density of vertebral bodies. The authors suggested a longitudinal study to determine whether exercises that strengthen spinal muscles can defer or reverse the postmenopausal loss of calcium in the vertebral bodies.

Dual-photon absorptiometry has been used in studying clinical conditions such as endocrine dysfunction (Seeman et al., 1982). DPA has shown significant bone loss from trabecular bone sites in hypoparathyroidism, whereas the SPA measurements in predominantly cortical bone did not demonstrate significant loss.

FRACTURE THRESHOLD

The use of dual photon absorptiometry in patients with osteoporosis indicates that lumbar spine bone mineral content values for osteoporotic individuals are better separated from normal individuals, as compared to studies of radius bone mineral content (SPA). DPA studies provide a means for defining a threshold for spinal compression fractures. Wahner has defined this threshold in patients with vertebral bone mineral values below 0.98 g/cm^2. For BMD values below this threshold, the risk of compression fractures is significantly increased (Wahner, 1984). Reported measurements on patients were expressed as spinal bone mineral relative to the normal range and corrected for age and sex. It is preferable to report the index for fracture risk and the rate of bone loss per year in follow-up studies in these patients.

RADIATION DOSE TO PATIENTS

The radiation dose delivered to patients undergoing the DPA procedure is the same order of magnitude as found in single-photon absorptiometry. Wahner (1983) has reported that the radiation dose is 18 mrad for a dual-photon scan of the lumbar spine using a 1.5-Ci gadolinium ^{153}Gd radionuclide source. This dose was determined by LiF thermoluminescent dosimetry (TLD-100). The radiation doses have been reported for another DPA device, in which the specific gamma-ray constant for gadolinium (^{153}Gd) has been determined as 0.0961 R/h/Ci at 1 meter within a 10-mil steel capsule. Neglecting self-absorption in the source and attenuation by the scanning table, the exposure rate at the entrance of the patient was measured as 0.22 mR/s for a 1.0-Ci source. The exposure rate was actually less than this value, since self-absorption by the source material and other factors were not taken into account. An exposure rate of 0.07 mr per second was measured by thermoluminescent dosimetry (TLD-100). Four TLD dosimeters were placed in the beam path for 100 minutes. The calculated dose rates at the table top for muscle and for bone were 0.20 and 0.61 mrad per second, respectively (for a 1.0-Ci source). A single point in tissue was irradiated for approximately 2.5 seconds during a scan. This resulted in a maximum radiation dose of 0.5 mrad to muscle and 1.5 mrad to bone. The skin dose was measured (TLD) and did not exceed 0.5 mrad (Peppler and Mazess, 1981).

The radiation dose was also determined for the DPA method using a 1.0-Ci

^{153}Gd source (Krolner and Pors Nielsen, 1980). Thermoluminescent dosimeters were placed in drilled holes of a phantom consisting of a human pelvis with lumbar vertebrae embedded in a body-shaped Perspex block. The skin dose per measurement of lumbar BMC carried out over L(3) was 0.10 mGy (10 mrad). The radiation dose to the ovaries per measurement was less than 0.02 mGy (2 mrad). The bone marrow dose in the irradiated area comprising 5% to 10% of the total bone marrow was less than 0.002 mGy (0.2 mrad).

Dunn et al., (1980) measured the DPA radiation dose using TLD on phantoms and patients. The dose was found to be dependent upon the strength of the source and the beam characteristics. The peak skin dose at the beam entrance for DPA ranged from 5 to 15 mrad (0.05 to 0.15 mGy); by comparison, the radiation dose associated with SPA of the radius was about 5 mrad (0.05 mGy).

5. QUANTITATIVE COMPUTED TOMOGRAPHY

Computed tomography (CT) scanners, which are primarily designed for imaging the human body, can be used to provide quantitative information regarding the composition of body tissues. Cross-sectional (transverse) images of the body tissues are produced. The quantitative data are the radiation attenuation coefficients of various tissues. CT scanning allows the separate determination of the attenuation coefficient values for trabecular bone and compact bone.

In addition, CT scanning provides a noninvasive method for the determination of the bone mineral content. It is a method that allows the evaluation of trabecular vertebral bone, which has been estimated to turn over at a rate eight times higher than cortical bone (ICRP 23, 1975). Therefore, it is believed that CT scanning provides a method for the assessment of a more sensitive measurement site in osteoporosis. High measurement precision and good sensitivity are required of the CT method for detecting small mineral changes in serial clinical studies, in evaluations of the efficacy of treatment regimens, and in the assessment of the progression of disease processes.

Computer tomography (CT) was first applied to the quantification of bone by Ruegsegger and coworkers (Hangartner et al., 1985), who developed a special-purpose CT scanner with a radioisotope (^{125}I) source — the gamma CT method. Rutherford et al. (1976) found that the absorption coefficients of bone could be precisely measured for small regions of tissue in vivo. It was further determined that the electron density and atomic number of tissues could be obtained by a computer algorithm that separates the photoelectric and Compton-scattered components of the attenuation coefficients, providing images containing additional information about the physical properties of the tissues. Separation of the CT data into these two components requires the performance of CT scans of the radius at two different x-ray energies (kVp's). The reproducibilities of the dual-energy scanning methods was about 2%.

Marschall et al. (1978) were the first investigators to report on CT densitometry in the human spine (Lampmann et al., 1984). They also demonstrated a linear correlation between the EMI (CT) numbers and the bone mineral content (BMC). CT bone densitometry was performed in the distal radius of patients (Isherwood et al., 1976), demonstrating the good reproducibility of the CT method. A study that compared the CT method with the radiographic microdensitometry method, as well as the SPA method, revealed that the CT method was the most sensitive (Pullan and Roberts, 1978). The trabecular bone mass of the radius measured by CT was found to correlate well ($r = 0.95$) with the concentration of trabecular bone as determined by histomorphometric methods (biopsy) of transiliac bone specimens (Jensen et al., 1979).

The advantages of the CT method in bone densitometry include the ability to obtain an image of the bone in which trabecular and cortical regions can be separately identified, while simultaneously obtaining quantitative values of mineral content. The CT image reduces the inaccuracy due to positioning of the spine and other bones. However, the CT method requires careful calibration with reference standards and highly reproducible positioning techniques (Genant et al., 1985). In addition, several limitations of the CT bone densitometry method have been noted and are discussed in this chapter.

MONOENERGETIC (GAMMA) CT

Ruegsegger designed and constructed a special forearm trabecular bone measurement device that provided careful positioning for studies of the appendicular skeleton. The radiation beam was produced by the monoenergetic radionuclide source iodine (^{125}I) having a primary energy of 29 keV. This system utilized a rotating sealed radiation source for scanning the extremities. The beam was highly collimated for good spatial resolution and for reduction of the radiation received by the patient. An image of the cross section of the forearm was generated by a computer algorithm, which assigned the attenuation coefficient values to all pixels in the image.

Exner et al. (1979) used the gamma-ray CT scanner to estimate the linear attenuation coefficients in compact and trabecular bone (Exner et al., 1979). The percentage of trabecular bone was evaluated in the tibia and the calcaneus using a gamma-ray CT scanner (Schneider et al., 1979). A similar ^{125}I CT scanner was built for monitoring the course of osteopenia and its treatment. The investigators reported a precision of 0.5% in measurements of the trabecular bone density of the distal radius in normal subjects and osteoporotic patients (Hosie, 1984). An important point, however, was the fact that CT measurements in the trabecular bone of the distal radius were profoundly affected by the layer of compact bone that surrounds the trabecular bone (Mazess, 1984).

It has been stated that commercial x-ray (polyenergetic) CT units are essential for measurements of the axial skeleton, while evaluations of the peripheral skeleton at low energy (29 keV) are less influenced by changes of the fat content in the marrow. In addition, the special purpose monoenergetic CT systems (figure 33) provide improved geometrical resolution (0.3 mm/pixel, figure 34) over commercial CT systems (0.8 to 1.5mm/pixel); and the monoenergetic CT systems are much less expensive (Hangartner and Overton, 1982). These investigators calculated the *relative bone content* (B) of each pixel, using the following formula:

$$B = \frac{\mu_B - \mu_M}{\mu_{CB} - \mu_M}$$

where μ_B is the linear attenuation coefficient of the pixel with unknown bone content, μ_M is the linear attenuation coefficient of bone marrow, and μ_{CB} is the linear attenuation coefficient of compact bone. The physical densities are calculated as follows:

$$\varrho_B = \varrho_{CB} \left[\frac{\mu_B - \mu_M}{\mu_{CB} - \mu_M}\right]$$

where ϱ_b is the physical density of bone corresponding to the linear attenuation coefficient μ_B, and ϱ_{CB} is the physical density of cortical bone. The reproducibility of this gamma-ray CT densitometer, using solutions of K_2HPO_4 in a phantom, is reflected by the coefficient of variation 0.04%. In clinical measurements, repositioning of the scan site (distal radius) was the largest source of error. The coefficients of variation for the clinical measurements of the linear attenuation coefficients for total bone, compact bone, and trabecular bone were 0.46%, 0.70%, and 0.57%, respectively.

In a study of the optimal CT settings for bone evaluations, it was found that the selection of optimal settings was dependent upon the object being imaged. The sensitivity (the change in the linear attenuation coefficient as the trabecular bone density changes) for detecting bone changes was dependent on the amount of bone present in the trabecular bone region. A nondivergent monoenergetic x-ray beam was used in a computer simulation of the CT scanner. A filtered backprojection technique was used for reconstruction of the images. It was shown that the sensitivity diminished gradually as the energy of the incident x-rays increased or as the density of the trabecular bone decreased. The investigators also determined the minimal dose per examination required to detect a relative change in trabecular bone density. It was concluded that peripheral bone measurements using a monoenergetic CT unit should be performed in the energy range 30 to 40 keV.

For energies below 30 keV, the sensitivity of the linear attenuation coefficient for changes of the trabecular bone density was higher, but the precision with which the linear attenuation coefficient was determined was much smaller. For energies above 40 keV, the precision was higher, but the sensitivity was diminished (Muller et al., 1985). The ^{125}I CT densitometry method meets the requirements for optimal CT settings and delivers a low radiation dose per examination.

PRECISION AND ACCURACY (GAMMA-CT)

The long-term precision of the system is reflected by the coefficient of variation of 0.6% for trabecular bone mineral measurements of the distal radius. This radionuclide method has demonstrated a good correlation (r = 0.9) between the bone mineral content of the radius and ashed specimens of vertebral bone (Ruegsegger et al., 1976). Clinical studies have been performed using this method in which patients with osteoporosis and other metabolic bone diseases were measured; other studies included information on fracture healing and immobilization. The ability of this method to provide a means of separating normal from osteoporotic populations may be superior to the single photon absorptiometry method (SPA) in radius bone mineral measurements (Wahner et al., 1984). A definitive study comparing the radionuclide CT method with the SPA method on the same population has not been performed. The radionuclide CT method has the advantage that it can assess not only the cortical bone (as does SPA), but it also assesses the trabecular bone, which is believed to reflect earlier changes in the quantity of bone mineral than compact bone.

Hangartner et al. (1985) measured bone density (BD) at the distal end of the radius with gamma-ray computed tomography (gamma-ray CT) in groups of postmenopausal women. The investigators refined the technology first introduced by Ruegsegger et al. (1976) to provide sensitive, high-precision measurements of trabecular and cortical bone densities in vivo (Hangartner and Overton, 1982). Individual BD values were found to have a standard deviation (SD) of ±0.6%. The standard deviation associated with the group of control subjects was ±1.25%. The gamma-CT method demonstrated a capability for monitoring small, rapid, transient changes in bone density in the peripheral skeleton. It was concluded that gamma-CT measurements may be of value in determining appropriate therapy and for assessing therapeutic responses to drugs.

Clinical studies have been performed using the miniaturized translational-rotational gamma-ray CT scanner (Ruegsegger et al., 1984). The clinical measurements were performed in the distal end of the tibia and in the distal end of the radius in normal and osteoporotic subjects. There was a good correlation between the trabecular bone parameters of the distal tibia and of the

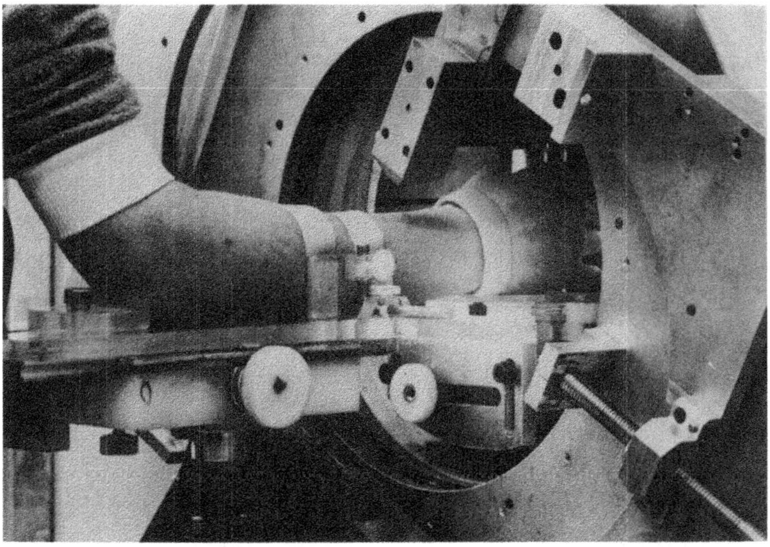

Figure 33. Gamma CT system and positioning devices (Courtesy: TN Hangartner)

distal radius in normal and osteoporotic subjects. The stated precision of the system was 0.3%.

Sambrook et al. (1985) compared ^{125}I CT measurements of bone mineral of the radius (trabecular bone index) with QCT and DPA measurements of the spinal vertebrae and found poorer correlation ($r = 0.65$) for patient studies than those yielded by the previous studies of Ruegsegger ($r = 0.924$) for macerated postmortem specimens. Sambrook stated that the relatively poor ability of all peripheral measurements to predict axial bone mineral reflects differences in the amount and nature of cortical and trabecular bone at different sites.

SINGLE-ENERGY X-RAY QUANTITATIVE CT

By 1985, there were approximately 2000 single-energy x-ray CT installations worldwide, of which 150 sites were using commercial CT scanners for quantitative vertebral mineral determination (Genant et al., 1985). X-ray CT scanners collect and store the x-ray intensities transmitted through the human body. Depending upon the design of the CT system, thousands of transmitted intensity values are collected as the x-ray tube revolves about the patient. Each of these transmitted rays is represented by an intensity equation, which contains mathematical terms describing characteristics of the tissues traversed by the radiation. The most important parameters contained in these equations are the *linear attenuation coefficients* for the various tissues through which the beam has

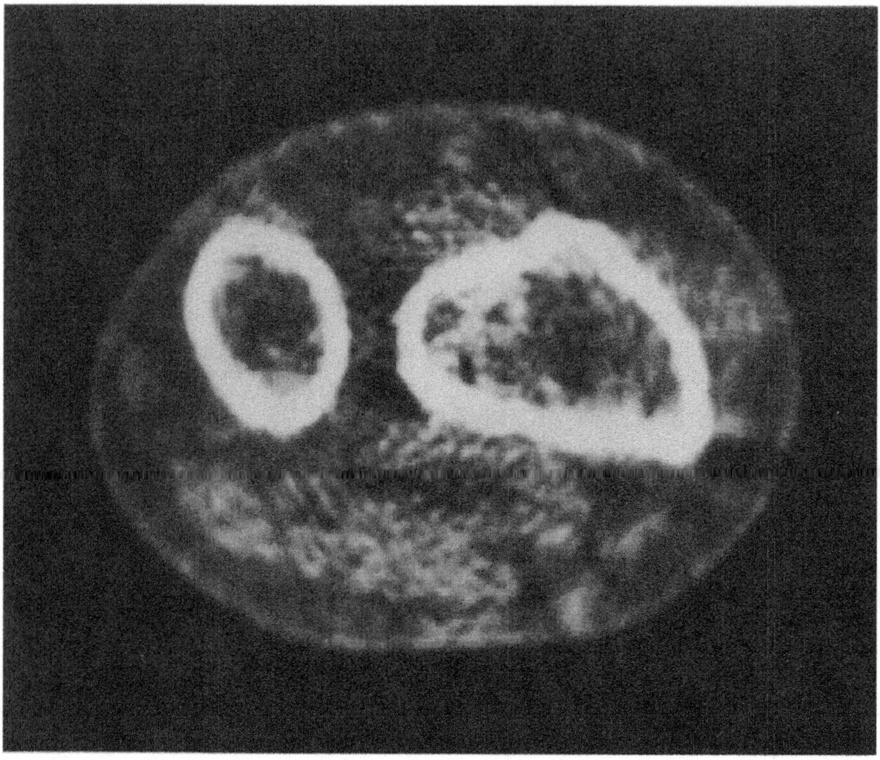

Figure 34. Gamma CT image of the forearm proximal to the radial styloid (Courtesy: TN Hangartner)

passed. These attenuation values are directly related to the *CT numbers* provided by the imaging system. The CT number represents an average of the attenuation coefficients of all the materials present, i.e., in the vertebral body, this includes mineral, collagen, soft tissue, and fat. However, for single-energy CT, a two-component mixture is assumed — soft tissue and mineral.

The values of the linear attenuation coefficients depend upon the energy of the x-rays; and each position in the CT image is assigned a CT number, which characterizes the linear attenuation coefficient value of the body tissue located at that position. The appropriate CT number is found following the determination of the attenuation coefficient for each location in the tissue cross section. These locations are referred to as *pixels* in a cross-sectional or transverse image; *voxels* represent the three-dimensional volume of tissue associated with each image pixel. An average linear attenuation coefficient value is computed for all tissues within the voxel, which often leads to CT numbers that represent a mixture of biological compounds. The computer solves a set of equations in order to assign the unique CT number to each pixel. The CT number H (Hounsfield units) is calculated from the linear attenuation coefficient as follows:

$$H_v = \frac{1000}{\mu_{W1}} (\mu_E - \mu_{W2})$$

where: μ_E is the linear attenuation coefficient of the substance in the pixel at the effective energy E of the x-ray beam, and μ_{w1} and μ_{w2} are linear attenuation coefficients chosen such that H is zero for water and -1000 for air.

The values of these CT numbers modulate the shades of gray assigned to each pixel, and this modulation provides the contrast between different types of tissues represented in the CT image. Since bone has large CT numbers such as 1500, and soft tissues have CT numbers near zero (water), one is able to depict the bone edges of the vertebra in the image. Using the single-energy CT method, the concentration of bone mineral within the vertebra is given by:

$$C_b = \varrho_b \left(\frac{H_V - H_{s,V}}{H_{b,V} - H_{s,V}} \right)$$

where H_{bV} is the CT number of bone mineral at the x-ray tube voltage V, H_{sV} is the CT number of soft tissue, H_V is the measured CT number of the bone/soft tissue mixture, and ϱ_b is the density of bone mineral. H_{bV} and H_{sV} are determined at the time of patient imaging, by scanning reference standards containing mineral and soft tissue components, respectively (Genant et al., 1981).

CT densitometry is performed with the patient in a supine position with the skeletal region of interest placed in the gantry. The body section to be scanned is selected by using a position alignment light through which the x-ray beam will pass in its rotational movement around the patient. In scanning the spine, it is often necessary to tilt the CT gantry in order to decrease lumbar lordosis. After aligning the patient, a scout view is performed, which provides a lateral view of the body trunk. This image is necessary for identifying the exact location of the CT cut. The motorized couch can be moved, as the digital position indicator is observed by the operator, to the chosen site in the spine.

The selection of slice thickness is important, since the vertebrae may contain multiple foci of trabecular bone loss. By using a CT slice thickness less than 5 mm in a vertebrae containing a focal lesion, the average mineral content may be misrepresented.

In one established clinical procedure, a lateral CT (scout view) is first obtained for localization, followed by single axial scans through the midplane of two to four lumbar vertebral bodies. A region of interest is selected and the CT number is averaged over 3 to 4 cubic centimeters of each vertebral body. The CT numbers of four reference solutions of the phantom are also obtained

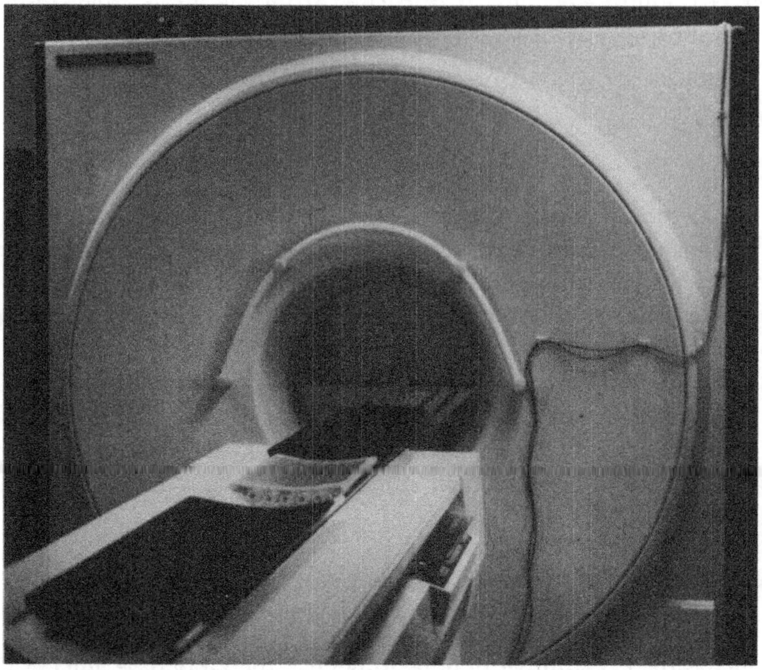

Figure 35. CT calibration phantom containing dipotassium hydrogen phosphate (Courtesy: HK Genant)

(figure 35). The readings are used to calculate the mineral density of the trabecular bone in mineral equivalents (mg/cc) of K_2HPO_4. The examination takes 10 to 15 minutes, and the radiation exposure is said to be one-tenth of that for a routine CT study (Richardson et al., 1985).

Window selection from the CT control console (figure 36) provides the operator with the means to select a range of CT numbers for image display. A center control is used to select the CT number to be placed in the center of the window. In this manner it is possible to separately view the range of CT numbers of interest, i.e., cancellous or cortical bone, marrow, or other soft tissues. Only the CT numbers included in the window are displayed over the range of the grey scale.

Lampmann et al. (1984) chose the transverse midplane of the fourth lumbar vertebral body as the CT scan site of the spine, tilting the gantry to select the midplane. This technique included a slice thickness of 6 mm and the scanning of three overlapping slices, each having a 3-mm overlap. The scan parameters for the Philips Tomoscan 300 CT unit were: 160-mm field of view, 120 kVp, and 450 mA. After these scans were completed, the gantry tilt was changed, and three additional scans were performed. Good visibility of the basivertebral

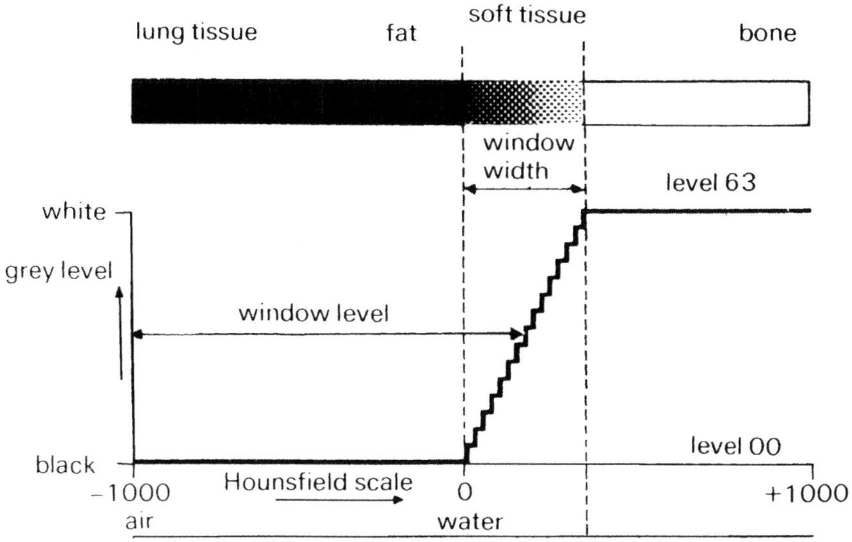

Figure 36. Principles of window width and window level in QCT (Courtesy: LEH Lampmann)

vein entrance indicated the exact middle of the vertebral body. A circular region of interest (ROI) was selected within the image of the vertebra; it contained 349 pixels, which provided a diameter of 13 mm of trabecular bone. The ROI was positioned well within the margins of the cortical shell. The mean CT density within the region of interest was determined. The investigators determined that measurements of the fourth lumbar vertebra provided the most reliable density values.

The region of interest selected by the operator must be carefully aligned within the trabecular region of the vertebrae for the clinical measurements (figure 37). The use of an elliptical region of interest has been investigated and found to be optimal. Phantoms containing excised vertebrae were used, and the effects of size and shape on the measured bone mineral densities were evaluated. For the elliptical ROI in each vertebra (figure 38), a change in position of the ROI of one pixel position in any direction in the transverse plane produced an average change of 0.8 Hounsfield units (HU: 1000 scale) in the mean CT number about an average of 240 HU for the spine specimen. It has been stated that the error in ROI positioning may contribute up to 15% of the overall error in the determination of vertebral mineral (Cann and Genant, 1980).

Ideally, x-ray CT methods should use monoenergetic x-ray sources and infinitesimally thin photon beams. Because these features cannot be completely achieved in commercial systems, artifacts are present in the reconstructed

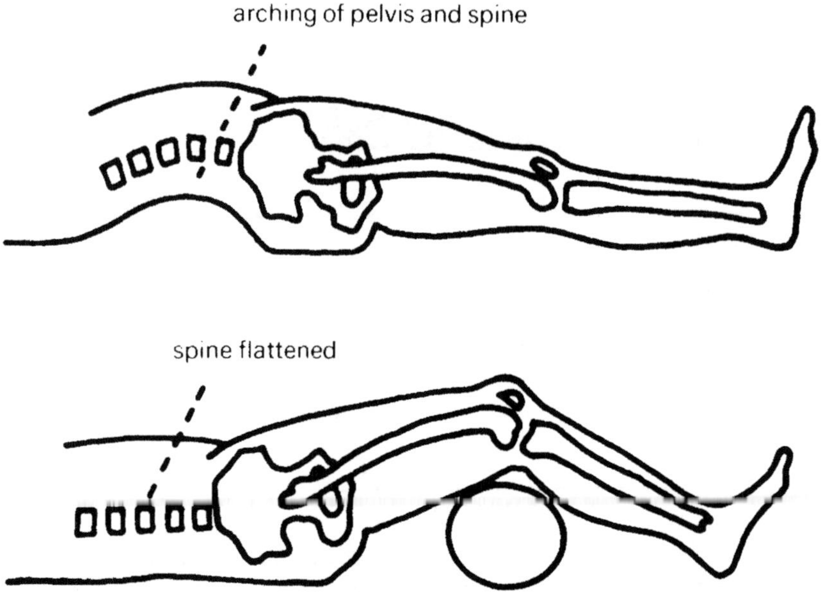

Figure 37. Positioning of the spine to minimize lumbar lordosis (Courtesy: LEH Lampmann)

images. The finite size of the x-ray beam is associated with linear and nonlinear degradations of the image (Verly and Bracewell, 1979; Glover and Pelc, 1980; Joseph and Spital, 1981).

Phantoms have been used to test the accuracy and precision of CT densitometry, such as the anthropomorphic phantom (Scanplas, Inc., Great Britain). This phantom (figure 39) consists of the actual anatomical and physical equivalent materials of the average human body and contains the fourth and fifth lumbar vertebral bodies. A cortical bone substitute (SB3) simulates cortical bone, containing 22.4% bone and 77.6% soft tissue by weight. The soft tissue substitute is a water substitute (WT1/35). The fake vertebrae contain thin walls of cortical bone substitute, an inner ring of cancellous bone substitute (1B7), and a central hole of 2.0 cm diameter. Polypropylene tubes are placed in the central hole, containing test solutions and calibration liquids of different concentrations. This phantom has been used to test the linearity of the CT numbers as a function of the concentration (Lampmann et al., 1984). Lampmann et al. demonstrated a very good correlation ($r = 0.99$) between the CT numbers (HU) and the concentrations (mg/ml) of K_2HPO_4 solutions using the Philips Tomoscan 300 CT unit.

In addition, calcium hydroxyapatite gel (commercially available as Bio-gel HTP, Biorad) was mixed in appropriate concentrations and scanned in the Scanplas phantom; a good correlation ($r = 0.99$) was found between the CT number (HU) and the concentration of hydroxyapatite (g/100 ml). Other

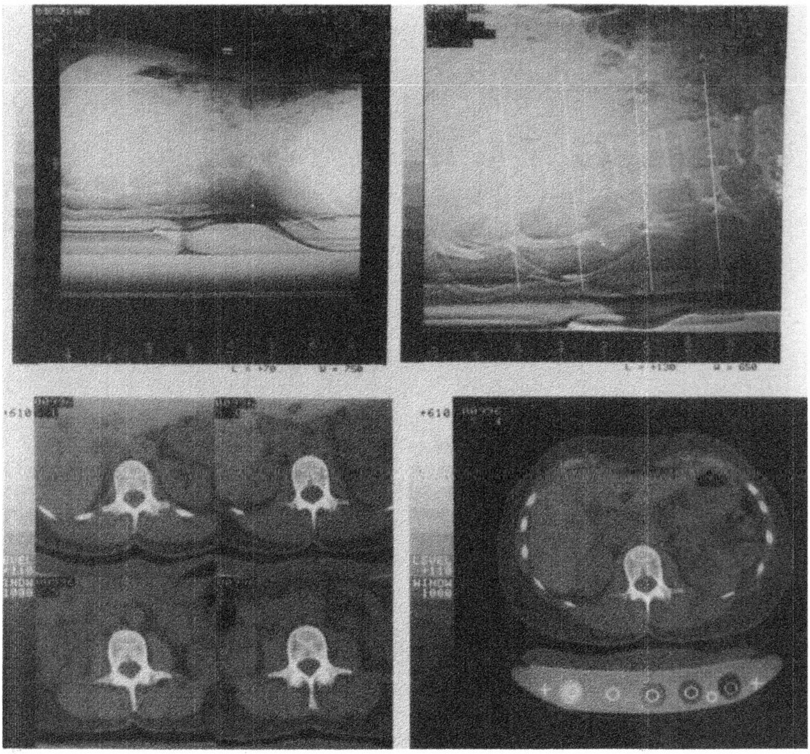

Figure 38. (Clockwise from upper left): lateral digital image of lumbar spine imaging planes through T12-L3, regions of interest in phantom and in vertebrae (Courtesy: ML Richardson)

investigators have used K_2HPO_4 and $CaCl_2$ as a substitute for calcium hydroxyapatite, since these solutions are readily available (Lange et al., 1978; Cann et al., 1979; Cann and Genant, 1980; Banzer et al., 1979).

Some investigators have reported that phantoms containing solutions are not stable enough to provide reliable calibrations, and solid phantoms have been substituted (Firooznia et al., 1986). There is a tendency for the K_2HPO_4 to recrystallize and settle out in the water solutions over a long period of time. The use of solid phantoms containing plasticized bone mineral substances was suggested as a more stable reference standard (Reiser and Genant, 1984).

A prototype phantom (ATS Laboratories, Inc., Bridgeport, Conn.) was described in which a flexible water-equivalent substance was used. Six tubes were inserted in the center of the phantom, three containing calcium hydroxyapatite with concentrations of 75, 150, and 250 mg/cc, two containing fat-equivalent and tissue-equivalent substances, respectively, and one containing water (Nickoloff and Feldman, 1984).

Nordin et al. (1985) investigated the absorption of calcium by the body.

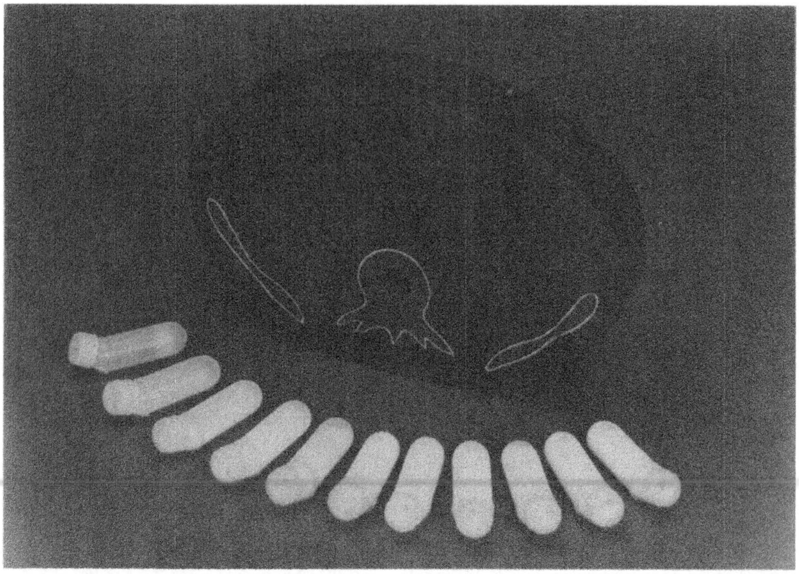

Figure 39. Tissue-equivalent materials and configuration of the Scanplas CT phantom (Courtesy: LEH Lampmann)

measuring the vertebral mineral density by quantitative computed tomography (Nordin et al., 1985). Vertebral densitometry was performed by the method of Cann and Genant, with minor modifications, using a GE 8000 scanner. A perspex phantom containing a water standard and potassium phosphate standards in concentrations of 50, 100, and 200 mg/ml was included beneath the patient during each scan.

A lateral scout view (120 kVp, 400 mA, 11 ms) of the lumbar spine was obtained and the linear cursors were positioned on the vertebral image to define transverse sections 10-mm thick through the centers of the first, third, and fifth lumbar vertebrae. Elliptical regions of interest were selected in the trabecular region of each vertebral body, and the average CT numbers were determined. The vertebral mineral density (VMD) of each vertebra was derived from the calibration curve of mean CT number versus milligrams of mineral per milliliter. Vertebrae that had been crushed were omitted from the determination. The accuracy error of the method was given as ±4.8 mg/ml (1 SD) or about ±5%. The radiation dose from the scout film was estimated as 3 mrem, and the marrow dose per scan was estimated as 470 mrem (for scan parameters: 120 kVp, 80 mA, 4.2 sec.).

Normal values of bone mineral concentrations in males and females were determined by CT densitometry of the lumbar vertebrae. The CT values were compared with bone mineral content of the radius obtained by single photon absorptiometry. The mineral loss after the age of 45 was found to be 1.5% to

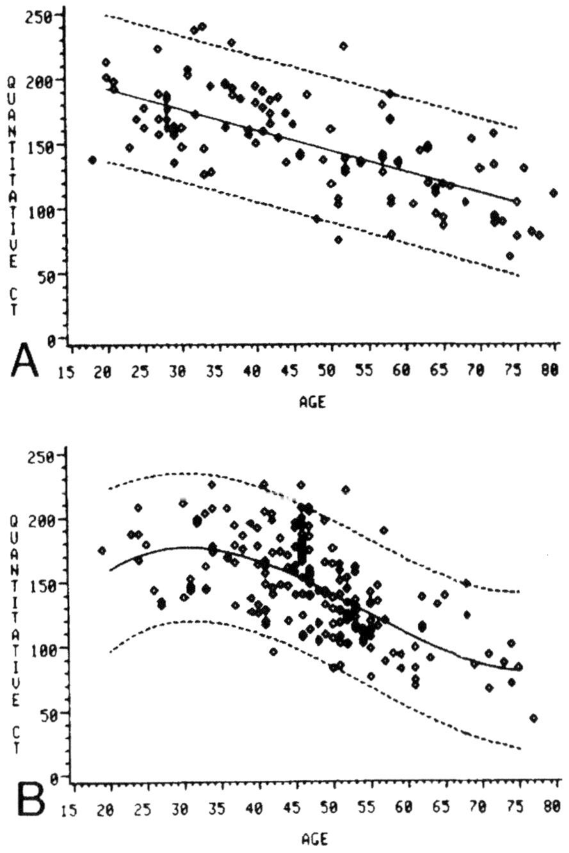

Figure 40. g/cc (QCT) versus age for (A) 120 normal men and (B) 203 normal women (95% confidence intervals) (Courtesy: ML Richardson)

2% per annum for normal males and 2% to 3% per annum for normal females over 45 years of age. The normal range for vertebral bone mineral of males and females in the age range of 25 to 45 years, was found to be 170 to 190 mg/cc K_2HPO_4.

Additional normal data is available, in which 120 men and 203 women between the ages of 20 and 80 years were scanned (figure 40). The normal mean value for young men and women is approximately 175 mg per cubic centimeter. It was reported that men lose an average of 0.94% of bone per year, whereas women lose an average of 1.2% per year (Genant et al., 1985; Cann et al., 1984).

PRECISION AND ACCURACY (SINGLE-ENERGY X-RAY CT)

In studying the sources of error associated with the clinical use of computer tomography scanning systems for bone densitometry, two main problems have been observed (Cann and Genant, 1980): (1) the ability to provide short-term and long-term stability of the CT number and (2) patient repositioning. As in the absorptiometry methods previously discussed, exact repositioning is extremely critical in CT bone mineral quantification. Repositional accuracy to within 1.0 mm is required. The midportions of the second or third lumbar vertebrae are the usual sites for spinal bone mineral determination (Wahner et al., 1984). Repositioning errors can be reduced to 1–1.5 mm if multiple slices of 5 mm through the vertebral body are made, followed by the reconstruction of a 10-mm slice through the midplane of the vertebral body (Cann et al., 1979). However, if the repositioning technique is not carefully followed, errors in the bone mineral content of up to 10% are possible (Cann and Genant, 1980). Care must be taken to avoid inclusion of the endplates in the scan. Angulations of the CT gantry of 5% to 7% may aid in repositioning.

CT number drift has been attributed to several factors including x-ray tube aging and self-filtration, radiation detector drift, and software and hardware modifications by the manufacturer. A precision of 1.5 to 2.5 HU has been observed for scans taken within a 1-hour period. It was noted that the day-to-day drift was about 8 HU, whereas the long-term drift caused differences of 30 to 40 HU. However, CT scanner drift can be corrected by simultaneously scanning a phantom containing reference standard solutions of known density (Cann et al., 1979). Improvements in standardization have been observed, and, with the usage of special phantoms, repeatability and accuracy have improved. Banks and Stevenson (1986) have stated that x-ray tube changes make little difference in the CT number. No significant change was noted following two x-ray tube replacements and a triode valve replacement.

A reasonable correlation ($r = 0.72$) between the single-photon absorptiometry method (SPA) and the single-energy CT method was found in patients, although a better correlation ($r = 0.92$) was found between the average CT numbers and the calcium content in cadaver bones (Reich et al., 1976). In another study the correlation between SPA and single-energy x-ray CT was found to be very good ($r = 0.9942$) (Posner and Griffiths, 1977); and the precision of repeated scans was 2%. A linear relationship was also found between the CT number and the calcium content of in vitro specimens of fresh cadaveric lumbar vertebrae (Huang et al., 1978). Wilson et al. (1978) found a high degree of correlation ($r = 0.994$) between the bone mineral content (BMC) of excised bone from the appendicular skeleton and the mass determined by the CT method. CT values for cadaver vertebrae also correlated well with the ash content ($r = 0.90$) (Banzer et al., 1979).

The accuracy of the single-energy x-ray CT method has been reported for measurements of test phantoms, animals, and human specimens (figure 41). The accuracy using solutions of K_2HPO_4 in the determination of the mineral concentration (mg/cc) was 1% to 2% (Genant and Boyd, 1977). The accuracy of the single-energy CT method for vertebral specimens (monkey) was determined as 5% (Cann et al., 1980). The accuracy of single-energy CT densitometry was reported as 4% to 10% for human vertebral specimens (preserved in sodium azide) for a population of large age range (Genant et al., 1984;

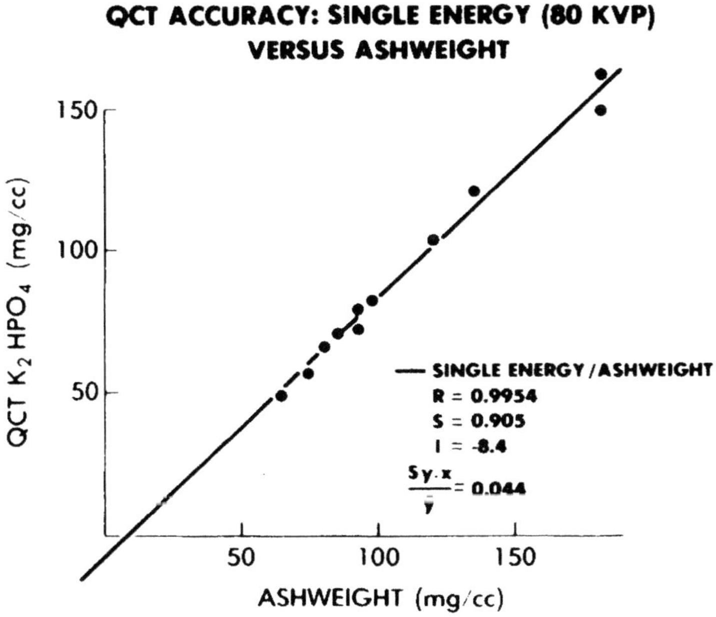

Figure 41. Correlation between measured concentrations and ash weight of human vertebral specimens (Courtesy: ML Richardson)

Genant et al., 1983; McBroom et al., 1984; Rohloff et al., 1982). In addition, vertebral strength and the *load at failure* have been found to correlate well with trabecular bone density determined by quantitative CT (Brassow et al., 1982; McBroom et al., 1984).

The precision of these measurements in humans was found to be 1% to 3% for single-energy (80 kVp) CT densitometry (Genant et al., 1982, Genant et al., 1983). The precision for repeated measurements of vertebral mineralization was earlier reported as 2.8%; the short-term variation in repeated measurements was given as 0.9% (Cann et al., 1979). It has been noted that patients scanned on one CT unit may not yield the same bone mineral density as that obtained on another CT unit. This was demonstrated by scanning two subjects using four different CT scanners of the same manufacturer. The coefficient of variation was found to be 3% to 4%, allowing the bone mineral values from one CT unit to be extrapolated to another unit (Genant et al., 1983).

A major disadvantage of the CT method in clinical densitometry is that in some demineralized patients with compression fracture, the CT values may be unexpectedly increased because of the compressed regions of bone. In addition, fat replaces bone in patients with severe osteoporosis, leading to lower CT values than expected. Dual-energy techniques can provide a correction for fat (Lampmann et al., 1984).

The ability of the CT scanner to separate the cortical bone mineral from the trabecular bone mineral is a significant advantage of the CT densitometry method. However, because the border between these tissue regions is irregular, any method that attempts to separate cortical and trabecular areas is subject to measurement errors. It has been shown that in long bones such as the femur, radiographs overestimate the actual cortical thickness. CT imaging systems blur the sharp edges from 1 to 4 mm because of inherent resolution limits, depending on the x-ray beam width and collimation, the reconstruction algorithm, and the displayed pixel element size (Koehler et al., 1979). When the reconstruction algorithm assigns a CT number to each pixel, an average CT number is given to the entire pixel. Because each pixel may include some cortex and some marrow and be presented as all cortex, the measured cortical thickness is greater than the actual cortical thickness. In a study of the cortical thickness of the femur, it was shown that the CT scan (GE 8800 CT/T whole-body scanner) overestimated the cortical thickness by 13.4% (±7.8%) as compared with caliper measurements of the excised femur (Smith et al., 1982). Inaccurate delineation of the cortex is well known (Jensen et al., 1980; Revak, 1980).

Firooznia et al. (1984) reported on the clinical use of a GE 8800 CT/T unit for quantitative BMC assessment. The patient was positioned as for a lumbar spine CT exam, and 10-mm thick axial slices through the midportion (spongiosum) of T-12, L-1, L-2, and L-3 vertebrae were reconstructed. The reference standards scanned simultaneously with the patients consisted of K_2HPO_4 solutions with densities equivalent to those of water, fat, and bone, respectively. The Hounsfield number of the vertebral trabecular bone was determined; the region of interest was adjusted so that the vertebral cortex and the basivertebral vein were excluded. The bone mineral content (BMC) was expressed in mg/cc of K_2HPO_4, as determined by comparing the CT numbers in the ROI with the corresponding calibration data generated from the CT numbers of the reference standards. The BMC of the four vertebrae were averaged and reported as spinal BMC. Care was taken to eliminate vertebrae containing fractures when serial studies were performed.

The accuracy of this method was determined by comparing the BMC values with those of ashed samples of fresh lumbar trabecular bone removed at autopsy. The ashed samples were scanned in a special human torso phantom designed for the insertion of the samples. The difference between the CT values of the fresh samples was 6% or less, while the precision of the measurement in these samples was 2% to 3%.

In a similar study using a GE 9800 CT/T unit, Firooznia reported the overall accuracy for vertebral specimens obtained from cadavers (ages 22 to 79 years) as 4% to 6% (Firooznia et al., 1984). The precision for vertebral specimens, which were measured 1, 2, and 3 months apart, was 1.4% for the GE 9800 CT/T unit. The precision for serial in vivo measurements on this CT unit was reported for three volunteer subjects as 1.8%.

Recent studies of postmenopausal women using single-energy CT densitometry have demonstrated the efficacy of the method and confirmed the reliability of the techniques introduced by Cann and Genant (1980). A Siemens Somatom 2 whole-body CT unit was used for bone mineral measurements (Banks and Stevenson, 1986). The ability to fully utilize the existing software of commercial CT units was emphasized, obviating the need to provide modifications in order to add this procedure to the regimen of clinical CT studies available within a radiology department. In all clinical studies, a lateral spine radiograph was performed in order to exclude women that demonstrated overt spinal osteoporosis. A phantom, following the design of Cann and Genant, containing dipotassium hydrogen phosphate, was scanned simultaneously during the patient scan. A slice thickness of 4 mm was taken through the midplane of the vertebrae, following a lateral scanogram (localization image). Additional scans at 4 mm above and below the midplane were performed. Three transverse scans per vertebra were therefore performed in L(2), L(3), and L(4).

The Siemens CT unit was operated at 125 kVp and 230 mAs, using a 10-second scan time. The complete bone mineral procedure required 25 minutes. The bone mineral content (BMC) was determined as mg/cc K_2HPO_4 equivalent. It was noted that the region of interest used in the method of Cann and Genant (1980) was too small to provide acceptable reproducibility of positioning, and it was recommended that the largest area of interest within the cortical margin be used. The high resolution of the CT software on the Siemens CT unit enabled the investigators to achieve the desired region of interest in the trabecular vertebral bone.

The precision of the method for phantom measurements was reported as 0.36% to 0.66%. The precision in patients was reported as 2.2%. The accuracy was given as 2.5% over the range of 50 to 200 mg/cc bone mineral equivalent; however, this percentage does not appear to be based on a comparison with biopsy specimens or other basic methods. The authors suggested that at least three separate vertebrae should be scanned in longitudinal studies, since vertebral compression and distortion (figure 42) will affect the reported bone mineral density (Banks and Stevenson, 1986).

In vivo CT densitometry has been performed in the peripheral skeleton (radius) to assess changes in cortical and trabecular bone mass (Jensen et al., 1979). The bone mass of the radius using CT correlated well ($r = 0.95$) with the trabecular bone mass as determined by quantitative histomorphometry of transiliac bone biopsy specimens. Bone mass by CT in the peripheral skeleton also gave a positive correlation with trabecular bone volume as determine by quantitative histomorphometry of transiliac bone biopsy specimens (Orphanoudakis et al., 1979).

BEAM-HARDENING EFFECTS

In clinical CT densitometry, the sources of error are generally related to: (1) beam-hardening software corrections; (2) software corrections for fat; (3) long-

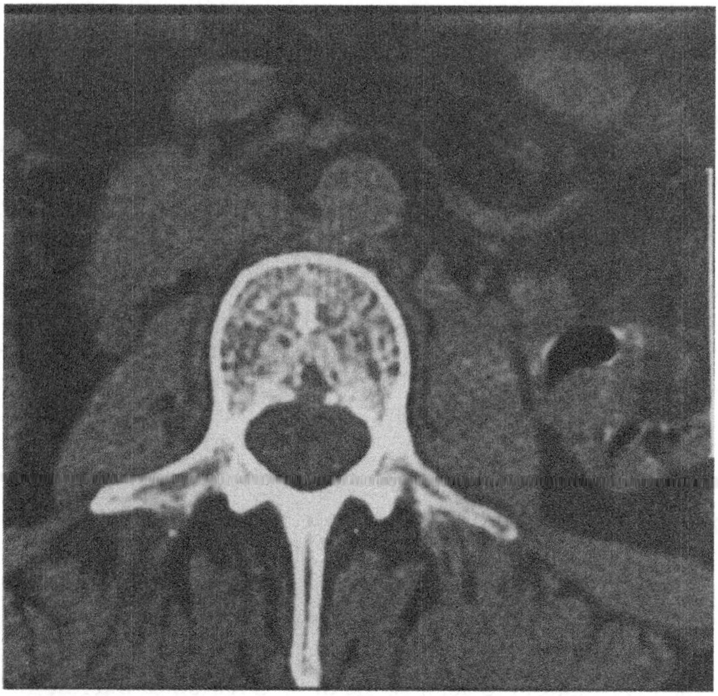

Figure 42. Sclerotic area on CT display within the trabecular bone of L3 (Courtesy: LM Banks)

term and short-term drifts in the CT scanner calibration caused by x-ray tube aging, detector drifts, and hardware and software changes; and (4) repositioning errors (Cann and Genant, 1980). In addition, motion artifacts and the partial volume effect limit the precision of CT densitometry (Lampmann et al., 1984).

The beam-hardening effect, a characteristic of all CT scanners, results from changes in the x-ray spectrum (figure 43) as the x-ray beam traverses the body tissues. Because the average energy of the beam increases as the spectrum changes, the linear attenuation coefficients decrease. The CT numbers are therefore also decreased, and the resultant CT image shows nonuniformities, especially in regions of highly dense tissues such as cortical bone. Beam hardening was significant in the first reported cases involving CT bone densitometry of the human spine (Marschall et al., 1978). A method was devised to correct for beam hardening in the reconstruction algorithms used to produce the final CT image (Joseph and Spital, 1978). Beam hardening (Stonestrom et al., 1981) and scattered radiation (Stonestrom and Macovski, 1976) can be significant in degrading CT images.

Imamura and Masamichi (1981) evaluated the effects of beam hardening in

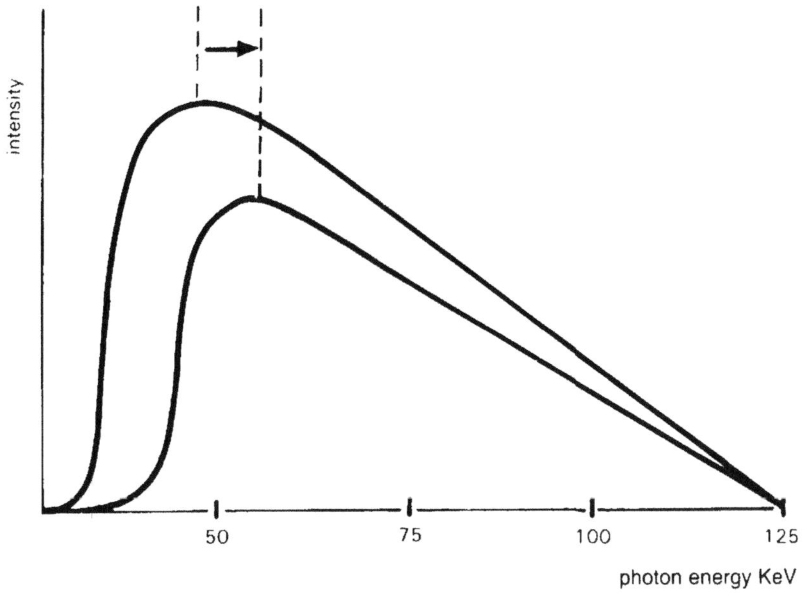

Figure 43. Beam hardening, shift of the average photon energy (Courtesy: LEH Lampmann)

the CT measurement of bone mineral content of the vertebrae. The part of the x-ray spectrum that has a lower energy is preferentially absorbed by soft tissue surrounding the axial skeleton, thereby changing the average energy of the transmitted beam; as a result, the CT number is altered. It was shown that a beam-hardening correction was required for the quantitative clinical study of bone mineral content. The authors described an empirical beam-hardening correction technique. The *beam-hardening index* was defined by the term:

$$e^{-\varrho^{21}} \cdot 10^7$$

where l is the x-ray path length. This term was used to estimate the beam-hardening effect on the CT number when converting the CT number of the vertebral body to calcium content. The beam-hardening index was linearly correlated with the CT number for homogeneous substances, as determined using a Varian 360 whole-body CT unit. The index clearly explained the decrease in CT number of a vertebral phantom, with the corresponding overall increase of x-ray absorption by the surrounding material. The physical density of the surrounding tissue was determined by the proportion of lean soft tissue to adipose tissue, and this proportion differed greatly among patients.

The beam-hardening index for patients ranged from 10 to several hundred, with an average of about 100 for adults. The CT number of the vertebral medulla had a standard deviation of ±10 to ±30, which corresponds to a

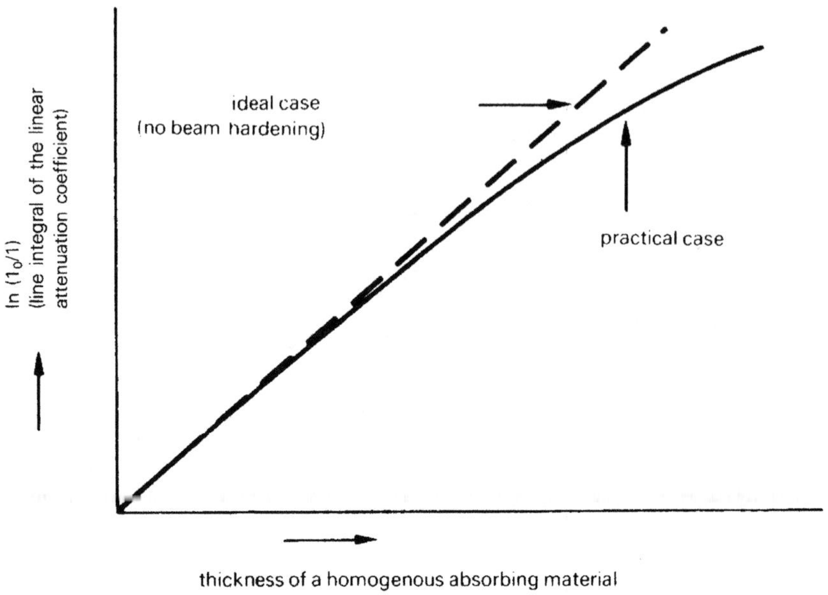

Figure 44. Beam hardening, nonlinearity with increasing absorber thickness (Courtesy: LEH Lampmann)

10% to 15% error. For normal subjects, beam hardening was not significant. However, the beam-hardening correction was found to be relatively large for subjects with low mineral concentrations. It was concluded that the beam-hardening index was needed to accurately determine mineral content of the vertebrae in cases of pathological mineral loss. Calibration curves of calcium concentration versus CT number were determined for various values of the beam-hardening index (figure 44).

PARTIAL VOLUME EFFECTS

The partial volume effect is observed in all CT scanners. It is the averaging of the calculated CT numbers over the volume of tissue defined by the slice thickness. Because the slice thickness may be varied, it is possible to choose a thin slice thickness, which reduces but does not eliminate the partial volume effect. The partial volume effect results from the fact that as the slice thickness is increased, more tissue is sampled. In the extreme case, soft tissue may be in the center of the slice thickness (voxel), whereas cortical bone may be at the very edge of the slice thickness. The average CT number for the voxel may reflect the presence of a small amount of cortical bone (high density), although most of the voxel contains soft tissue (low density). This average CT number will be artificially high and may not be representative of the soft-tissue nature of the region of interest. Instead, the CT number is higher due to the partial inclusion of bone. Thinner slices (1.5 mm) have the advantage of reducing partial volume effects and thereby increasing the spatial resolution of the CT scan, although an increase in the image noise is also present.

EFFECTS OF MARROW FAT

The errors associated with bone mineral determinations using single-energy CT have been investigated with regard to the effects of marrow and bone composition (Mazess, 1983). Bone has a variable composition in the human body (figure 45). The normal range for trabecular bone volume (TBV) in humans is 15% to 25%, while osteopenic bone volumes are less than 12% (Meunier et al., 1973). However, about 25% to 75% (by volume) of the marrow is adipose tissue (Hartsock et al., 1965). The quantity of adipose tissue in marrow increases from 30% in young adulthood to perhaps 60% in the elderly. For normal subjects, the magnitude of adipose tissue is 50 ± 25%, and for subjects with osteoporosis, 70 ± 15% (Johnell, 1980).

Marrow is one of the most labile tissues in the body (Custer, 1974); immobilization produces a rapid but transient increase of marrow fat (1%/week) in the body (Minaire et al., 1974). Mazess has noted that the relatively large density variations that are observed as a result of variations in bone and marrow composition affect the linear attenuation coefficients that are the basic parameters determined by the CT method. Substantial errors have been found in conventional CT scans using both polychromatic (x-ray tube) and monoenergetic (^{125}I) beams (Genant and Boyd, 1977; Rosenfeld et al., 1980). Genant and Boyd reported a 30% error associated with a 20% change of fat using phantoms of very low bone concentration. Rosenfeld predicted an error of about 10% for a 20% change of fat content in normal bone. The magnitude of the error due to marrow and bone composition is excessive for the accurate determination of bone mineral content in some patients.

Other errors in CT imaging, such as partial volume effects, reconstruction artifacts, scanner drift, and calibration, are generally smaller errors; beam hardening, however, may lead to larger errors (10%) in low-density bone (Imamura and Fujii, 1981). Jensen et al. (1980) have demonstrated in renal patients, that osteoid proliferative tissue states involve the overestimation of bone using CT. Weissberger et al. (1978) found that x-ray CT had low sensitivity for demonstrating changes in trabecular bone, which obviated the clinical advantages.

The use of dual-energy CT scanning has the potential of eliminating the problem of marrow variability. However, the precision of dual-energy CT (about 14%) is approximately five times worse than that of single-energy CT (Tofts, 1981; Abols et al., 1980). It has been shown that dual-energy CT, when using preprocessing or postprocessing of the CT image, reduces the magnitude of errors produced by fat in bone mineral studies. Although unnecessary for most clinical applications, this correction may reduce the fat error to 2% to 4% in elderly subjects (Genant et al., 1985).

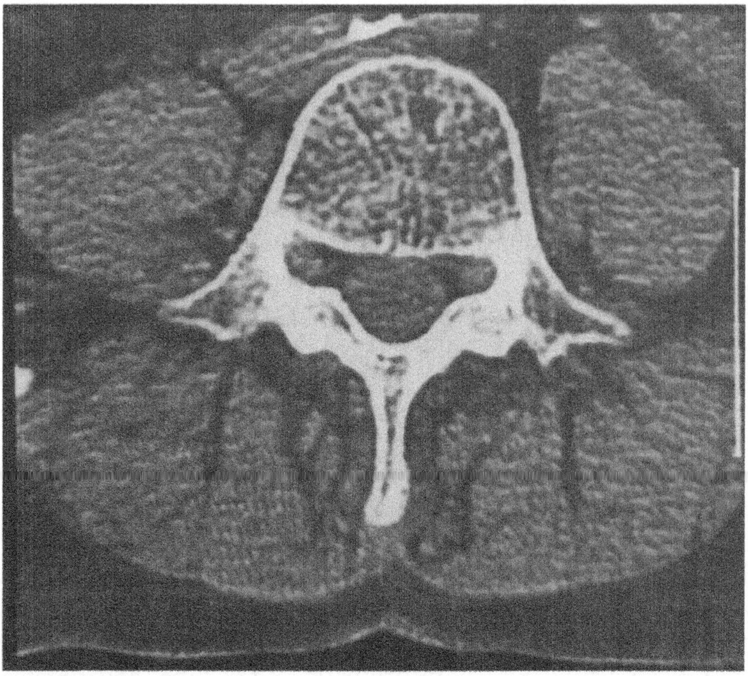

Figure 45. Fatty deposit on CT display within the vertebra L4 (Courtesy: LM Banks)

The accuracy for quantitative CT densitometry is said to decrease to 20% to 25% in the elderly population; this decreased accuracy also occurs in dual-photon absorptiometry of the spine. This is the result of many factors, such as the presence of fatty yellow marrow, which reduces the measured spinal mineral equivalent by 7 mg per 10% fat by volume (Faul et al., 1982). By applying a fat correction, the underestimation of the mineral content may be corrected with a residual uncertainty of 4 to 5 mg/cc, one standard deviation (Dunnill et al., 1967; Richardson et al., 1985). For single-energy CT measurements, the errors due to fat content are minimized by the use of lower kVp; however, even low kVp scans have substantial errors due to the fat. One percent of fat (by volume) results in a decrease of the CT number by 0.8 to 1.5 HU, or a 0.4% reduction of the bone mineral value (Nickoloff and Feldman, 1984).

DUAL-ENERGY X-RAY QUANTITATIVE CT

The dual-energy CT densitometry method utilizes two transverse scans of the vertebra instead of one. The energies (kVp's) of the x-ray beams are separated as much as possible in order to provide greater differences between the attenuation coefficients of the tissues of interest. The Hounsfield numbers are related by the following equation (Genant et al., 1981):

$$H_V - H_{s,V} = \frac{c_f}{\varrho_f}(H_{f,V} - H_{s,V}) + \frac{c_b}{\varrho_b}(H_{b,V} - H_{s,V})$$

where H_V = CT number of interest;
$H_{s,V}$ = CT number of soft tissue at energy V;
$H_{f,V}$ = CT number of fat at energy V;
$H_{b,V}$ = CT number of bone at energy V;
c_f, c_b = concentration of fat, bone, respectively (g/cc); and
ϱ_f, ϱ_b = mass density of fat, bone, respectively (g/cc).

Two linear equations are formed upon scaning at two different energies (kVp's). By simultaneously solving these two equations, the computer calculates the bone mineral concentration for each image pixel.

The dual-energy CT densitometry method was used to assess the bone mineral content of the lumbar vertebrae of patients (Nickoloff and Feldman, 1984). A Siemens DR3 CT unit operated at 96 kVp (680 mAs) and 125 kVp (520 mAs) was used. The difference between the CT numbers of the two separate scans in which the same region of interest was used, was proportional to the bone mineral content. Both prereconstruction and postreconstruction processing were used in the studies. Calibration phantoms modeled after the design of Cann and Genant were used, and the bone mineral was determined in terms of mg/cc of K_2HPO_4.

A dual-energy CT densitometry method has been proposed in which the x-ray tube is replaced with two monoenergetic radioactive sources, ^{241}Am and ^{125}I. This technique offers the advantages of high stability, low overall weight, and no need for a high-voltage supply for the sources. Beam hardening is not as significant since the ^{125}I is nearly monoenergetic and may be filtered to produce a monoenergetic beam. Although this design may be useful in the peripheral skeleton, it is limited by the available source activities and the photon-counting statistics when proposed for use in the axial skeleton (Larsson et al., 1978).

A method for reducing the effects of beam hardening in CT imaging by 60% to 90% was introduced by Hemmingsson et al. (1986). Using a Siemens Somatom DR2 alternately pulsed at 96 kVp and 125 kVp, respectively, post-processed images were generated in which image noise was also reduced. Dual-energy images were separated into osseous and soft-tissue components in both phantom and clinical CT studies (Hemmingsson et al., 1986). The evaluation of bone mineral by CT densitometry may be improved by the application of this technique.

PRECISION AND ACCURACY (DUAL-ENERGY CT)

Dual-energy CT densitometry of the radius was found to have higher accuracy than single-energy CT densitometry (Orphanoudakis et al., 1979). Single-energy CT densitometry, on the other hand, was found to have a higher degree of precision. Dual-energy CT densitometry (80 kVp/140 kVp) has a reported precision of 3% to 5% (Genant et al., 1982; Genant et al., 1983).

The dual-energy CT method was used to quantitate bone mineral in patients using calibration curves generated for each patient during each scan. A set of calibration curves was generated by simultaneously scanning a set of mineral equivalent solutions, which were determined to be linear within 2% to 3% for K_2HPO_4 solutions below 400 mg/cc (Crouch et al., 1980).

The precision of single-energy CT scans for bone mineral measurements was found to be 10 times better than that of the dual-energy CT scans (approximately 2% for single-energy versus 21.2% for dual energy). It has been found, however, that dual-energy CT scans are less susceptible to inaccuracies in bone mineral values due to fat content.

Dual-energy CT. densitometry has been investigated with regard to the determination of the electron density and atomic number of bone. The potential accuracy of the method was evaluated by scanning a 5% $CaCl_2$ solution. The calculated electron density of the solution was 3.44×10^{23} electrons per milliliter, whereas the calculated effective atomic number was 8.75. The solution was scanned on a EMI 7020 CT unit at energies corresponding to 100 kVp and 140 kVp. A region of interest of area 3.49 cm^2 was used for determination of the CT number of the solution at each energy. The electron density and atomic number, which were calculated from the CT scan data, were 3.41 ± 0.07 (SD) $\times 10^{23}$ electrons per milliliter and 8.72 ± 0.40(SD), respectively, resulting in a difference of less than 1%. Patients were also scanned using dual-energy CT, although the accuracy and precision in patients was not reported. The major sources of error in dual-energy CT densitometry, and in the determination of the electron density and atomic number of the vertebrae, were the inability to accurately reposition the exact scan plane after the first scan, as well as patient motion during the scan (Dunscombe et al., 1984). It has been suggested that the problem of movement between scans may be eliminated by using a split filter technique (Rutt et al., 1980).

CLINICAL MEASUREMENTS

A CT study of oophorectomized women, using L(1) and L(2), has suggested that CT is a more sensitive indicator of bone mineral change than single-photon absorptiometry. The cortical thickness proved to be the least sensitive indicator (Ettinger et al., 1979).

CT densitometry was used to measure the bone mineral content of the spinal trabecular bone in osteoporotic women. Eighty-five percent of those with vertebral fractures had bone mineral content values below the fifth percentile

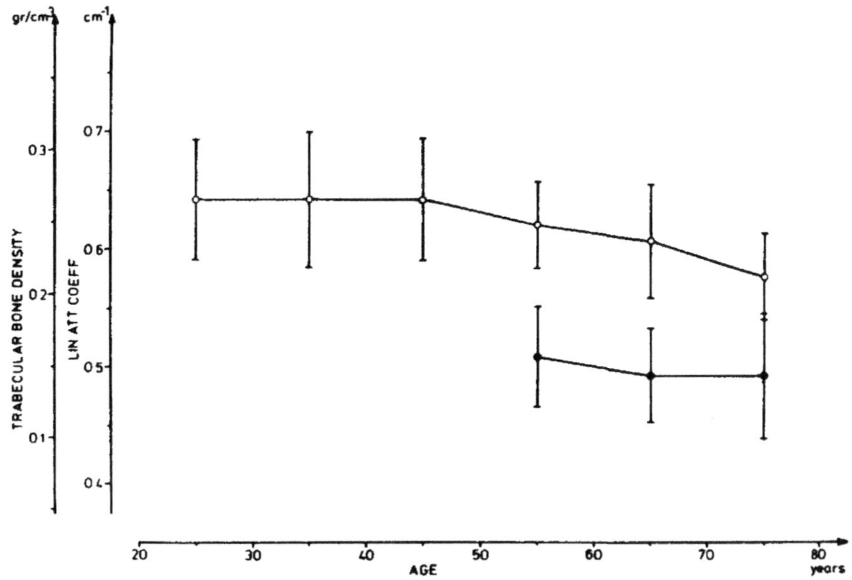

Figure 46. Mean trabecular bone density versus age for normal females (circles) and for osteoporotic females (dots) (Courtesy: P Ruegsegger)

for normal premenopausal women; this level of mineralization was considered a fracture threshold. The investigators suggested that diagnosis of osteoporosis be made when the spinal bone mineral content value is below the fracture threshold (Firooznia et al., 1984). It was stated that quantitative CT is a simple and highly reliable procedure that can accurately determine the BMC of spinal trabecular bone. In addition, the CT method was found to be useful in establishing the diagnosis of osteoporosis, in predicting spontaneous vertebral fractures, and in evaluating the treatment of osteoporosis.

A fracture threshold has been proposed in which patients with vertebral mineral densities below the threshold have a significant probability of bone fractures. The relationship between fracture and vertebral bone mineral density has been examined in males and females. Vertebral mineral density was well correlated ($r = 0.74$) with the prevalence of fracture (Richardson et al., 1985). The fracture threshold value of approximately 110 mg/cc represents the vertebral bone mineral density below which fractures may occur and above which fractures are rare (Cann and Genant, 1983; Genant et al., 1983).

Firooznia et al. have reported the spinal trabecular BMC (mg K_2HPO_4 per cc) in 316 normal men and 132 normal women. BMC in men was seen to decline over their lifetime by about 30%; whereas, in women, BMC was seen to decline by 45 to 50% over their lifetime. These data indicate that in women there is an accelerated rate of bone loss following the menopause. It was noted that the accuracy of the CT method is affected by biological variations in the vertebral body composition, particularly the quantity of fat tissue. The CT values may be lowered by one Hounsfield unit per 1% fat by weight.

Ruegsegger et al. (1984) have measured the trabecular bone density of the distal end of the tibia of healthy and osteoporotic women using the gamma-ray CT method. The osteoporotic patients had considerably less trabecular bone than those of the normal population (figure 46).

Computed tomography has been used to evaluate the status of the vertebrae following total hip arthroplasty (Black, 1985). CT densitometry was used to assess the vertebral bone density of postoperative patients, preoperative patients, and controls. A single-energy CT unit (Philips Tomoscan 300) operating at 118 kVp was used for the patient studies. Density changes of 5% were detectable in serial testing. The average CT numbers were determined in the central vertebral bodies of T(12), L(1), and L(2), using 6-mm thick slices. A significant loss of vertebral bone density was found in the physically inactive postoperative patients. The precision of the measurements was 1.1% despite the potential repositioning errors and the machine variability.

RADIATION DOSE TO PATIENTS

The radiation dose to patients undergoing CT densitometry depends upon the following factors: (1) scan parameters — kVp, mAs, (2) patient size, (3) x-ray source/detector geometry, and (4) detector collimation and calibration. Because the x-ray beam of the CT system has a slice thickness in the range 1 to 10 mm, the radiation received by the patient is limited to a narrow band. The biological effects of irradiating this small volume of tissue become more significant as adjacent slices are imaged in the patient. The benefit of such radiation is the valuable diagnostic information obtained. CT radiation doses from abdominal procedures may be in the range 1 to 5 rads to the surface of the patient, while the internal radiation dose is much less.

The radiation dose with QCT is in the range of 200 to 250 mrad and is greater than that of the dual photon absorptiometry method (5 to 15 mrad). By comparison, a lumbar spine series in radiography delivers a radiation dose of about 600 mrad (Davies and Saha, 1985).

Some early investigations of CT densitometry in patients were reported to give radiation doses of 450 mrem using 450 mAs exposures; it was stated that the patient dose could be reduced to 100 mrem per study if 50 mAs were used (Cann et al., 1979). In another study, Mazess and Wilson (1979) reported that the patient dose in single-energy CT was 3.0 rems per study, and that dual-energy CT provides a lower patient dose of 1.0 rem per study. The results of a later comparison of CT densitometry methods, including the monoenergetic source (^{125}I) techniques, indicated that the UCSF GE 7800 system delivered a radiation skin dose of 200 mrad per CT slice, whereas the ^{125}I methods delivered a radiation skin dose of 4 to 80 mrad per CT slice (Hangartner and Overton, 1981). In a study of the optimal CT settings for monoenergetic CT densitometry, it was found that a dose below 150 μSv is sufficient to detect a change of 1% in the trabecular bone density (Muller et al., 1985).

The use of low-dose CT techniques in quantitative spinal mineral analysis has been investigated (Cann, 1981). The determination of the radiation dose was made using TLD (dosimeters). The average dose within the body during the spinal mineral analysis was determined by placing the TLDs at five positions within a simulated human torso scanned at 80 kVp using contiguous slices of 5-mm slice thickness. The average dose was reported as 375 mrem (3.75 mSv). It was determined, however, that a dose of 100 mrem (1.0 mSv) was adequate to produce an image of acceptable quality, which would allow calculation of the vertebral mineral (mineral equivalent in mg K_2HPO_4) with a satisfactory statistical precision. The author did not state the skin dose, although the gonadal dose in men and women is believed to be extremely small.

In a clinical study of postmenopausal women using single-energy CT (GE 8800 unit), following the method of Cann and Genant (1980) with minor modifications, the estimated radiation dose from the scout (localization) film to the bone marrow was 3.0 mrem (120 kVp, 400 mA, 11 ss). The bone marrow dose received by the patient as a result of the vertebral mineral scans (120 kVp, 80 mA, 4.2 ss) was estimated as 470 mrem (Nordin et al., 1985).

Lampmann et al. (1984) conducted a study of patient dose, using a method suggested by Yalcintas et al. (1979). Thermoluminescent dosimeters (TLD chips) made of lithium fluoride (LiF) trap the energy absorbed by x-rays and release that energy upon heating the chips. TLD chips were sealed in plastic (two TLD's per container) and positioned on the surface of the Scanplas phantom. TLD containers were arranged in a clockwise pattern, 45° apart, along the centerline of the scan path of the x-ray beam. In another set of measurements, the TLD sets were placed on the surface of a patient at 5.0-cm intervals along the midline in a cranial-caudal direction. The TLDs were read out with a Harshaw TLD reader. The maximum skin exposure was found on the posterior of the patient (spine) with a value of 5.2 rem. The authors also reported the following absorbed doses for a CT scanogram (for localization and positioning) plus one transverse slice (for CT densitometry):

A. female gonadal dose (max) = 600 μGy (60 mrad)
B. male gonadal dose = negligible
C. female bone marrow dose = 110 μGy (11 mrad)
D. female total body dose = 40 μGy (4 mrad)
E. male total body dose = 60 μGy (6 mrad)
F. male and female thyroid dose = negligible

The CT total-body dose was compared with that for a conventional lumbar spine (lateral) radiograph and found to be an order of magnitude lower. The scattered radiation to various organs outside the transverse slice is minimized because of the highly collimated x-ray beam. Other investigators have reported the radiation dose to the upper abdomen from four axial slices obtained through the selected vertebrae as 200 to 250 mrem. The scattered radiation to the ovaries and the testes, in phantom studies, was given as about 11 mrem and 4 mrem, respectively (Firooznia et al., 1986).

Banks and Stevenson (1986) have reported the approximate mean surface-radiation dose (multislice; 125 kVp, 230 mAs) as 16 mGy, with the dose to the spine of 3 mGy, as determined using the method of the CT Working Party of the Hospital Physicists' Association (H.P.A., 1981). Dual-energy CT, while overcoming the inaccuracies related to marrow fat, has the disadvantage of increasing both the scanning time and radiation dose while decreasing the precision of bone mineral measurements.

6. SCATTERING METHODS IN DENSITOMETRY

All of the previously described densitometric methods are based on the use of transmitted x-rays or gamma rays. The radiographic methods utilize radiographic films for the detection of x-rays. Single-photon absorptiometry requires the use of scintillation detectors for determining the gamma-ray transmission through bone and soft tissue, as does the dual-photon method. CT densitometry is based upon the detection of the transmitted x-rays or gamma rays at multiple angles about the body by an array of scintillation or gas detectors. The basic interaction upon which these transmission methods depend is the photoelectric interaction between the incident x-ray or gamma ray and electrons of the affected atoms of the tissues. The energy range for tissue densitometric transmission methods is generally below 100 keV, where the photoelectric effect is the most dominant of the possible x-ray interactions. The scattering methods, by contrast with these transmission methods, rely upon two additional fundamental types of photon interactions: (1) elastic (coherent) scattering and (2) inelastic (incoherent) scattering of x-rays and gamma rays.

The inelastic scattering of x-rays by the electrons of an atom was first satisfactorily described by A.H. Compton in 1923 (Compton, 1923). When an x-ray or gamma ray is scattered in a substance, it is scattered in a definite direction, giving up part of its energy to the electron (recoil electron). The energy of the scattered x-ray is less than that of the incident x-ray; and the quantity of energy carried off by the scattered x-ray depends upon the angle of scatter. The fundamental theory of Compton scattering is reviewed elsewhere (Williams, 1977).

The investigation of the Compton-scattering interaction later led to the determination of the electron densities of various substances, based upon measurements of the intensities of scattered photons at selected angles. Odeblad and Norhagen (1956) published the first article on electron density measurements, in which they used a ^{60}Co source (20 mCi) to irradiate various substances (brass, water, benzene) including some biological specimens. In vitro experiments were performed in which the relative 90° scatter intensities were determined in liver, fat, and lung tissues. In vivo experiments were performed in two subjects in which the electron densities relative to water were determined for the human lung and knee. It was proposed at that time to study diseased tissues in vitro and in vivo using the Compton-scattering method.

COMPTON-SCATTER IMAGING METHODS

Lale (1959) introduced the concept of a scanning Compton-scatter densitometer for the in vivo determination of the electron densities of human tissues. The process of measuring Compton scatter is inherently insensitive when compared with direct beam (transmission) measurements by a factor of 100. However, this disadvantage may be less important than the fact that the measurement of Compton-scattered photons allows the determination of the electron density of the substance, which cannot be determined by the technically simpler transmission techniques.

The experimental system used by Lale (1950) utilized an ^{192}Ir source of gamma rays. A highly collimated beam 3 mm in diameter was directed at the specimen (small animals); the axis of the detector (perspex crystal and photomultiplier tube) was positioned at 90° to the axis of the gamma-ray beam. Scattered gramma rays were collected using a collimator system focused on a small volume of tissue. Lale proposed an in vivo system based upon these preliminary experiments. A system for scanning the human body was suggested in which the scattering of high-energy x-rays (about 1 Mev) was envisaged using a linear accelerator as the source. A focused collimator and detector, made up of a number of lead cones, would allow the determination of the scatter intensity from a small, well-defined volume of tissues positioned at a fixed distance along the detector axis. Lale's proposed device would provide resolution of density differences as low as 1%, with a radiation dose of 100 mrad.

Lale (1968) described further work using x-rays from a 5.6 Mev linear accelerator. A collimated x-ray beam of 3 mm diameter was passed through the patient. The *scattering volume* was defined as a small volume of tissue, which was delineated by the incident beam diameter and the focusing characteristics of the detector collimator. The x-ray beam was moved across the patient by an elaborate system consisting of rotating source and detector collimators; the tissue region of interest was selected by moving the patient couch. In this way, a two-dimensional image of the density distribution within the patient was created. The lateral spatial resolution of the system was 3.0 mm, while the tissue thickness sampled was effectively 2.5 cm. The average radiation exposure at the body surface was 20 mR (scan time: 50 seconds).

Several problems were associated with this scatter imaging system: (1) background radiation, which required the use of extra lead shielding; (2) variations in the photon energy and dose rate of the linear accelerator; (3) variations in the mechanical alignment of the source/detector collimator system; (4) absorption and scatter by tissues outside the plane of focus; (5) patient motion; and (6) artifacts in the image display. Because of these limitations, the reported density resolution was 4%, while the detection of 1% density differences was desired.

Clarke (1965) investigated the feasibility of the scattering methods in medical diagnosis. The scattering system consisted of a highly collimated source and detector system maintained at a fixed scattering angle. The source/detector system was fixed relative to the patient, and the patient couch was moved in a rectilinear fashion so as to intersect different volumes of tissues during the scan. The scatter intensities for each point in the scan were found to be proportional to the electron densities of the tissues present.

Clarke and Van Dyk (1969, 1974) further reported on the development of a high-energy Compton-scatter imaging system, using a 600 Ci ^{60}Co source. The collimated beam was 1.75 cm in diameter. A focused collimator (15.2 cm thick) and a sodium iodide crystal (and photomultiplier) detector were used. The scattering volume was an ellipsoidal region defined by the intersection of the focused collimator holes and the incident gamma-ray beam. The spatial resolution of the imaging system was about 0.5 cm (for a density difference of 13%). The density resolution possible with this system was better than 5%. The radiation dose to the patient was estimated as 30 mrad. In imaging human subjects, two main problems were encountered: (1) reduction in image contrast and (2) reduced tissue density resolution due to multiple scattering and attenuation artifacts (Clarke, 1974). Multiple scattering from regions between the surface of the patient and the scattering volume of interest contribute to the lack of density resolution possible with a scatter imaging system of this design.

A Compton-scatter system was developed for the determination of the density distribution of body tissues, which could be utilized in treatment planning in radiotherapy (Farmer and Collins, 1971). The system consisted of a monoenergetic ^{137}Cs radionuclide source (50 Ci), which produced a horizontal gamma-ray beam through the patient. The detector system included a high resolution germanium Ge(Li) detector, with which it was possible to discriminate between the scatter energy peaks at different scattering angles. A general disadvantage of this detector is that it requires a supply of liquid nitrogen and a reservoir attached directly to the crystal for cooling the detector; cooling reduces the electronic noise. The detector was positioned at 90° to the horizontal incident beam and below the patient couch. Scattered radiation entering the detector was collimated to reduce unwanted scatter (from other directions); the scatter intensities were collected from each point on the horizontal line traversed by the incident beam (662 keV).

The range of scattered photon energies (226 to 402 keV) corresponded to a range of scattering angles from 60° to 120°. Therefore, each energy channel observed on the multichannel spectrum analyzer corresponded to a particular horizontal location in the patient and a particular scattering angle. The intensity associated with each energy channel corresponded to the electron density value at a specific location.

The spatial resolution that was attainable was based upon a compromise between the thickness of the germanium crystal and the incident beam diameter. If the crystal thickness was large (efficient for stopping gamma rays), the spatial resolution was decreased because of the increased scatter within the crystal. If the beam diameter was large (increasing the detector sensitivity), the spatial resolution was also reduced. However, the spatial resolution obtained was approximately 0.5 cm, adequate for treatment planning purposes. As the horizontal beam was raised vertically, a two-dimensional distribution of electron densities was obtained, forming the basic data array for a transverse image of the body. The scanning time per line in the image was about 10 seconds. The radiation dose for an average patient was about 1 rad.

It was later reported (Farmer and Collins, 1974) that the background radiation intensities were considerable and were mainly due to multiple scattering in the patient. Farmer and Collins experienced similar restrictions on image quality to those of Clarke (Battista et al., 1977). Because this system was strongly dependent on the energy resolution capability of the germanium crystal, scattering within the crystal itself presented problems in discriminating peaks corresponding to specific scattering angles; however, background subtraction by the computer improved the images. The scan time for the thorax was reported to be about 20 minutes and for the head was about 10 minutes; the radiation dose was less than 2 rads. It was noted that improvement of the counting statistics was not possible, because of the limited specific activity of the ^{137}Cs source. The limited resolution of this scatter imaging device precluded its use in diagnostic imaging, although the method may be used successfully for radiotherapy treatment planning.

A computer-controlled tomographic imaging device that utilized Compton scattering (figure 47) was later developed for clinical testing (Clarke et al., 1976). Using an 800 Ci ^{60}Co source, which provided a 1.0 cm diameter beam at the position of the scattering volume, focused collimators were used to detect scatter in the forward direction at the scattering angle of 45°. The detection system utilized four large plastic scintillators. The radioactive source was positioned above the patient, and the detectors were placed below the patient and scanning table. The patient was moved through the fixed vertical

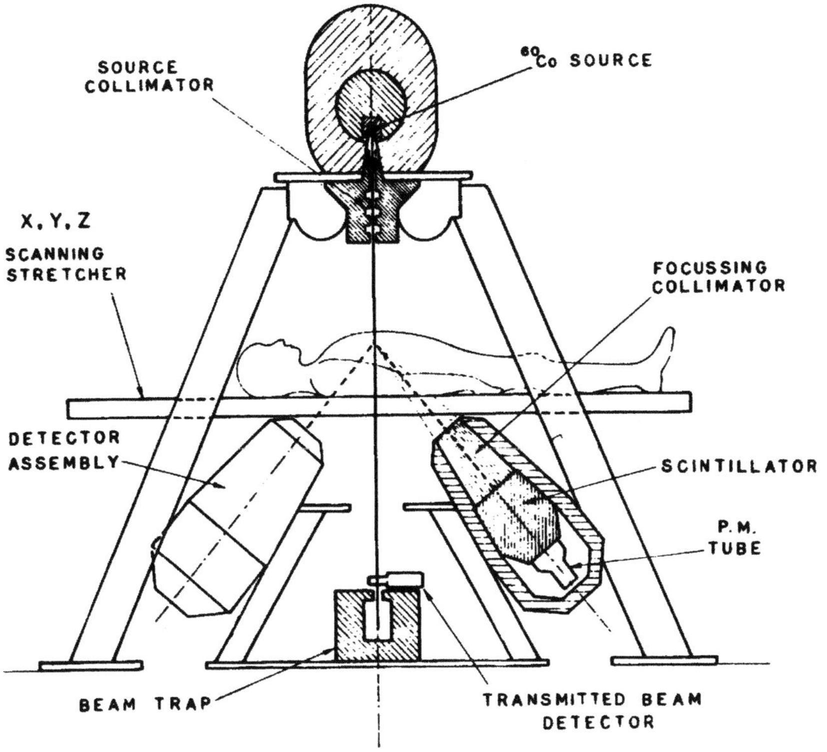

Figure 47. Compton-scatter imaging system (Courtesy: RL Clarke)

primary beam, using a motorized couch. An additional detector measured the transmitted intensity of the primary beam and was used as an aid in repositioning. The effective scattering volume was 1.0 cc of tissue.

The authors reported a density resolution of 1% in test specimens at a spatial resolution of 5 mm in the scan plane; however, the vertical spatial resolution was about 1.2 cm. The radiation dose was 0.25 to 1 rad. The scatter images of anaesthetized dogs suffered image resolution losses due to respiratory motion. In studies on patients, however, the density resolution was 2 to 4%. However, the lack of density resolution may have resulted from an oversimiplified correction for tissue absorption (Conrad, 1979).

Battista and Bronskill (1978) investigated the design and imaging characteristics of the Clarke tissue density scanner. Using various models involving both analytic and Monte Carlo calculation methods, the problem of multiple scattering was studied. The investigation included incident monoenergetic photon energies in the range 300 to 2000 keV and scattering angles of 30° to 130°, using a focused detector and a uniform water phantom. It was demonstrated that multiple scatter contamination can be minimized but not eliminated by using a detector of superior energy resolution. It was found that the ratio of multiple scatter to single scatter decreases with increasing incident photon energy. In the energy range used, this ratio decreased from 64% to 35% as the energy was increased, using a mean scattering angle of 40°.

The radiation dose to the patient (per measurement) increased from 1.0 to 4.1 rad over this energy range. Thus, the radiation dose is decreased at the lower energies, but at the expense of increased multiple scattering. It was shown that the selection of a forward scattering angle minimizes both the radiation dose and multiple-scatter contamination. The multiple-to-single scatter ratio decreased from 122% to 27% and the dose from 14.3 rad to 1.2 rad as the mean scattering angle was decreased from 130° to 30° (for the incident energy 1.25 MeV). For ^{60}Co energies and a mean scattering angle of 40°, the multiple-scatter contamination of the measured scatter intensity was 51%. Battista and Bronskill concluded that a spatial resolution of better than 1.0 cm and an electron density accuracy of about 5% for a radiation dose of about 5 rad was feasible with the Clarke scanner.

Battista and Bronskill (1981) later presented clinical images of patients scanned (figure 48) using the Compton scatter imaging method developed by Clarke et al. (1976). The scanner used a 700 Ci source of ^{60}Co, having a collimated beam of rectangular cross section 0.5 cm × 12 cm, located 80 cm from the source. Two focused detector collimators (45 cm from the scattering volume) were provided below the patient to accept forward scatter at angles of 32° to 48° to the incident beam direction (Clarke et al., 1976); sodium iodide detectors were used. Dual-channel photon spectrometry was used to discriminate between the single scatter and the multiple-scatter intensities (Battista et al., 1977). The subtracted multiple-scatter contamination was 30% of the total-scatter intensity. A third sodium iodide detector with a single-slot collimator was added to detect primary beam transmission through the patient; the transmitted intensity was used to verify the attenuation corrections of the scattered beam intensities. The background count rate was found to be typically 5% of the total scatter intensity and was the result of leakage radiation through the source shield.

A computer-controlled couch was used to scan the patient in a rectilinear fashion at a speed of 1.2 cm per second; the scan time was 15 minutes. The radiation dose to the patient was reported as 0.055 Gy (5.5 rad) for a spatial resolution of 1.0 cm. In order to increase the spatial resolution to 0.5 cm in the x-y plane, a radiation dose of 0.11 Gy (11 rad) was necessary; however, the spatial resolution in the z direction was still 1.0 cm. Comparing the Compton-scatter imaging system with that of a CT scanner, the CT imaging system gives better spatial resolution (0.17 cm) with a radiation dose of 0.046 Gy (4.6 rad). The CT scanner also permits scan times as short as 1 second, due to the high flux x-ray tube; this is an advantage in reducing respiratory and patient motion artifacts. It was stated that for both high resolution and low resolution imaging, Compton-scatter systems require much higher radiation

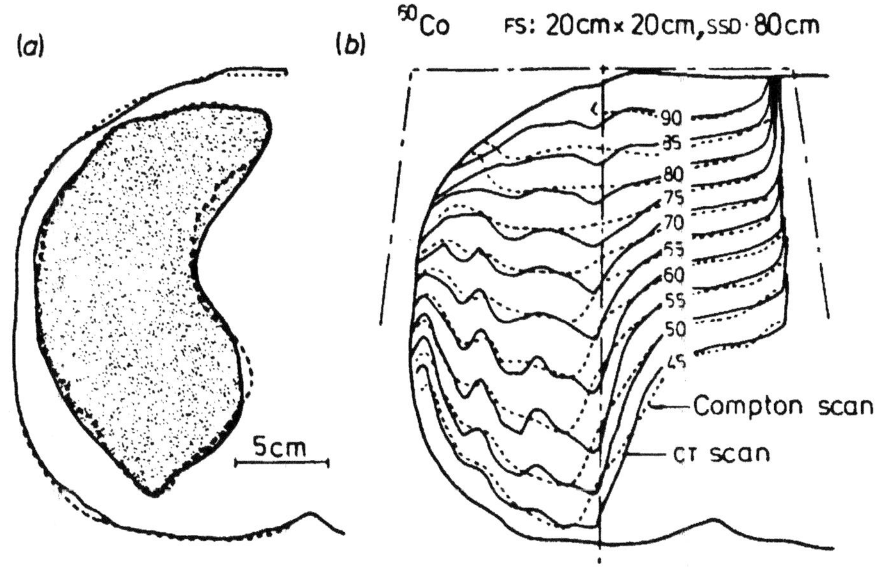

Figure 48. Anatomical (a) and isodose (b) contours using CT scan data (lines) and Compton scan data (broken lines) (Courtesy: JJ Battista)

doses than transmission (CT) imaging systems. The reason for this result is the inherently low probability for Compton interactions, as well as the poor photon detection efficiency for scattered photons. Battisa and Bronskill (1981) have concluded that there is little potential remaining for Compton-scatter imaging as a tool for clinical diagnosis.

Tomographic (scatter) images (figure 49) of the chest were obtained using a conventional large-field gamma camera (Pistolesi et al., 1978). Ninety degree scattered radiations (181 keV) were detected with a slit collimator (3 mm width × 80 mm length). The radioactive source was ^{203}Hg (279 keV; half-life, 46.9 days) and was constructed as a collimated linear source of 80-cm length. It was determined that a minimum source activity of 500 mCi was required for this system (Guzzardi et al., 1978). The intensities of scattered photons originating from points along the axis of the incident beam were proportional to the electron densities of tissues at those locations. The scan time was 3 minutes when a 1 Ci source was used; and the radiation dose was estimated as 90 mrad. The resolution using a chest phantom was 1.0 cm., which is typical of nuclear medicine images.

A problem with this method was that tissues farther from the source produced fainter images because of the greater attenuation of the radiation beam; in addition, the beam broadened at greater distances unless sufficient source collimation was provided. Multiple-scatter contamination was reduced through energy discrimination and by the use of an 8 cm thick parallel-hole collimator.

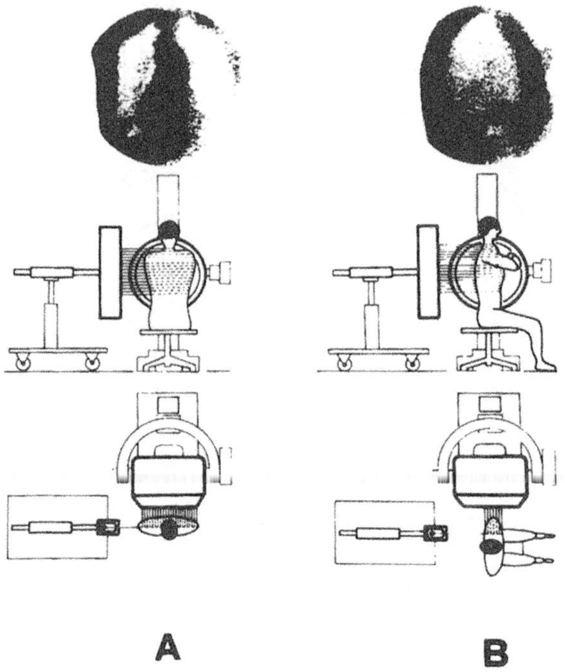

Figure 49. Compton-scatter imaging using a gamma camera and an external source for frontal chest (left) and sagittal (right) tomograms (Courtesy: M Pistolesi)

In order to overcome the problem of decreased contrast of the image caused by attenuation, two solutions were possible: (1) use of two gamma-ray sources on opposite sides of the patient, (2) a computer correction for nonuniformities (Giuntini et al., 1979). The authors demonstrated chest images having resolutions similar to that of conventional nuclear medicine images obtained with the gamma camera.

Guzzardi and Mey (1981) later determined that the smallest visible separation distance observed using a high-contrast bar phantom was 3.5 mm. Zito et al. (1982) introduced the concept of two ^{192}Ir linear sources used in conjunction with the conventional gamma camera and computer for chest imaging by scattering.

Later developments by this group demonstrated that two 5.0 Ci ^{192}Ir sources permitted a scan time of less than 1 minute per slice; an increase in activity was proposed to reduce the scan time to 15 to 20 seconds. The collimated line sources were positioned opposite each other and on the sides of the patient; the conventional gamma camera was placed over the patient and perpendicular to the irradiation plane. The source collimator slits were 40 cm × 3 mm; and two 90° scatter photopeaks of 191 keV and 245 keV were detected, corresponding to the incident energies 317 keV and 468 keV, respectively. The spatial resolution was given as 7 to 10 mm. It was indicated that further improvements were being made to reduce the scanning time and to reduce the effects of attenuation by increasing the source activity. A mobile support and scanning mechanism were being developed to increase the ability to scan more sections of the patient and to provide a unit that would be used at the bedside for acute patients (Guzzardi et al., 1985).

A Compton-scatter brain imaging system using a conventional scintillation camera was described by Mirell et al. (1976). The patient was positioned as for a vertex scan of the head. A conventional parallel-hole collimator was used on the gamma camera. A planar beam produced by either a rotating fan beam or a planar collimated ring source was used for scanning. This system was characterized by the movement of the source, while the detector and the patient remained in fixed positions. The planar source was positioned to provide a cross-sectional scatter image of any selected plane of the head. A collimated ring source containing 5 Ci of ^{99m}Tc and distributed in a circular tube, produced a 1-cm wide radiation field, and the scan time was several minutes. It was later found that ^{99m}Tc, because of its short half-life, was not a practical choice, and other sources were investigated.

Sources with high energies provided the advantage of reducing the attenuation artifacts, although collimation and shielding became more problematical. Low-energy sources, however, were reported to increase patient dose due to increased photoelectric absorption and increased multiple scattering. The artifacts produced by this planar imaging method were seen as nonuniformities in the brain images. However, a computer interfaced to the gamma camera enabled corrections for these artifacts and for the inherent scintillation camera field nonuniformities and attenuation effects.

It was further suggested that a dual-energy source would allow another means for determining and correcting for the attenuation artifacts. The authors found that densiy differences of 1% could be seen with a resolution area of 0.25 cm^2. The patient radiation dose was given as 0.5 rad. The authors suggested that this Compton-scatter imaging method might become an alternative to CT imaging in patients. However, Guzzardi and Mey (1981) have stated that for 90° scatter imaging off the brain, the gamma camera is not suitable because of the requirements for greater resolution.

A novel Compton-scatter imaging system has been described that provides two-dimensional scanning with very short scan times (milliseconds). Harding (1982) suggested that the most likely x-ray photon interaction at 60 keV is a scatter event and he designed a simple scatter imaging system. It was suggested that a system for measuring backscatter in the spine and in other tissues results in lower radiation doses than transmission methods such as CT and absorptiometry. This two-dimensional scatter imaging system, with stationary x-ray source and detector, included a small diaphragm, which was designed to sweep the primary beam across the patient.

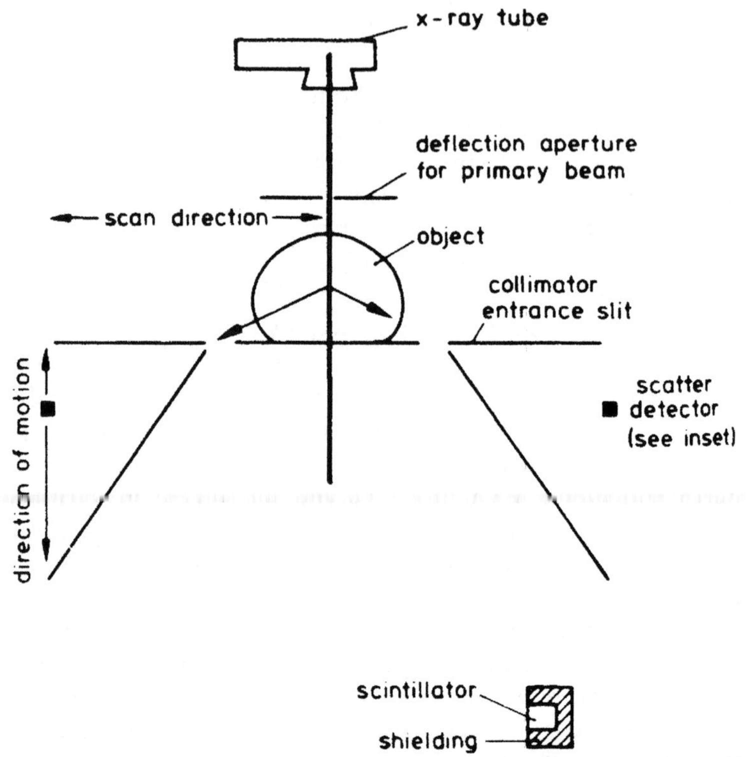

Figure 50. Cross-sectional scatter-imaging device (Courtesy: G Harding)

The experimental system (figure 50) used a 320 kVp (Philips MCN 320) x-ray generator and a beam-defining aperture (1 × 3mm^2). The two scatter detectors consisted of shielded NaI(Tl)/photomultiplier combinations. Specially shaped lead slits and steel multislit collimators with large scatter acceptance angles were used. The two detector systems were symmetrically placed to record the forward scatter from within the patient. The collimator was focused and was movable in a direction parallel to the direction of the primary beam; this allowed imaging with 1 mm resolution from any scattering volume element (voxel) in the path of the primary beam. The lamellar collimation discriminated against the effects of multiple scattering. The primary beam was scanned using a rotating disc aperture and provided for millisecond scanning of the patient.

The scattered-photon intensity produced from a point along the primary beam within the patient was measured and a standard scattering object was used for calibration. A correction was made for the primary beam attenuation (above the voxel of interest) and for the attenuation along the scatter path. A corrective term was added for multiple scatter. A set of equations was solved that yielded the electron density distribution within the scanned area. The author obtained images of a test phantom in which backscatter was measured at an angle of 140°. The radiation dose was 4 rads, and the images of 1% sugar solutions were resolved by the device.

Harding and Tischler (1986) explored a dual-energy Compton-scatter-imaging method (Comscan) that had applications to the imaging of bony structures and densitometry. The method allowed the determination of the photoelectric attenuation factors for the primary and scattered radiations. The method also provided Compton-scatter images that were corrected for attenuation using dual-energy measurements (figure 51).

Harding has stated that Compton systems employing forward-scatter geometry have no geometrical advantage relative to transmission radiography, whereas backscatter methods have no direct analogue in transmission imaging. The Comscan device employs backscatter geometry as described in the work by Harding et al. (1983). The radiation source of the Comscan system constisted of an x-ray tube and generator (Philips MCN 165, 3 kW, 160 kVP (max)). The x-ray beam was filtered by a 150-micron copper foil. The 1 mm × 1 mm beam was collimated with an eightfold slit collimator positioned coaxially with the primary beam for receiving backscatter over 360°. The slit collimator focused the primary beam onto eight detector arrays. The scattering angle from a point 30 mm deep in the object was chosen as 140°. Steel lamellae were interposed between the collimator slits and the detector arrays to absorb the multiply scattered radiation; the ratio of multiple-to-single scatter was on the order of 20%. The detectors consisted of BGO scintillators coupled to photomultiplier tubes.

The flux of the x-ray beam was such that the statistical precision was 1% for a measurement time of 10 ms. The radiation dose (surface) was given as 1.5 mSv for this exposure time. The tomographic slice thickness was determined as 7.5 mm. The x-ray generator was switched between 100 kVp and 160 kVp, providing the incident beams required by the dual-energy method. Dual-energy scatter images of the skull were performed in which the measurement time for 16 slices was 20 minutes and the skin dose was approximately 20 mSv. The electron densities of objects contained in the AAPM-computed tomography phantom were determined using the device, and these values were compared with the calculated electron densities. The dual-energy Compton-scatter imaging technique using an x-ray generator eliminates the need for higher photon fluxes as desired in radionuclide techniques. This method has the additional advantage of detection of a greater fraction of the scatter radiation. The effects of multiple scatter and the presence of artifacts in the image were being investigated.

An x-ray tomographic system was developed for assessing biological materials and for use in medical diagnosis (Yoneda and Chikaura, 1982). This device consisted of a collimated pencil beam incident on the sample and two combined circular slits adjusted such that only forward-scattered x-rays with a particular scattering angle were detected. An x-ray tube and generator (40 kV,

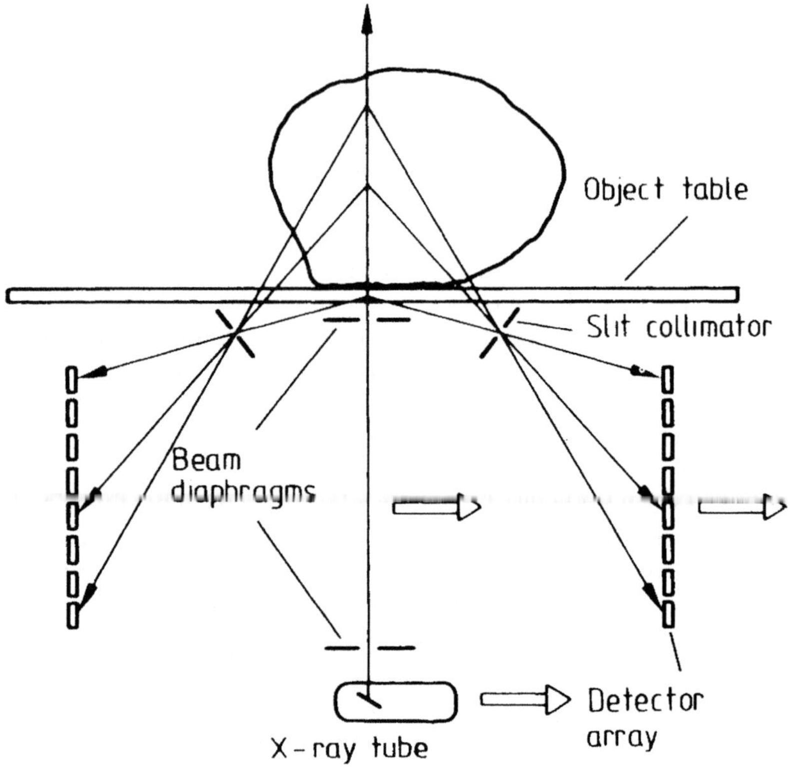

Figure 51. Comscan system showing the primary and scatter-beam geometry (Courtesy: G Harding)

20 mA) was used as the radiation source. In vitro studies were performed on specimens of biological materials. The level of the tomographic slice was selected by the movement of the slits along the axis of the pencil beam. The samples were moved in a plane perpendicular to the pencil beam in order to select points lateral to the beam. Alternatively, the source/detector system could be moved, while maintaining the sample (or patient) in a fixed position. A unique aspect of this system was the color image displayed on the TV monitor; three colors (blue, green, or red) assigned to each spot on the screen corresponded to the scatter intensity in one of three energy ranges as detected by three separate pulse-height analyzers.

The spatial resolution was found to be dependent upon the circular slits and was better than 0.1 mm. Tomographic sections as thin as 0.5 mm were possible. By changing the separation of the circular slits, it was possible to select either a small, medium, or large scattering angle for imaging. It was noted that scattering by air and absorption in the sample (bone and other soft tissues) sometimes caused artifacts in the image; this was due mainly to inadequate photon counting statistics. The scan time was typically several minutes (sometimes several tens of minutes) with a spatial resolution of 0.2 mm. The advantages of the design included: (1) identification of biological materials using the scatter data, (2) multicolored image display, and (3) variety of imaging modes easily obtained by changing the geometric and electronic parameters.

FIXED-POINT COMPTON-SCATTER METHODS

Fixed-point tissue densitometers are distinguished from Compton-scatter, imaging devices because they are designed primarily for the quantitative assessment of the electron density or mass density of a specific point or a specific type of tissue (i.e., lung, bone, etc.). Fixed-point systems do not generally include optimization of the image, although an image display of the quantitative data distribution may be provided.

The determination of the density of a selected volume within an irregular object by radiological methods involves the use of a set of equations in which the unknown variable represents the electron density of the region of interest and the coefficients are the attenuation factors of the incident and scattered photon beams. A solvable set of equations can be found, provided measurements can be made along the same path through the substance by both the transmitted and the scattered beams.

Clarke and Van Dyk (1973) have proposed two methods (figures 52 and 53) by which the absorption characteristics of the scattered and transmitted beams along the same path are determined. The *high-energy method,* which requires two radiation sources, provides that the energy of one source, after Compton scattering through a given angle, must equal the energy of the incident beam of the second source. After the initial transmission and scatter measurements are performed, the sample is rotated about the centerpoint of the volume of interest, and additional transmission and scatter measurements are performed. Because the attenuation factors are identical for the transmission and scatter beams, they cancel and do not appear in the density calculation.

The *low-energy method* is based upon the assumption that for incident energies much less than 0.511 MeV, the energy shift due to Compton scattering of the incident photon is negligible. This means that the scattering angle is not selected on the basis of matching the scatter energy of one source with the incident energy of the second source; this angle may be selected on the basis of other reasons. In the low-energy method, a single source (incident beam) is moved from the first location to the second, removing the requirement for using two radiation sources. This method does not require that the sample be rotated, as in the high-energy method; instead, the source is rotated about the region of interest. The scattered and transmitted intensities are determined with the source sequentially facing one fixed detector and then a second fixed detector. Investigations of both the low-energy and high-energy Compton-scatter methods have been reported in the literature.

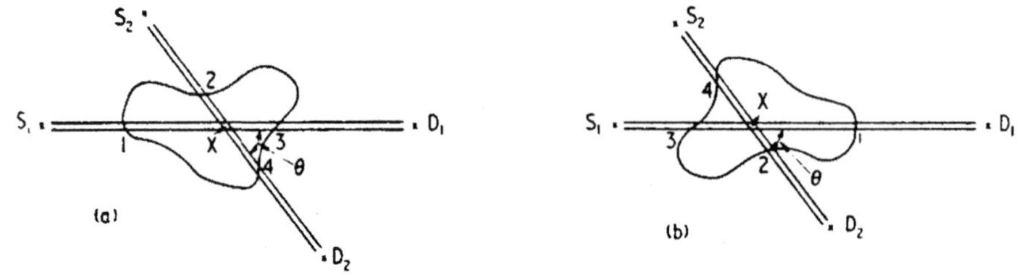

Figure 52. Fixed-point Compton-scatter (high-energy) method: (a) initial configuration and (b) sample rotated 180° (Courtesy: RL Clarke)

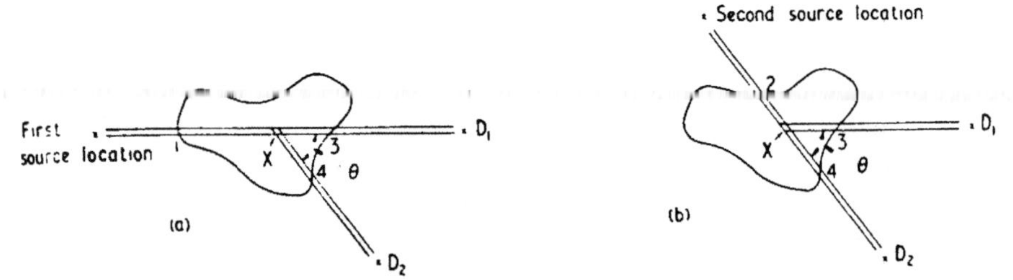

Figure 53. Fixed-point Compton-scatter (low-energy) method: (a) initial measurement configuration and (b) second measurement configuration (Courtesy: RL Clarke)

DUAL-SOURCE/DUAL-DETECTOR METHODS

The number of scattered photons detected N, is proportional to the intensity of the source I, the cross section for Compton scattering, and the electron density, as follows:

$$N = \text{constant} \cdot I\sigma_e \cdot \frac{\varrho Z N(a)}{A}$$

where the last term is the electron density (electrons per cc), N(a) is Avogadro's number (atoms/M), ϱ is the mass density (g/cc), and A is the atomic mass (g/M). When the scattering material is a mixture of elements, the term Z/A is replaced with a term representing the weighted amounts of each element.

Garnett et al. (1973) introduced a technique for the in vivo measurement of absolute bone density (figure 54). It was noted that no previous method measured bone density directly in terms of mass per unit volume. The method required two radionuclide sources and two detectors. A 400 mCi ^{198}Au source (412 keV) and a source of ^{203}Hg (279 keV) were used. The scattered photon

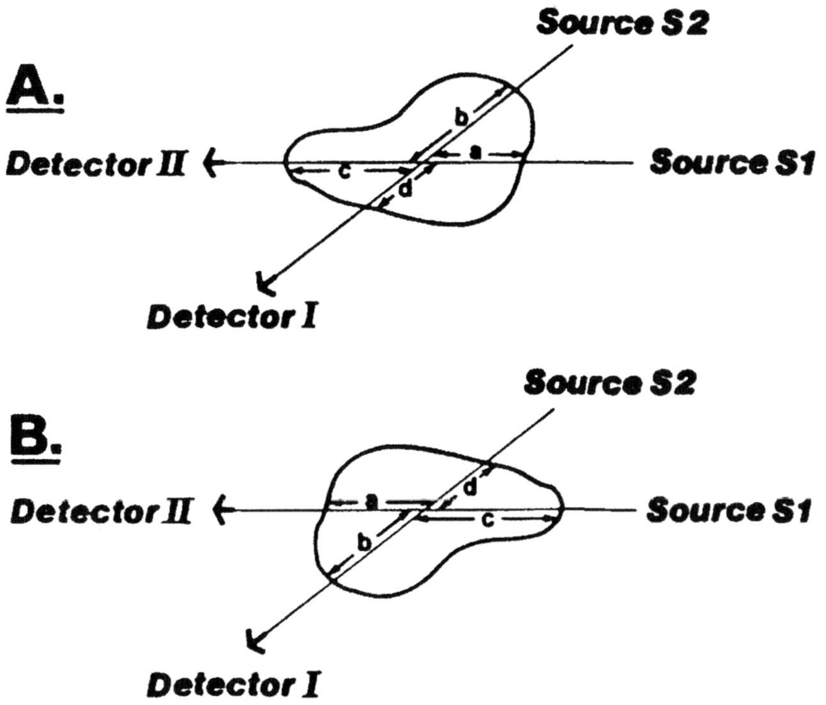

Figure 54. (A) Compton-scatter geometry for attenuation correction and (B) sample rotated 180° (Courtesy: ES Garnett)

energy for the ^{198}Au source was matched to the incident energy of the ^{203}Hg source by the choice of a 67° scattering angle. This matching of energies provided a means for correcting for the attenuation along the scatter and incident paths of the sample. The following sequence of measurements was performed: (1) two measurements (transmission and scatter, respectively) using the ^{198}Au source, (2) one transmission measurement with the ^{203}Hg source, followed by a 180° rotation of the sample, and (3) one scatter measurement using ^{203}Hg. The density relative to water was determined as follows (Kennett et al., 1972):

$$\varrho = \text{constant} \cdot \left(\frac{N_1 N_1''}{N_2 N_1'}\right)^{\frac{1}{2}}$$

where N_1 is the scattered intensity from ^{198}Au, N_2 is the transmitted intensity from ^{198}Au, N_1' is the transmitted intensity form ^{203}Hg, and N_2'' is the scattered intensity from ^{203}Hg. The constant in the equation was determined by performing the measurements in a water phantom.

The reproducibility of the density determination in samples of lumbar vertebrae was ±2%. A good correlation between the density by Compton scattering and the density measured by the Archimedes principle was reported. The radiation dose was stated as 10 rads. Garnett proposed that the optimal energy for the high-energy source was approximately 90 keV and that the use of this energy would result in a lower radiation dose and a shorter scan time (a few minutes). The main advantages of this measurement scheme were (1) the resulting density values were independent of the soft-tissues attenuation surrounding the bone, (2) the method provided a direct determination of the physical density in units of g/cc. A disadvantage, in addition to the high radiation dose, was the necessity for rotation of the sample, which increased the repositioning errors and is a complication for in vivo human measurements.

Using the method described by Garnett et al. (1973), Webber and Kennett (1976) designed a system (figure 55) for the in vivo measurement of the human os calcis (heel of the foot). ^{153}Sm (half-life, 47 hours; activity, 1.7 Ci) and ^{170}Tm (half-life, 129 days, activity, 450 mCi) were selected for the dual-source, dual-detector (NaI) arrangement. The incident energy of the ^{153}Sm beam was 103.2 keV and the scattered photon energy for the 90° scattering angle was 85.9 keV. The incident energy of the ^{170}Tm beam was 84.3 keV, which nearly matched the scattered photon energy of the ^{153}Tm as desired. Although a source of ^{153}Gd with a half-life of 242 days was considered, the investigators had access to a reactor facility in which a ready supply of ^{153}Sm was available. A cerium filter was used in the beam of the ^{153}Sm source for removal of the unwanted europium K x-rays (41.5 keV), which would have added unnecessary patient dose. Similarly, a gadolinium filter was used in the beam of ^{100}Tm source for removal of the unwanted 52.4 keV ytterbium characteristic x-rays. The source holders were positioned 90° apart, with the detector holders directly opposite each source.

The 90° scattering angle was selected because it provided the most symmetrical scattering volume (8.3 cc) within the os calcis of human subjects. For in vivo measurements, the foot was restrained such that the os calcis was positioned at the intersection of the two photon beams. The incident beams from each source were exposed in sequence. The transmitted and scattered intensities were determined for the first source (^{153}Sm), and only the transmitted intensity was determined using the second source (^{170}Tm). Following the 180° rotation of the foot, the scattered intensity from the second source (^{170}Tm) was measured.

The density of the trabecular bone of the os calcis was determined using the previously mentioned equation, which included a correction for the difference in the ratio (Z/A) between bone and water (reference standard). The exposure time was 3 minutes, and the standard error in the density measurement (due to counting statistics) was 1.0%. The calculated absorbed dose was 160 m. It was noted that the use of ^{153}Sm instead of ^{198}Au resulted in a reduction of the radiation dose by a factor of approximately 50. The precision of the density measurement for a simulated foot phantom was 1.5%. The measured range of densities of the os calcis in 12 human subjects was 1.11 to 1.53 g/cc. Webber

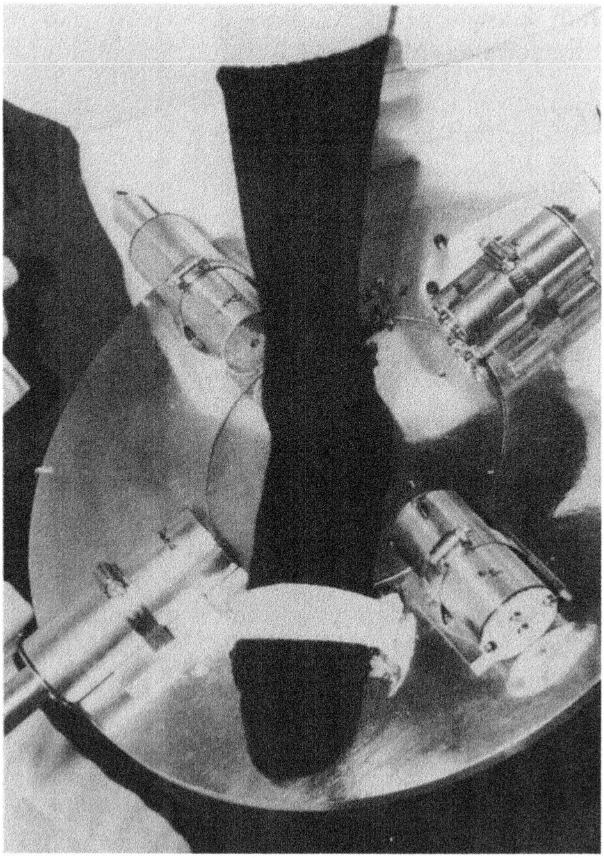

Figure 55. Bone density apparatus (Courtesy: CE Webber)

and Kennett concluded that this Compton scatter system was simple in design and use, and would be an ideal method for the accurate in vivo detection of small serial changes in bone density of the human os calcis.

A Compton scatter densitometer was specifically designed for the measurement of in vitro specimens of human tissues (Shrimpton, 1981). The system followed the design of Clarke and Van Dyk (1973) and Garnett et al. (1973), except that the radionuclide sources chosen were ^{57}Co (half-life, 270 days; energy, 122 keV) and ^{153}Gd (half-life, 242 days; energy, 100 keV). The 86° scattering angle was chosen to match the scattered photon energy of the ^{57}Co source with the transmitted energy of the ^{153}Gd source; the scattering volume defined by the collimators was 0.5 cc. Two transmission and two scatter measurements provided the corrections for attenuation, as well as the quantities needed to calculate the electron densities of the samples. Various solutions were used to establish the correlation between the measured and theoretical electron densities. The number of electrons per unit volume of a material ϱ is calculated from knowledge of its mass density (ϱ) and its composition according to the formula (Murty, 1965):

$$\varrho_e = \frac{N(A)\varrho Z}{A_{eff}}, \text{ electrons per unit volume,}$$

where

$$\frac{Z}{A_{eff}} = \sum_i P_i \frac{Z_i}{A_i},$$

N(A) is Avogadro's number and P_i is the fraction by weight of the ith element (atomic number Z_i and mass number A_i in the material). The uncertainty associated with this in vitro Compton-scatter densitometer was less than ±2% for biological specimens. The results of experiments with several human tissue types (table 3) showed that most normal healthy soft tissues have electron density values in the range of ±5% around 3.4×10^{23} electrons per cubic centimeter (except for lung tissue). As a result, it was concluded that the electron density alone may be a poor clinical parameter for in vitro tissue analysis.

A similar method was developed by Piper and Preuss (1976) in which the radionuclide sources ^{153}Gd (half-life, 242 days; activity, 100 mCi; energy, 100 keV) and ^{170}Tm (half-life, 131 days; activity, 500 mCi; energy, 84 keV) were used. An extensive study and comparison of dual-source combinations was performed in which the patient radiation dose, cost of the sources, source dimensions (specific activity), and primary photon energy were considered to be ideal for the ^{153}Gd/^{170}Tm and ^{144}Ce/^{57}Co combinations (Preuss et al., 1975).

In the experiments, the two radionuclide sources were placed in parallel with the opposing NaI(Tl) detectors; the sources and detectors remained fixed in position throughout the measurement procedure. The scattering angle (angle between the axes of the source/detector combinations) was 86°. The incident beam of the ^{153}Gd source was exposed while the ^{170}Tm source remained off, during which time the transmitted and scattered intensities through the sample were measured. In sequence, the ^{170}Tm source was exposed while the ^{153}Gd source remained off, and the transmission of this beam was measured. The beam of the ^{170}Tm source was matched to provide an energy in transmission nearly equal to that of the scatter energy of ^{153}Gd at the 86° scattering angle.

Following the 180° rotation of the sample, the ^{153}Gd source was again exposed, and a second scatter intensity was measured. Solving the four equations that describe the transmission and scatter intensities under these mea-

Table 3. Electron densities of human tissues: sample measurements and calculated values (Courtesy: PC Shrimpton)

Sample	Mass density range (g cm^{-3})	Calculated range for electron density $\times 10^{23}$ (cm^{-3})	Observed electron density $\times 10^{23}$ (cm^{-3})
Adipose tissue	0.92–0.93	3.08–3.13	3.10 ± 0.02
Brain	1.03–1.04	3.41–3.47	3.43 ± 0.02
Breast	0.97–1.05	3.21–3.46	3.40 ± 0.03
Kidney	1.05	3.41–3.48	3.43 ± 0.05
Liver	1.05–1.07	3.49–3.57	3.50 ± 0.05
Lung	0.26–1.06	0.86–3.48	2.29 ± 0.03
Muscle	1.04–1.06	3.41–3.50	3.51 ± 0.04
Pancreas	1.02–1.05	3.38–3.51	3.48 ± 0.02
Spleen	1.05–1.06	3.47–3.52	3.46 ± 0.02
Thyroid	1.04–1.07	3.45–3.55	3.61 ± 0.04

surement circumstances, the electron density was calculated. The densities of 20 ox bone samples, as determined by this scattering method, were well correlated ($r = 0.977$) with the densities determined by Archimedes' principle. The accuracy was determined as 3%, as measured for materials of known density. In vivo densitometry in the human os calcis using this method was estimated to require sources having greater activities, resulting in a radiation dose of 330 mrad. It was suggested that a cerium filter be used to eliminate the low-energy gamma-rays of ^{153}Gd, thereby reducing the estimated patient dose.

Duke and Hanson (1984) investigated the use of commercial x-ray tubes as a replacement for the radionuclide sources in Compton-scatter densitometry. Because of their increased photon flux as compared with radionuclide sources, x-ray tubes might provide improved spatial resolution, precision, and counting times. Commercial x-ray tubes with 1 to 2 mm focal spots offer photon fluxes equivalent to radionuclide sources with activities of 10 to 80 TBq, whereas present radionuclide sources used in Compton-scatter densitometry have activities of only 5 to 100 GBq.

Duke and Hanson estimated that a measurement precision of 1% could be obtained with x-ray tubes, while reducing the counting times to under 10 seconds with a spatial resolution of better than 1 cc. The difficulty with the use of polychromatic sources (x-ray tubes) is that the beam attenuations in the sample no longer cancel. The polychromatic beam may be considered as a set of monoenergetic beams that undergo different amounts of attenuation because of their different energies. Correction factors for beam hardening, attenuation differences due to the Compton energy shift, and polychromaticity of the beam have been predicted on the basis of an analytic model in which published x-ray spectra were used. Multiple scattering was not included because of the complexities encountered in analytic models of multiple scattering.

In addition, numerical analyses were performed for hypothetical samples including biological samples. The results indicated that the biases due to polychromaticity of the beam were not substantially more problematic than those that arise in the case of monoenergetic beams using radionuclide sources. It was expected that the multiple scatter errors were an order of magnitude greater than the investigated biases for both polyenergetic and monenergetic beams. The same types of bias corrections were found possible for densitometers using x-ray tubes. It was concluded that the use of x-ray tubes in Compton-scatter densitometry may provide better economy, convenience, safety, accuracy, and precision than the densitometers using radionuclide sources.

Hanson et al. (1984) designed a system for densitometry of the human lung in which the measured density was directly related to the presence of fluid in the lung (figure 56). The source was a conventional x-ray tube. This fixed-point Compton-scattered system used the principles of the dual-source/dual-detector design. Two conventional rotating anode x-ray tubes and two sodium iodide detectors were mounted on an adjustable C-arm mechanism, with source-detector distances of 60 cm. Each x-ray tube faced a detector, and the scattering angle was fixed at 40°. The C-arm was mounted on a mobile x-ray generator for use at the patient's bedside. The detectors were collimated with a bundle of small-diameter tantalum tubes. The x-ray tube collimators and the detector collimators provided a scattering volume of 45 cc in the shape of a prolated ellipsoid (approximately 9 cm × 3 cm).

The patient was initially centered at the intersection of the two source-detector axes. Both x-ray tubes were fired simultaneously and continuously; however, during each measurement, the shutter blocked one of the beams so that only one beam was transmitted. A density determination required measurements in two phases. When the first beam was turned on, the transmission through the lung was measured; during this time, the scattered intensity at 40° was measured. In the second phase, the other x-ray tube was fired and the transmitted and scattered intensities were measured. The density was calculated as follows:

$$\varrho = K\left(\frac{S_1 S_2}{T_1 T_2}\right)$$

where S_1 and S_2 are the scatter intensities; T_1 and T_2 are the transmitted intensities in the lung; and K is a constant determined by calibration with a known density substance. The scan time was 1.0 second (0.5 second for each phase) using 100 kVp and 40 mA as exposure factors. Each x-ray tube contained lead or aluminum filtration to reduce the incident beam intensities to levels that would not overload the detector electronics (dead time). The filters were removed when the detectors measured the scattered photon intensities.

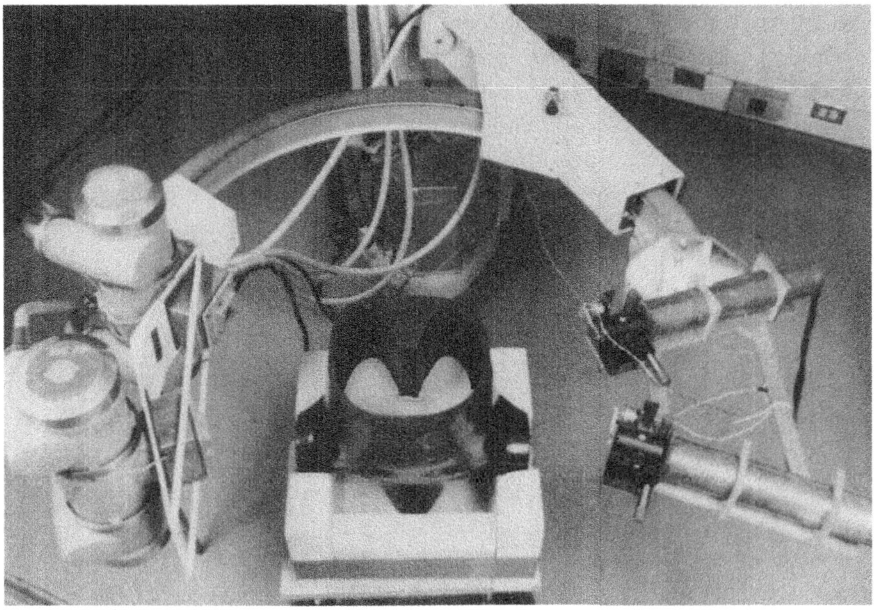

Figure 56. Lung densitometer and anthropomorphic phantom (Courtesy: JE Hanson)

It was found that multiple-scatter contamination was the principal source of error in this system, leading to a possible error in the density of 10% at high lung densities (>0.5 g/cc), although the standard error of the estimate was 2.4%. The authors did not specifically mention the problem of x-ray generator stability, although this error may be included in the error assessment. The radiation exposure (skin) for a 1-second measurement was 400 to 600 μGy. The reported precision was 5%, and the accuracy was 2% to 3%. On the basis of these short exposure times, dynamic studies of lung function have been proposed.

DUAL-SOURCE/SINGLE-DETECTOR METHODS

A densitometry system using the dual sources ^{60}Co (1.25 MeV) and ^{137}Cs (662 keV) was described by Clarke and Van Dyk (1973). The development of this high-energy method required the use of an 80 Ci ^{60}Co source for scatter measurements (50° scattering angle) and 100 mCi ^{60}Co and ^{137}Cs sources for transmission measurements. A single NaI(Tl) detector was rotated to the appropriate positions for the transmission and scatter measurements, yielding a scattering volume of 1 cc. The relative electron densities of various solutions were found to be in good agreement with calculated values. However, this simplification in the requirement for detectors is counteracted by the addition of errors in repositioning of the detector during in vivo densitometry.

SINGLE-SOURCE/SINGLE-DETECTOR METHODS

Olkkonen and Karjalainen (1975) described a Compton-scattering technique (figure 57) for the determination of bone density in which a single radionuclide source, ^{170}Tm (half-life, 130 days; activity, 650 mCi; energy, 84 keV) was fixed relative to the sample, and a single NaI (Tl) detector was rotated for measurements at three locations around the sample. The effective scattering volume of bone was 1 cc. The first of two transmission measurements was performed with the detector aligned parallel with the incident beam. The second transmission measurement followed the rotation of the sample through an angle equal to the scattering angle (30°). The first scatter intensity measurement was performed on the unrotated sample at a scattering angle of 30° to the incident beam. The second scatter intensity measurement was performed on the unrotated sample at a 30° scattering angle, but on the opposite side of the incident beam in the same plane as the first scatter measurement.

Four equations involving the attenuation factors for the transmitted and scatter intensities and the path lengths were solved simultaneously to yield an expression for the electron density of the substance. The method used the assumption that because the scattering angle is much less than 90° and the incident energy (E) is much less than 0.51 MeV, the energy of the scattered photons (E′) is approximately equal to the incident energy; therefore, it was assumed that the linear attenuation coefficients in transmission and scatter were approximately equal.

The method was tested for samples of acrylic, polystyrene, muscle, fat, and bone; the results were compared with those based on the Archimedes principle. A good correlation ($r = 0.94$) was found between these results. The precision of the method was 2%. The densitometer as designed was useful for measurements of the peripheral skeleton only. However, it was concluded that since this scattering method was not affected by the tissues surrounding the volume of interest, it could be successfully applied in the determination of the densities of the spinal vertebrae and femoral neck.

A single-source low-energy Compton-scatter densitometer was developed by Huddleston and Bhaduri (1979). The radionuclide source was ^{153}Sm (half-life, 47 hrs; activity, 1.2 Ci; energy, 103 keV), which was produced in a local reactor facility. A cerium foil was used to filter out the low-energy europium K x-rays. The source was fixed in position, and the NaI(Tl) detector was rotated to three locations about the sample. The scattering angle was chosen as 30° (scattered photon energy, 100.5 keV), and the source and detector were collimated using cylindrical collimators.

The choice of the scattering angle was based upon the assumption that the Compton energy shift of the scattered photons does not significantly alter the attenuation coefficients of the substances surrounding the scattering volume. This assumption simplifies the calculation of the electron density. The measurements were performed in the following sequence: (1) transmission, with

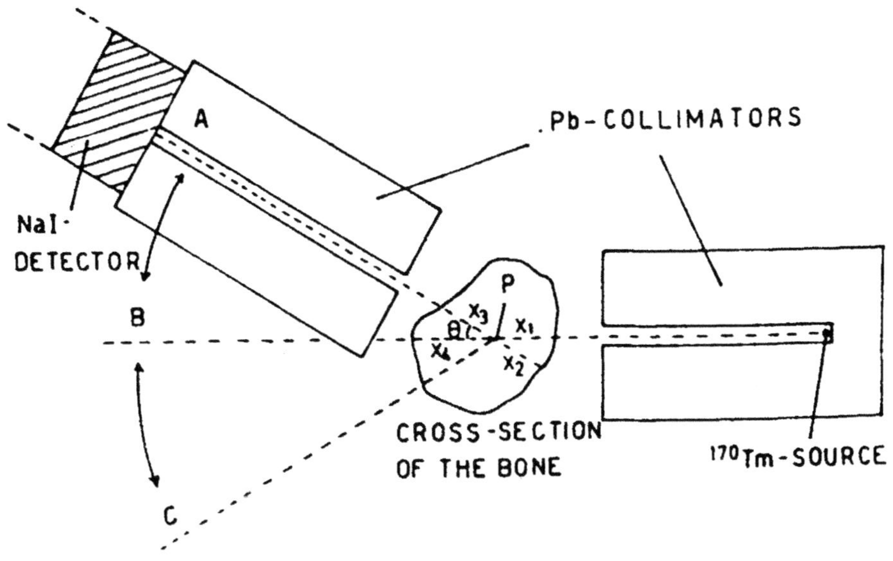

Figure 57. Compton-scattering technique (Courtesy: H Olkkonen)

the detector at 0°; (2) scatter, with the detector at 30° (sample is, then, rotated clockwise through an angle of 30°); (3) scatter, with the detector rotated clockwise to a position 30° on the opposite side of the incident beam direction; and (4) transmission, with the detector at 0°. These intensities were utilized in the four equations that describe the attenuation properties for each geometry. The density of the sample was calculated using the relationship:

$$\varrho = \varrho_e \left(\frac{Z}{A}\right)$$

where ϱ_e is the electron density of the sample relative to water determined by solving the four simultaneous equations. The ratio of Z to A corrects for the difference between the Z/A for water and the Z/A for the sample material. The theoretical considerations of this method are found in the literature (Huddleston et al., 1978). The mass densities for homogeneous chemical solutions, obtained using the single-source/single-detector low-energy Compton-scattering method, showed good correlations (r = 0.99) with the densities as determined by the Archimedes method.

In addition, the bias due to multiple scattering was determined by measuring the densities of increasing diameters of the solutions. This bias was not significant for samples of diameter less than 4.5 cm. Bias corrections were applied to the density values and were found to be in agreement with the magnitude of bias corrections reported by Kennett and Webber (1976). Final-

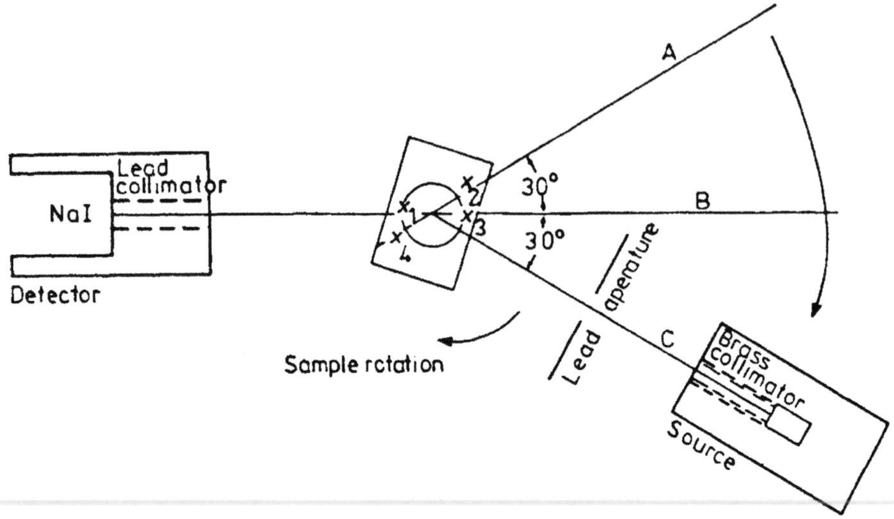

Figure 58. Single-source low-energy Compton densitometer (Courtesy: AL Huddleston)

ly, intact human femoral heads removal at surgery were placed in a water phantom, and the relative electron densities (corrected for multiple scatter bias) were determined. The densities of the femoral head samples, obtained in vitro, were well correlated ($r = 0.94$) with the bone mineral content as determined by single-photon absorptiometry (Norland-Cameron device).

Huddleston et al. (1979) later substituted the ^{153}Sm source with ^{153}Gd source because of the longer half-life, which provided additional long-term stability to the measurements (figure 58). The uncertainty of the single-source/single-detector low-energy Compton-scatter method was 1% to 3% when the bias corrections for multiple scatter were included. An empirical equation from which the density bias can be predicted was determined from the experimental results of this investigation.

The single-source dual-energy Compton-scatter method (Huddleston and Weaver, 1983; Huddleston and Sackler, 1985) has several advantages when compared to the dual-source methods (figure 59). The single source (^{153}Gd or ^{192}Ir) was fixed in position, as was the single NaI(Tl) detector. The method did not require the rotation of the sample. Corrections for attenuation along the scatter and transmission paths were not required because the density calculation relied upon previously determined attenuation coefficients and an approximate knowledge of the path lengths in tissues. The equations describe the number of photons scattered to the detector from the volume element of interest, corresponding to the two incident photon energies.

The effective linear attenuation coefficient, μ(EFF), was determined by measuring the scattered intensities for cylindrical specimens of excised bone

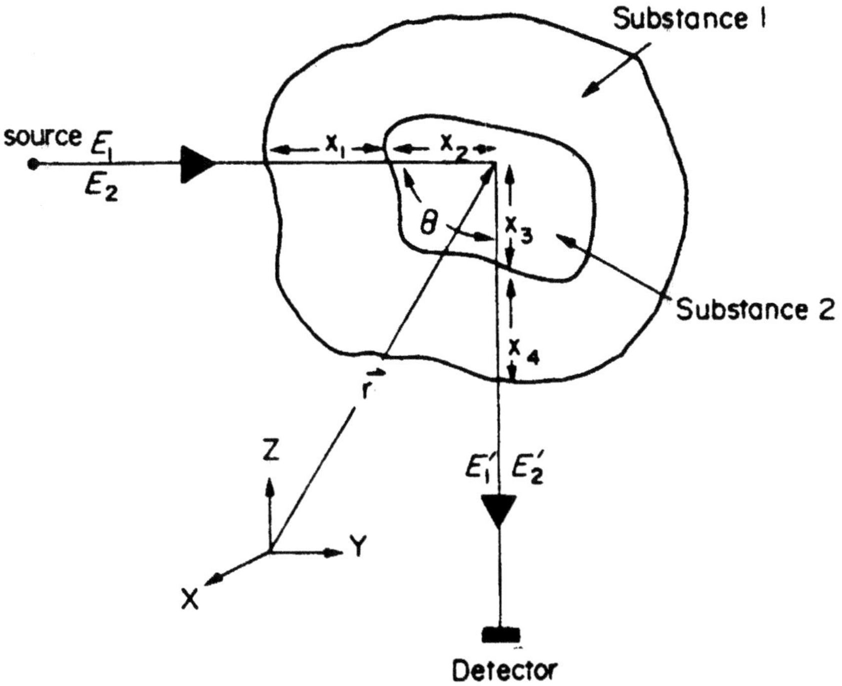

Figure 59. Dual-energy Compton-scattering method (Courtesy: AL Huddleston)

and soft tissue at the selected scattering angle. The scattered-photon intensities were plotted as functions of the increasing diameters of the cylindrical specimens, and the effective linear attenuation coefficients were derived from the curve using an exponential curve-fitting procedure (Huddleston and Weaver, 1983).

For the ^{153}Gd source (energies, 41 keV and 100 keV), the energies of the scattered photons at a scattering angle of 90°, were 38 keV and 84 keV, respectively. The activity of the ^{153}Gd source was approximately 1 Ci for the experiments using samples of known densities (K_2HPO_4, $CaCl_2$, polystyrene, and plexiglass). The source and detector were placed in the horizontal plane and were collimated to provide a scattering volume of diameter 1.0 cm in a water phantom. The samples were placed in cylinders at the intersection of the source and detector collimator axes. The 90° scattering angle was chosen because the scattering volume was more symmetric and easily contained within the sample cylinders. Different collimators were used to provide a second geometrical configuration. For both experimental geometries, good correlations were found between the electron densities determined using the Compton-scatter method and those calculated on the basis of known elemental composition ($r = 0.991$ and $r = 0.985$, respectively). The uncertainty of the method (using ^{153}Gd) was 1% to 3%.

In a later study, Huddleston and Sackler (1985) evaluated the dual-energy Compton-scatter method, using a medium energy source (^{192}Ir: half-life, 74 days; activity, 7.4 × 10^{10}) Bq; energies, 317 keV and 468 keV). The scattered photon energies for the 90° scattering angle were 195.6 keV and 244.3 keV, respectively. Experiments were performed in samples of known densities on a prototype clinical Compton-scatter densitometer. A three-dimensional positioning system was used as a rigid support for the source and detector (fixed at a 90° scattering angle) and for accurately positioning the scattering volume within the samples. The system was designed for usage below a patient couch (backsactter geometry) in which the scattering volume could be positioned at any location within the patient's spinal vertebrae.

Three scattering geometries were investigated, and the optimal geometry for in vivo densitometry was determined for a scattering angle of 90°. The in vitro experiments in phantoms showed that the uncertainty in the electron density measurements was 1% to 2%. These experiments also showed that the 2 to 3% uncertainty in the determination of the effective linear attenuation coefficients was sufficient for the dual-energy Compton-scatter method. The method was believed to be the most convenient as well as accurate method for in vivo electron density measurements, with a radiation dose of less than 1 rad.

The advantages of the method included: (1) only one scatter intensity measurement was required for the determination of the electron density in a clinical study, (2) no rotation or movement of the source/detector system or the sample (patient) was required. These advantages together provided a reduction in the errors due to repositioning of the patient. The mechanical and geometrical simplifications provided by the fixed angle-source/single-detector method were similarly found in the design by Hazan et al. (1977). In addition, the use of a dual-energy source increased the accuracy and precision, since the attenuation coefficients of bone were measured instead of estimated from values in the literature.

Lung densities have been determined using a fixed-point Compton-backscatter densitometer, incorporating a rigid single-source (^{137}Cs)/single-detector arrangement. Reiss and Schuster (1972) developed a system (Siemens AG, Erlangen, Germany) for the determination of the density of lung tissues in subjects with pulmonary diseases. The system included a patient table having motions in three dimensions. A fluoroscopic x-ray unit mounted below the table allowed the precise selection (using a TV monitor) of the lung volume to be measured. Although the source activity was not stated, the exposure rate in the lung for a 10-second measurement was given as 0.42 R/min. The densities at various points in the lung were determined under conditions of expiration and inspiration. It was stated that unwanted multiple scatter reaching the detector was below 10%.

Dohring (1979), using Reiss' backscatter design, also reported on the measurement of lung densities in patients. The radioactive source was ^{137}Cs (activity, 10 Ci; half-life, 30 yrs; energy, 662 keV); a scintillation crystal (5-

inch diameter × 2-inch thick) and photomultiplier tube were used for detection of scattered radiation. Both the source and detector were stationary, placed below the table, and adequately shielded with lead. The source was angulated at 50° to the vertical, and the detector was aligned to give a mean scattering angle of 110°. The scattering volume defined by the gamma-ray beam diameter and by the focusing characteristics of the detector collimator were given by the following dimensions: 1.7 cm (longitudinal), 1.5 cm (transverse), and 2.7 cm (vertical). This scattering volume could be positioned at any location within the patient by using the motorized table. The radiation exposure was reported as 1 R/min/cm^2. The equations used for calculating the lung densities at specific points within the patients are given in the papers by Reiss and Schuster, and by Dohring (1979).

SINGLE-SOURCE/DUAL-DETECTOR METHOD

Another system designed for lung density studies used a single source that was sequentially positioned at two different angles, providing two scatter intensity measurements in the lung (Kaufman et al., 1976). Two cadmium telluride (CdTe) solid-state detectors with multihole (parallel) collimators were positioned in a plane opposite the source (^{153}Gd: energies, 100 keV and 41 keV; half-life, 242 days; activity, 10 Ci). With the source in the first position, the transmitted beam intensity through the lung was measured by the first detector. The scattered intensity was measured at the scattering angle of 20° by the second detector. The source was then moved for alignment with the second detector, and a second transmission measurement was made. The second scatter intensity measurement was made using the first detector. It was assumed that the energies of the transmitted the scattered beams were not significantly different and that the attenuation along the exit paths was the same for both transmitted and scattered photons. The density of the lung, relative to that of water, was determined by calculation using an equation relating the incident and scattered attenuation characteristics. The accuracy of the lung density determination was reported as 2% to 5%. The density was found to be linear over the range of 0.1 to 1 g/cc.

FINITE GEOMETRY EFFECTS

Several problems inherent in Compton-scatter methods have been described (Kennett and Webber, 1976). One problem results from the finite geometry of the incident and scattered photon beams. During the transmission measurement, the volume of substance viewed by the detector is defined solely by the incident beam size. However, for the scatter measurement, the volume of substance viewed by the detector (from which single scatter is received) is defined by the detector "field-of-view" as well as by the incident beam size. The geometries for the transmission measurement and for the scatter measurements are therefore 'nonidentical' (Kennett and Webber, 1976). It is evident that the photons of the incident beam interact at different positions within and outside the scattering volume (Kennett and Webber, 1976).

Thus, the total (incident plus scatter) path lengths are not the same for all photons in the beam. Those photons that are scattered at sites in the scattering volume nearest the detector have shorter path lengths than those scattered from the far side of the scattering volume. The attenuation correction, when taking into account all possible paths through which single-scattered photons arrive at the detector, does not equal that for a photon scattered from a point along the central ray of the incident beam. Since the attenuation correction theoretically represents photons along the central ray, an attenuation error is introduced that increases the measured density. Kennett and Webber found an increase in the os calcis densities of about 1%. However, this error was neglected since it was within the overall precision of the measurement.

MULTIPLE SCATTERING

Kennett and Webber (1976) investigated the effects of multiple scattering on Compton-scatter density measurements. This effect caused a positive bias in the measured densities in the human os calcis in the range of 5% to 11% using their densitometer design. A correction for multiple scattering was suggested in which the density bias was expressed as a function of the ratio of the natural logarithms of the transmissions for the sample to that of the standard substance. It was found that the multiple-scatter bias increased as the density of the sample was increased. A theoretical analysis showed that the magnitude of the multiple-scatter bias was dependent on both the density and the size of the object. Multiple scattering is also dependent upon sample diameter, scattering angle, and scattering geometry (figure 60).

CLINICAL MEASUREMENTS

Webber and Garnett (1976) performed measurements in human subjects using the Compton scatter densitometer described by Kennett et al. (1972). The densities of the right and left os calcis in 52 subjects were measured, having a standard deviation in the measurements of ±1.5%. In this study of limb dominance, the investigators found that there was a significant difference between the density of the right and left os calcis in 90% of the subjects using this method.

A simplified method for in vivo Compton-scatter densitometry of the peripheral skeleton was developed by Hazan et al. (1977). The system (figure 61) was designed specifically for the determination of the density of the human distal radius. The radioactive source was ^{137}Cs (half-life, 30 years; activity, 0.5 Ci; energy, 662 keV). The scattering angle was 90°, and the energy of the detected scattered photons was 288 keV. A parallel-hole collimator with rectangular cross section was used to collimate the incident beam. A focused collimator of 37 holes and focal length of 6.3 cm was used with the NaI(Tl) detector; the scattering volume was not calculated, but the detector field-of-

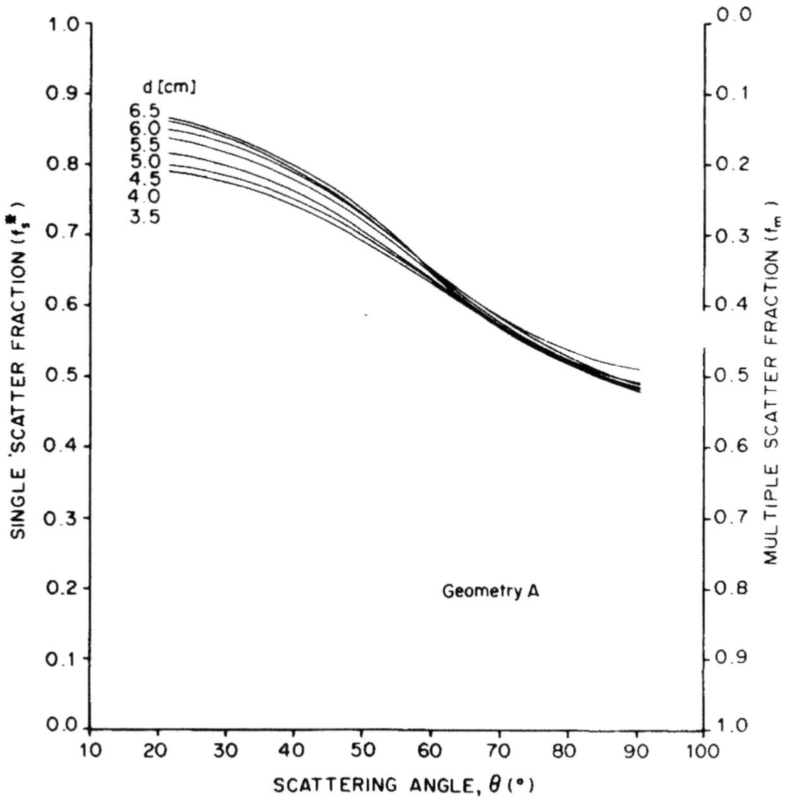

Figure 60. Single-scatter fractions and multiple-scatter fractions of total scatter as functions of scattering angle and sample diameter (Courtesy: AL Huddleston)

view in the focal plane was 2.0 cm in diameter. A single-channel analyzer was used in the scatter measurements. The forearm of the patient was positioned below the detector collimator and in the same horizontal plane with the source. The distal radius was positioned such that the maximum scatter intensity was detected. The radiation dose for a series of 10 measurements, each of 30-seconds duration, was about 2 rads in a tissue volume of 2.5 cc.

A population of 45 subjects suspected of bone mineral loss and five young normal adults were studied. The left radius (3 cm proximal to the distal tip) of each subject was examined by Compton scattering, following a radiographic exam (film) of the radius. This skeletal site was chosen because only a thin layer of cortical bone surrounds a larger region of trabecular bone. All subjects in which the radial diameter was found to be less than the scattering volume diameter (2 cm) were excluded; this ensured that tissues surrounding bone were not included in the scattering volume. The attenuations of the incident beam and the scattered beam were taken into account by performing measurements on a water phantom in which lucite rods simulated bone. The scattered intensity was not corrected if the soft-tissue layer was between 0.6 cm and 1.0 cm; the reason for this approach was that attenuation losses would be compensated by the detection of secondary photons (multiple scattering).

The experimental data in materials of different densities demonstrated that the magnitude of the bias due to multiple scattering were within the range of error of the density measurement and required no correction. An attenuation correction was made, however, for soft-tissue thicknesses in excess of 1.0 cm. A calibration curve was determined from measurements in materials of known density and a simple relationship between the scattered counts and the density (g/cc) was derived following corrections for background. The density of the distal radius was determined from this calibration line. The average long-term precision of the method was 3.3%, although repeated measurements in some subjects gave a precision of 7.4%. Careful repositioning of the radius using the method of maximizing the scattered intensity resulted in an improvement in the average precision (1.56%) for some of the subjects. It was stated that even slight rotation of the forearm may significantly change the result. Positioning of the patient was therefore very important in long-term studies with this method.

The density as measured by Compton scattering was compared with the clinical diagnosis made from radiographs of the spine using a grading system that described the degree of osteoporosis. In addition, the cortical index of the third metacarpal of the nondominant hand was measured from the radiograph. A very low correlation was found between the cortical index and the bone density of the radius by Compton scattering ($r = 0.462$). Nearly all the subjects with measured bone densities of the distal radius less than 1.25 g/cc showed definite signs of osteoporosis on the spinal radiographs. Density values less than 1.2 g/cc were believed to indicate advanced osteoporosis. It was concluded that the bone density as measured by Compton scattering provided a useful tool in the diagnosis of osteoporosis.

Stein et al. (1983) used the Compton-scatter method developed by Hazan et al. (1977) for the investigation of the density of the lower tibia in normal subjects and in patients with knee or calf injuries, osteoporosis, or chronic renal failure. The Compton-scatter densitometer incorporated a ^{137}Cs source (500 mCi), which directed a beam of gamma rays of energy 662 keV at an area of the tibia. A multihole collimator was used to detect photons at the 90° scattering angle. The precision of the Compton scatter density (g/cc) measurements was ±2%.

In addition, the bone mineral content was determined in these subjects by the single-photon absorptiometry method (Norland-Cameron bone mineral analyzer). However, a poor correlation was found between the Compton densities and the BMC values (g/cm^2); this was expected since the BMC of the tibia included cortical bone, whereas the Compton density was confined to the trabecular bone only. The Compton-scatter densities of the tibia were better

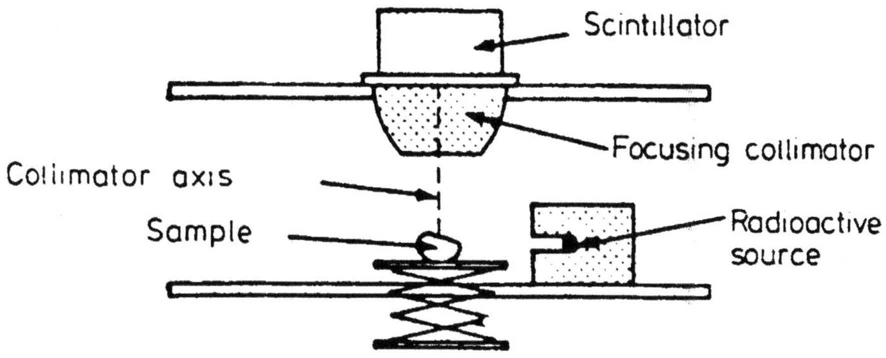

Figure 61. Compton-scatter system for forearm measurements (Courtesy: G Hazan)

correlated with the radiographic diagnosis and provided better differentiation between osteoporotic individuals and normals individuals than the single-photon absorptiometry method.

The Compton-scattering method described by Webber and Kennett (1976) was used in a study comparing the calcaneal morphologic index, determined from radiographic trabecular patterns of the os calcis, with density measurements of the os calcis (Cockshott et al., 1984). Using lateral radiographs of the foot, the method of Jhamaria et al. (1983) was used to score the trabecular patterns on a five-point scale. The grading system was found to fail, however, as it showed no correlation with the actual bone density of the os calcis. A similar comparison for the Singh Index, used for grading the trabeculae of the femoral neck, showed a poor correlation with ^{125}I single photon absorptiometry (Khairi et al., 1976).

Roberts et al. (1982) reported on the study of the density of trabecular bone in the os calcis of 321 human subjects, using the Compton-scatter densitometer of Webber and Kennett (1976). The system was calibrated using a water standard and the long-term precision of the system was 1.6%. The radiation dose received by the subject was reported as 1.5 mSv per measurement. A good correlation between the trabecular bone density of the os calcis and the weight and age of the subject was found; the measurements in normal subjects were predicted with a standard error of 5.6%. It was concluded that Compton-scatter densitometry of the os calcis was capable of detecting the effects of metabolic stresses such as high-dose corticosteroid therapy, anticonvulsant drug administration, and physical activity in human subjects.

Roberts et al. (1984) studied a population of normal postmenopausal women using the Compton-scattering method of Webber and Kennett (1976). Measurements of the calcaneal bone density demonstrated a significant reduction with age in the normal postmenopausal women, while the osteoporotic women treated with combination (estrogen) therapy demonstrated increased calcaneal density. Therapy was shown to prevent the expected age-dependent reduction of bone density in osteoporotic males. The in vivo short-term precision was 1.6%, and the long-term precision obtained from foot-phantom measurements was 1.6%. It was concluded that the method (in the calcaneous) was useful in monitoring changes in the mineral status of the skeleton.

COHERENT/COMPTON-SCATTER METHODS

A new technique was introduced by Puumalainen et al. (1976) in which both coherently scattered and Compton-scattered photons were detected. The probability for the emission of coherent radiation from an atom is given by:

$$P_1 = \varrho k f(\theta) \frac{\overline{Z}^3}{E^3}$$

where ϱ is the density of the medium, k is a constant, $f(\theta)$ is a function depending on the scattering angle, $\overline{Z}$ is the mean atomic number of the medium, and E is the energy of the scattered photons. The probability for the emission of Compton-scattered photons from an atom is given by:

$$P_2 = \varrho k' \sigma (\theta, E) \frac{\overline{Z}}{\overline{A}}$$

where ϱ is the density of the medium, k′ is a constant, (θ, E) is a function depending on the scattering angle and the energy, $\overline{Z}$ is the mean atomic number of the medium and $\overline{A}$ is the mean mass number of the atoms. The ratio of the coherent and Compton scatter intensities for a fixed energy and scattering angle is:

$$\frac{P_1}{P_2} = \text{constant} \cdot \frac{\overline{Z}^3}{\overline{Z}} \cdot A$$

The ratio of the coherent and Compton scatter intensities is, therefore, dependent upon the average atomic number (i.e., the elementary composition) of the medium. An advantage of this method is that the attenuation of the incoming beam by soft tissues surrounding the volume of interest is the same for both components of the scattered radiation, and the attenuation factors appearing in the ratio P_1/P_2 cancel. The ratio is, therefore, independent of attenuation effects.

One of the problems associated with the coherent/Compton ratio method of bone mineral density determination is the low count rate for the detected coherent photons. The intensity of the coherent peak, as seen in the scatter energy spectrum, is significantly smaller than that of the Compton peak. This effect results from the rapidly decreasing differential atomic cross section for coherent scattering as the scattering angle is increased in the range of 0 to 90° degrees. As a result, it is generally accepted that small scattering angles are preferred (Karellas et al., 1983).

The Z dependence exhibited by the differential coherent atomic cross section is different for small and large scattering angles (Roy and Reed, 1968). Since the momentum transferred to electrons during the scattering process is higher for larger scattering angles, the inner electrons, which have higher binding energies, dominate the process. For small scattering angles, it is the outer electrons of the atom that dominate the scattering process. These different scattering mechanisms, therefore, depend on different exponential powers of the atomic number (Kissel and Pratt, 1978; Jauch and Rohrlich, 1955). Webster and Lillicrap (1985) have stated that the value of the coherent/Compton ratio R falls rapidly with increasing scattering angle; the choice of scattering angle is, therefore, a compromise between a good separation of the coherent- and Compton-scatter peaks and a high probability of coherent scatter.

Karellas et al. (1983) used theoretical calculations and experimental measurements to investigate the dependence of the coherent/Compton ratio (R) upon the scattering angle. They showed that the sensitivity of the coherent/Compton-scatter method for bone mineral density is increased as the selected scattering angle is increased, over the atomic number range $Z = 2$ to 25 and the scattering angle range $\theta = 30.2°$ to 93.6°. Experimental studies using aqueous K_2HPO_4 solutions yielded good correlations ($r = 0.99$) between the coherent/Compton ratios (relative to that of water) and the densities of the solutions for all scattering angles investigated.

Since the exponential power of the atomic number was found to increase with increasing scattering angle, it was seen that the sensitivity of the method improved with larger scattering angles. In addition, it was shown that the uncertainties of the density determinations decreased for the larger scattering angles. The optimization of the selected scattering angle enhances the usefulness of the coherent/Compton ratio methods. It was further noted that measurements based on the detection of coherent scatter alone are expected to have superior sensitivity to any change in the effective atomic number compared to the coherent/Compton scatter ratio methods.

Cesareo (1981) described a coherent/Compton-scatter ratio method for the analysis of metal alloys. The radionuclide source ^{241}Am (activity, 200 mCi) was used in a backscatter arrangement (scattering angle, 155° ± 12°). A high-resolution silicon semiconductor detector was used for detection of the scatter spectra from Ag-Cu samples. A 0.2 mm thick copper filter was placed over the face of the detector to remove the Cu x-rays in an effort to increase the detectability of the elastic and inelastic scatter intensities. The energy range of the detected Compton-scattered photons was 48.3 to 49.2 keV. Good separation of the coherent and Compton energy peaks was observed in the spectrum. The precision of the measurement was 0.9%. This was compared with the precision obtained by the use of other methods: gravimetric analysis (0.6%), gamma-ray transmission using a ^{57}Co source (0.95%), and Compton scattering (1.7%). It was noted that the Z dependence of the coherent/Compton ratio disagreed with the theoretical dependence (Z squared). The exponent n was found to be 2.4 instead of 2.0. This disagreement regarding the Z dependence was also found by Schatzler (1979) and by Puumalainen et al. (1979) for biological specimens of low mean atomic number.

Holt et al. (1983) investigated the coherent/Compton ratios in small tissue specimens (liver, breast cyst fluid) from rats. The elastic and inelastic scatter measurements were performed on the Compton spectrometer at the University of Warwick, Coventry, England. The spectrometer utilized a 5 Ci annular ^{241}Am radionuclide source and had a fixed angle of 171° for Compton scattering. A high-resolution germanium detector was linked to a multichannel analyzer and a microcomputer. The system was calibrated with saline solutions of varying concentrations, giving a precision of ±1%. The coherent and Compton energy peaks were well separated in the spectra, and the ratio of the two scatter intensities showed a good correlation. The scattering angle (171°) was not ideal because of the asymmetry of the scattering volume, which is defined by the source and detector collimation; the irradiated volume of the sample was about 1 cc. Multiple scattering was also ignored in the calculations.

The measurements of breast cyst fluid yielded intensity ratios that were significantly different from those of pure water and from those of the saline solutions. It was shown that a change of 0.2% in the concentration resulted in a measurable 2.5% change in the coherent/Compton ratio. The ratios for intact liver tissue and homogenized liver tissue exhibited detectable differences. These in vitro experiments demonstrated the sensitivity of the coherent/Compton ratio method in biological tissues, although the spectrometer was not designed for in vivo tissue densitometry.

Puumalainen et al. used the radionuclide source ^{241}Am (half-life, 458 yrs; activity, 500 mCi; energy, 59.5 keV). The 90° scattering angle (figure 62) was chosen for the detection of both coherently-scattered and Compton-scattered photons. A high resolution germanium semiconductor detector was used because of the need to separate the coherent and Compton-scatter peaks in the detected spectrum (figure 63) displayed on a multichannel analyzer. The energy of the Compton-scatter peak was 53.4 keV, whereas the energy of the coherent-scatter peak was 59.5 keV, a separation of only 6.1 keV. The difference in the attenuation factors for the scattered beams, therefore, was considered negligible. The ratio P_1/P_2 was determined by dividing the area under the coherent peak of the spectrum by the maximum intensity (height) of the Compton peak. The area under the Compton peak was not used because it included the effects of multiple scatter. The multichannel analyzer provided the total area by spectral integration. The relative P_1/P_2 ratio was calculated by dividing the ratio for the substance by the P_1/P_2 ratio for water.

The relative coherent/Compton ratio was well correlated ($r = 0.96$) with the mineral content of standard samples (calcium hydroxyapatite in paraffin solutions); the accuracy (and precision) of the measurements was 2%. The radiation absorbed dose was less than 100 mrem. The advantages of the coherent/Compton method in clinical measurements included the following: (1) slight movement of the patient was permissible, since the calculated ratio provides a

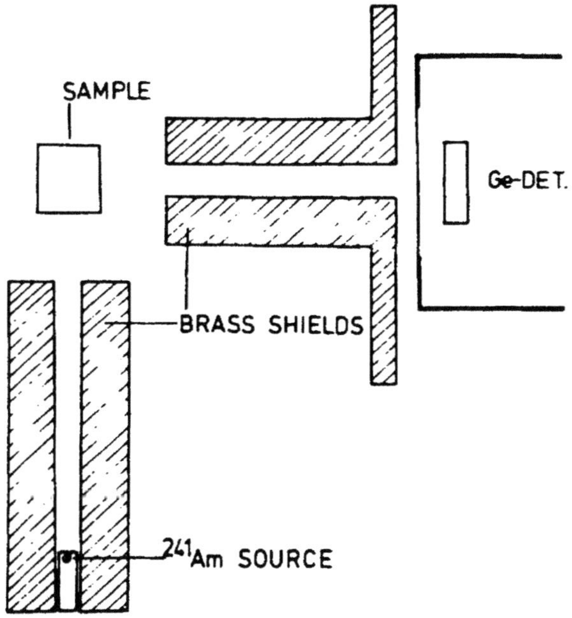

Figure 62. Coherent/Compton-scatter ratio measurement geometry (Courtesy: P Puumalainen)

cancellation of the changes in the two intensities; (2) the method permitted determinations in cancellous bone as well as cortical bone; (3) the method enabled the evaluation of osteoporosis in the proximal femur; and (4) a comparison between the in vivo densities of the axial skeleton and the peripheral skeleton using the same measurement method was made possible.

The coherent/Compton ratios R, derived from theoetical considerations, are only valid for pure elements. For a composite material of known composition, a value of R can only be calculated by averaging the coherent and Compton contributions from component elements; the relative contributions vary with the selected scattering angle and the incident photon energy (Webster and Lillicrap, 1985). However, for a fixed scattering geometry and incident photon energy, an empirically determined value of the effective atomic number (e.g., for bone) is a reliable indicator of composition, even though a different value is obtained for a different geometry and energy.

Puumalainen et al. (1977) later utilized the coherent/Compton-scatter ratio method for the in vitro determination of the fat content of human liver specimens obtained at autopsy (figure 64). It was shown that fatty liver specimens had significantly lower coherent/Compton ratios compared to normal liver specimens. In addition, a device was developed for in vivo measurements of liver fat in humans. An annular source of ^{241}Am (activity, 500 mCi) was used, and the scattering angle was 90°. The system was tested using a simulated liver

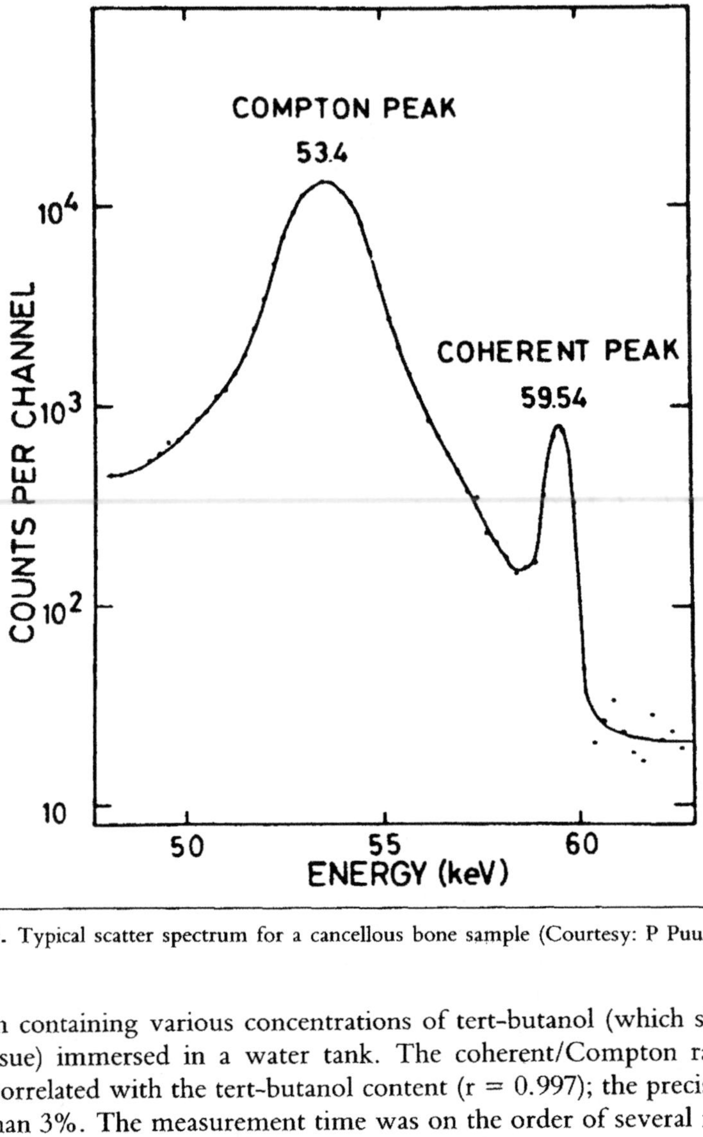

Figure 63. Typical scatter spectrum for a cancellous bone sample (Courtesy: P Puumalainen)

phantom containing various concentrations of tert-butanol (which simulates fatty tissue) immersed in a water tank. The coherent/Compton ratio was highly correlated with the tert-butanol content (r = 0.997); the precision was better than 3%. The measurement time was on the order of several minutes, and the radiation dose was about 10 mrem for the in vivo system.

Leichter et al. (1984) further investigated the sensitivity of the coherent/Compton method, with emphasis on its dependence upon the incident photon energy. Three radionuclide sources were separately used in the experimental studies: (1) ^{241}Am (half-life, 458 yrs; activity, 44 GBq; energy, 60 keV), (2) ^{133}Xe (half-life, 5.4 days; activity, 1.18 GBq; energy, 81 keV), and (3) ^{99m}Tc (half-life, 6 hrs; activity, 8.51 GBq; energy, 140 keV). The system (figure 65) consisted of an intrinsic germanium detector; and a scattering angle of 47° was maintained. The coherent/Compton ratios R were determined for aqueous

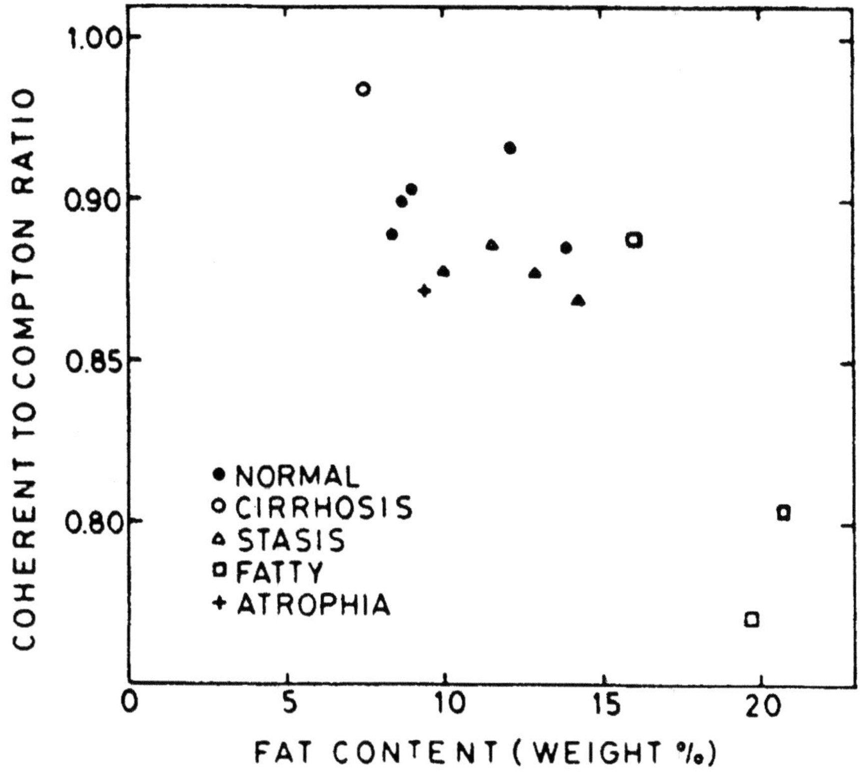

Figure 64. Coherent/Compton-scatter ratio as a function of the chemically analyzed fat content of liver (Courtesy: P Puumalainen)

solutions of K_2HPO_4. Very good linear correlations (r = 0.99) were obtained between the log (R/R_w) and the log $(\bar{Z})$, where R_w is the coherent/Compton ratio for water and $\bar{Z}$ is the effective atomic number for the solutions. The slopes of these lines increased with increasing incident energies.

The intrinsic sensitivity of the measurement was defined as the change in the coherent/Compton ratio R for a given change in the atomic number. It was demonstrated that an increase in the photon energy or in the scattering angle results in a higher sensitivity but also reduces the counting statistics. However, it was stated that the increase in sensitivity more than compensates for the loss of precision due to reduced coherent scatter counts. It was emphasized that sensitivity was another important characteristic in the design of the system.

Stalp and Mazess (1980) suggested an improvement in the coherent/Compton density method using optimization of the scattering angle and higher incident beam energy. They compared ^{241}Am (activity, 4.07×10^8 Bq; energy, 60 keV) and ^{153}Gd (activity, 2.48×10^9 Bq; energies, 103, 97 keV) as radionuclide sources, using an intrinsic germanium detector with good energy resolution.

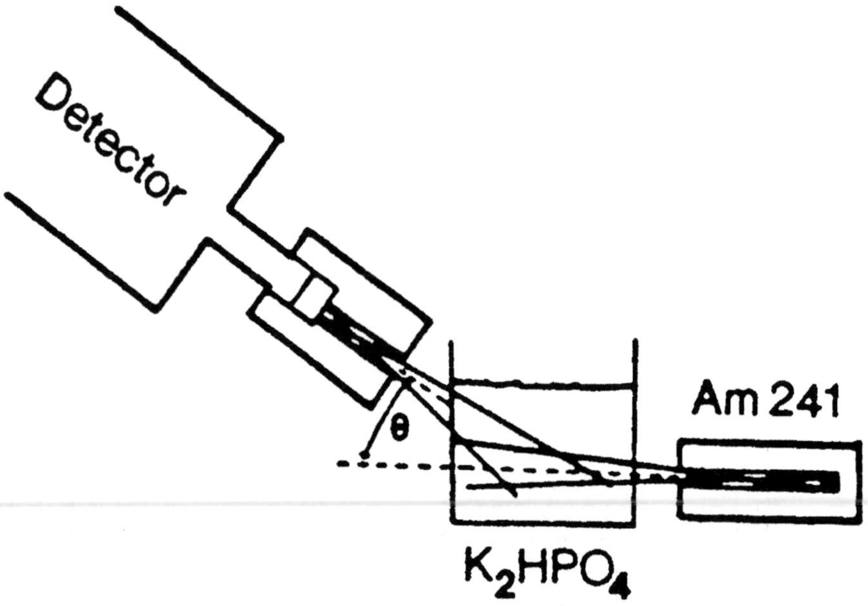

Figure 65. Coherent/Compton-scatter ratio method (Courtesy: I Leichter)

The coherent/Compton ratios were determined for various concentrations of aqueous K_2HPO_4 solutions. A high correlation (r = 0.97) was found using the ^{241}Am source and a 60° scattering angle; the separation between the coherent peak and the Compton peak was adequate, although the scatter intensities were not optimal. A repeat study with a scattering angle of 30° increased the scatter intensities, but the energy separation of the peaks was small and the peaks were difficult to resolve. The correlation between the coherent/Compton ratio and the density was not as good (r = 0.94), due to the poor resolution of the two peaks.

The ^{153}Gd source was introduced in order to increase the Compton energy shift at the 30° scattering angle. The 103 keV and 97 keV peaks were not resolved in the spectrum, although the coherent and Compton peaks were well resolved. A high correlation (r = 0.99) was obtained for the K_2HPO_4 solutions at the 30° scattering angle. A counting precision of 1% was found for an exposure dose of 14 cGy, while the dose required for a counting precision of 3% was 1.5 cGy (0.6 cGy, with filtration of the low-energy gamma rays). It was noted that radionuclide sources with higher energies were not considered because of the reduced counting efficiency of the germanium detectors and the decrease of both the Compton- and coherent-scattering cross sections at high energies. The ratio of coherent- and Compton-scatter intensities provides a means of determining the density without attenuation corrections. Also, the effects of multiple scattering are essentially the same for both the coherent and

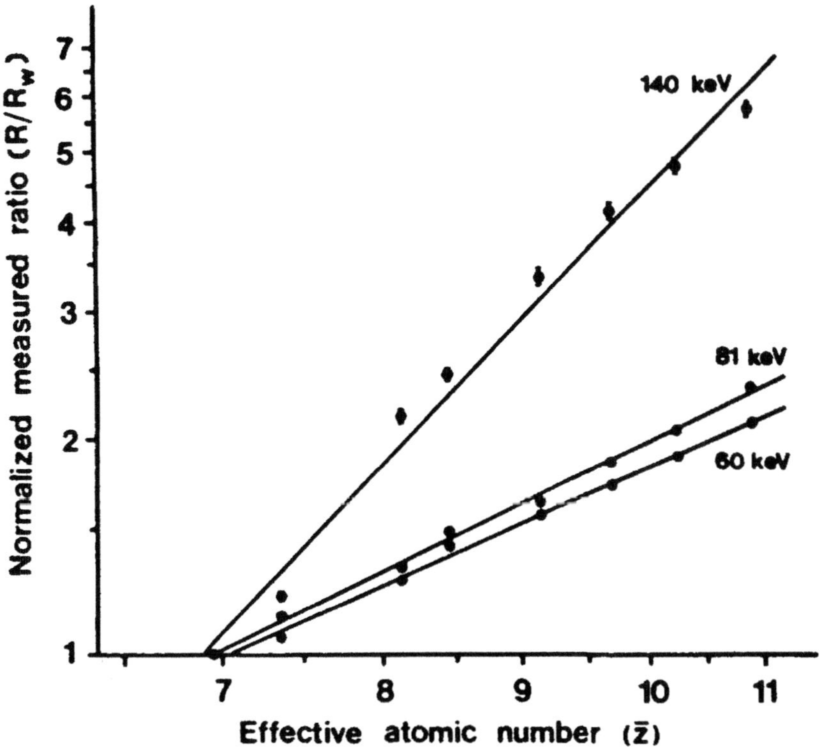

Figure 66. Coherent/Compton ratio normalized to water as a function of the effective atomic number of aqueous dipotassium hydrogen phosphate, for scattering angle 47° (Courtesy: I Leichter)

the Compton processes, and the multiple-scatter effects cancel when computing the ratio.

Kerr et al. (1980) investigated the feasibility of using the coherent/Compton-scatter ratio method in the human os calcis. Their studies showed that the system design should incorporate the use of small scattering angles, realizing that as the scattering angle is reduced, the difference in energies between the coherent- and Compton-scattered photons becomes smaller. Because detection systems are limited in energy resolution, the system may not be able to separate the two energy peaks sufficiently for counting. The experimental arrangement included the radionuclide source ^{153}Sm (half-life, 47 hrs; activity, 40 GBq (1 Ci); energy, 103.2 keV), an intrinsic germanium detector, and parallel collimation using tantalum tubes. A simulated foot phantom was positioned for measurements in the os calcis.

Experiments for three scattering angles (15°, 23°, and 28°) demonstrated the strong dependence on the separation of the coherent- and Compton-energy peaks in the scatter spectrum; the peaks were well resolved for the 28° scatter-

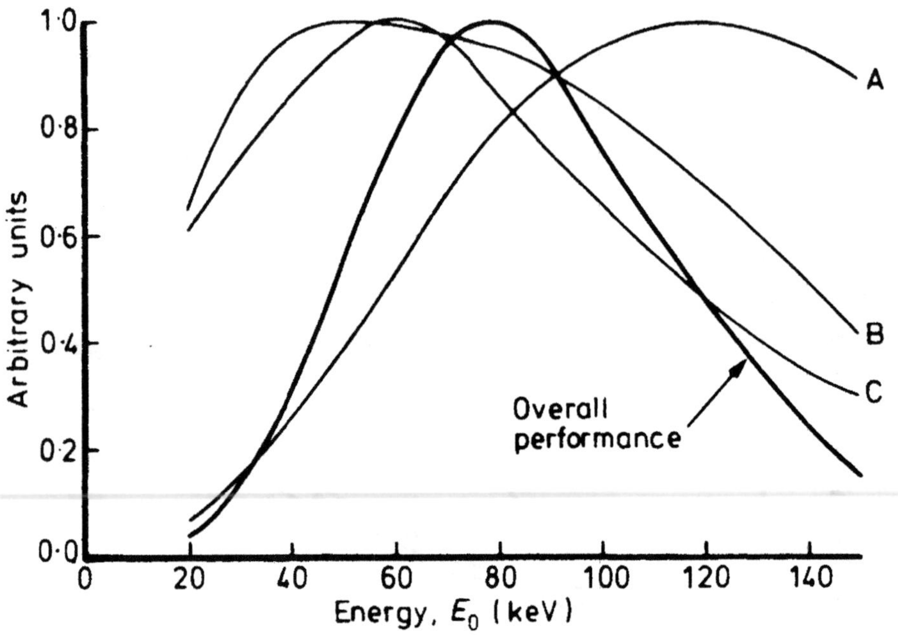

Figure 67. Overall system performance as a function of energy for the coherent/Compton method. Curves A, B, and C are, respectively, the number of coherently scattered photons per unit dose, the detector counting efficiency, and the calculated mass attenuation coefficient for coherent scattering (Courtesy: SA Kerr)

ing angle. However, the coherent scatter peak had greater intensity at 15°, but seriously overlapped the Compton peak. The 23° scattering angle represented the acceptable compromise between the necessary coherent-scatter intensity and the problem of spectral overlap.

In a study using autopsy specimens of human feet and a scattering angle of 22.5°, a strong linear correlation was found between the os calcis densities and the coherent/Compton ratios over the range of densities for the os calcis 1.00 to 1.31 g/cc. The coherent/Compton ratio was found to be a good indicator of the density, with clinical implications in the evaluation of skeletal status. It was further stated that the determination of the coherent/Compton ratio produced similar results to that of the Compton-scatter method alone for a given biological change. It was noted that calculating the ratio of the two scatter measurements in effect reduces the sensitivity for detecting changes in density.

Kerr et al. have recommended the use of a technique in which only the coherent scattering was measured, thereby improving the sensitivity. This idea was later supported by Karellas et al. (1983). Kerr et al. (1980) suggested that the design of a system based upon the measurement of coherent scatter alone could be optimized for overall performance (figure 67) by considering (1) the energy dependence of the number of coherently scattered photons per unit

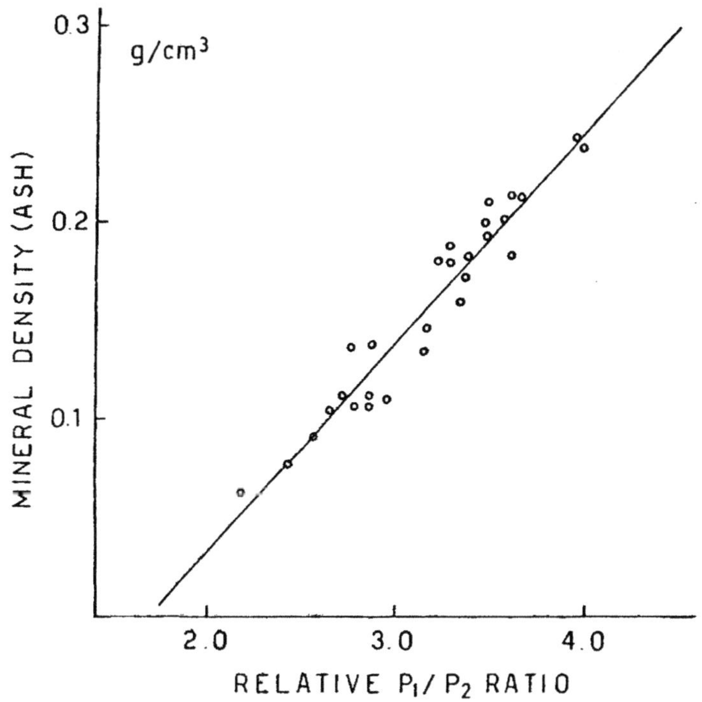

Figure 68. Correlation between bone ash density (g/cc) and the relative coherent/Compton ratio for the distal radius (Courtesy: H Olkkonen)

radiation dose, (2) detector counting efficiency, and (3) the calculated mass attenuation coefficient for coherent scattering. The optimum incident photon energy was found to be near 80 keV, and the corresponding scattering angle was 25°. Use of the coherent-scatter intensity alone necessitates the addition of a transmission measurement to correct for beam attenuation. It was suggested that a precision of 3% could be obtained for a radiation dose of 4 mSV (400 mrem) to the heel in clinical studies of the os calcis.

Olkkonen et al. (1981) further investigated the use of the coherent/Compton ratio in autopsy specimens of human distal radii. Using a scattering angle of 90°, the germanium detector, and an ^{241}Am source (40 mCi), 10-minute scatter counts were collected with a multichannel analyzer. The volume of trabecular bone was about 1 cc. No scanning procedures were used. The P_1/P_2 ratios (figure 68) were well correlated with the ash contents (g/cc) of the trabecular bone (r = 0.96). The trabecular bone mineral density (TBMD) showed a correlation (r = 0.75) with the bone mineral density (BMD) obtained by the single-photon absorptiometry method. Because the values of $\overline{Z}$ and $\overline{A}$ are considerably greater for the bone mineral than for the soft tissues contained in bone, changes in the coherent/Compton ratio reflect the changes in the bone mineral density as bone mineral is resorbed in the skeleton.

Puumalainen et al. (1982) later introduced the use of an x-ray tube (59 kVp, 1 mA) as the primary radiation source in coherent/Compton scatter measurements. Two source/detector arrangements were investigated in which (1) an intrinsic germanium detector was used and (2) two NaI(Tl) detectors were used. In the first arrangement, a filter (CsCl) in the primary beam produced a nearly monoenergetic beam with a peak energy of about 36 keV; a scattering angle of 60° yielded the greatest net coherent scatter intensity. The second method was unique because separate detectors were used to measure the coherent- and Compton-scatter intensities; NaI(Tl) detectors have an inherently lower energy resolution than the germanium detector, but they are more convenient to use in a clinical environment. In the second method, the primary beam was filtered with a lanthanum oxide pellet (figure 69). The scattering angle was selected so that only the coherently scattered radiation (38.9 keV) could excite the Cs K-alpha x-ray fluorescence radiation in a CsCl target (K-absorption edge, 36.0 keV); the Compton-scattered photons penetrated the target. The CsCl target was placed between the bone sample and the NaI (Tl) detector measuring the Compton-scatter intensity. The scattering angle in the bone sample was 107°, providing the Compton-scatter energy of 35.4 keV. The NaI(Tl) detector used to measure the coherent-scatter intensity was aligned facing the CsCl target and perpendicular to the Compton-scatter photon path.

Both systems were tested using paraffin cubes of approximately 1 cc volume containing calcium hydroxyapatite in varying concentrations. The first method showed a good correlation between the coherent/Compton ratio ($r = 0.96$), as did the second method ($r = 0.90$). The coefficient of variation for repeated measurements using the first method (Ge detector) was less than 2%, while the coefficient of variation using the second method (two NaI(Tl) detectors) was 8%. The greater uncertainty of the second method resulted from the use of the x-ray fluorescence target, which produced insufficient counting statistics. The lower resolution technique using NaI(Tl) detectors, therefore, was not considered adequate for further study.

The first method was used to determine the coherent/Compton ratio for samples of trabecular bone taken from the spine, femoral neck, and patella of oxen. The trabecular bone mineral content (TBMC) was well correlated ($r = 0.97$) with the ash content of the bone specimens, and the precision was better than 5%. The radiation dose was measured as 100 mrad per exposure. Fluctuations of the x-ray tube output did not significantly affect the coherent/Compton ratios. It was suggested that a higher x-ray energy would be required for measurements of larger bones such as the femoral head.

Ling et al. (1982) described a coherent/Compton-scatter device for the in vitro measurement of trabecular bone mineral density (TBMD). The system used an ^{241}Am (activity, 200 mCi) source and a scattering angle of 90° (figure 70). The coherent/Compton ratio R in fresh trabecular bone samples (human femoral heads) showed a linear correlation ($r = 0.94$) with the ash densities. These authors investigated the effects of (1) overlying soft tissue, (2) self-attenuation by the trabecular bone and cortical layer, and (3) marrow fat of the

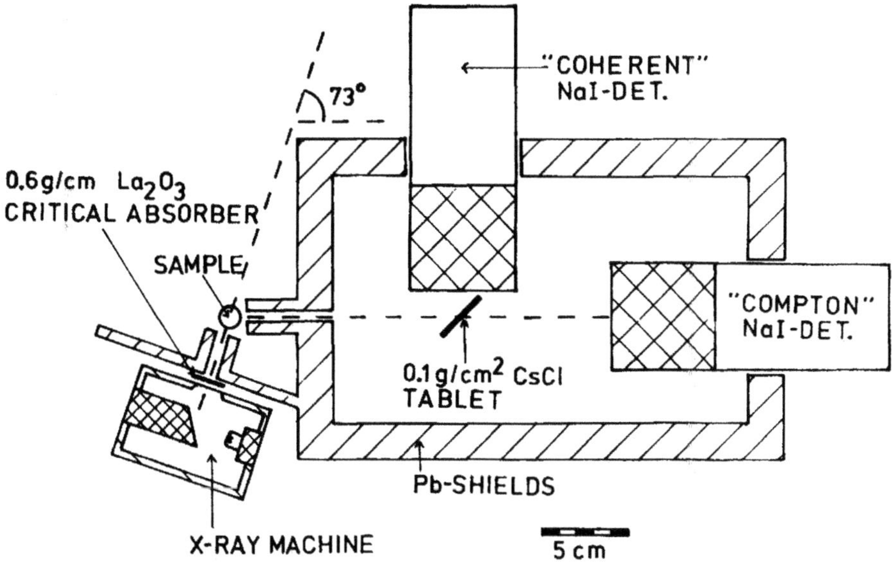

Figure 69. Coherent/Compton-scatter method employing two NaI detectors (Courtesy: P Puumalainen)

interstices of trabecular bone. A high-purity germanium crystal detector provided good separation between the coherent- and Compton-scatter peaks of the energy spectrum (figure 71).

The statistical precision of the measurements was found to be strongly dependent upon the lower count rate of the coherent peak, and therefore the total area under the Compton peak was not determined. Instead, a curve-fitting routine was used to fit the upper energy side of the Compton-scatter energy peak. The Compton contribution was then subtracted from the total area to yield the coherent peak. The effects of the overlying cortical layer and the attenuation within the trabecular bone were insignificant (within the range of uncertainty of the method, ±3%). However, the effect of overlying soft tissues (0.6% to 7.2%) was significant; a correction for this effect was suggested.

Varying concentrations of tert-butyl alcohol were used to estimate the effect of fat within the marrow of the bone. It was found that a 10% increase in the trabecular fat content corresponded to a 2.5% decrease in the coherent/Compton ratio R. The authors suggested that the lack of knowledge of the exact fat content may be overcome by selecting bone sites that contain only yellow marrow of which 80% is fat; the magnitude of variations in fat between individuals is expected to be reduced, thus minimizing the errors due to the marrow fat. The calcaneus of the adult may be a suitable site, since it does not contain a significant amount of red marrow. The estimated radiation dose to the bone marrow was 139 mrad.

Gigante and Sciuti (1985) evaluated the sensitivity of the coherent/Compton

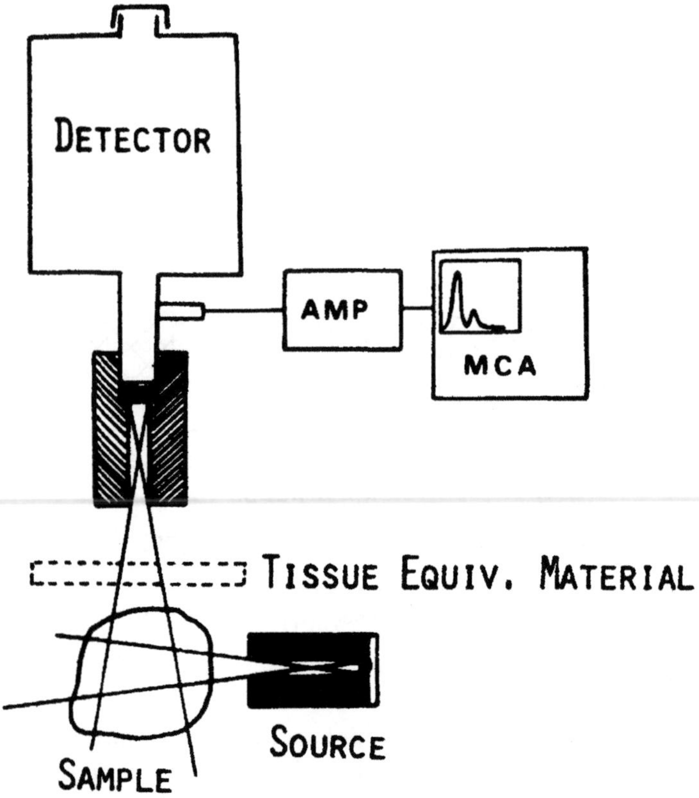

Figure 70. Germanium detector/^{241}Am source configuration for coherent/Compton-scatter ratio measurements (Courtesy: SS Ling)

ratio method using an experimental arrangement in which ^{241}Am (activity, 7.4 GBq (200 mCi)) was used to provide the incident beam. The scattering angles 45°, 90°, and 135° were used, and an x-ray hyperpure germanium detector and multichannel analyzer were used to collect and analyze the scatter intensities. This study showed that the relative sensitivity of the 135° scatter method was 1.7 times that of the 90° scatter method and six times that of the 45° scatter method.

A prototype system (figure 72) was designed for in vivo measurements using the back-scatter angle (135°) and calibrated using aqueous K_2HPO_4 solutions. A good correlation ($r = 0.999$) was demonstrated between the coherent/Compton ratio and the concentrations of the solutions. The advantages provided by the use of the backscatter design include (1) small overall dimensions to allow better positioning of the source/detector arrangement, (2) short source-sample and sample-detector distances for maximizing the scatter intensities, and (3) use of two or more radionuclide sources surrounding the

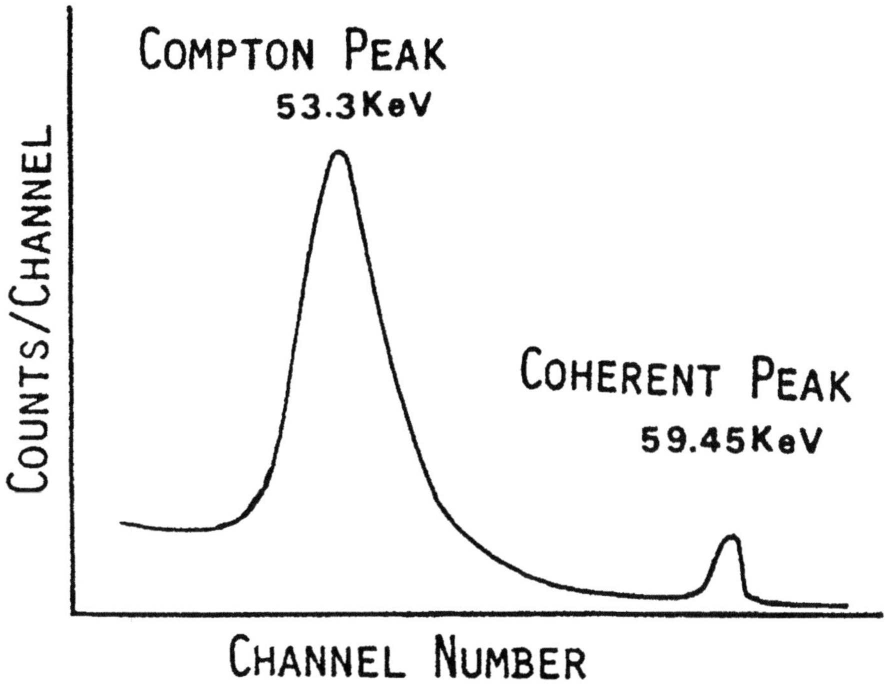

Figure 71. Typical 90° scatter spectrum from a trabecular bone sample in a narrow beam geometry (Courtesy: SS Ling)

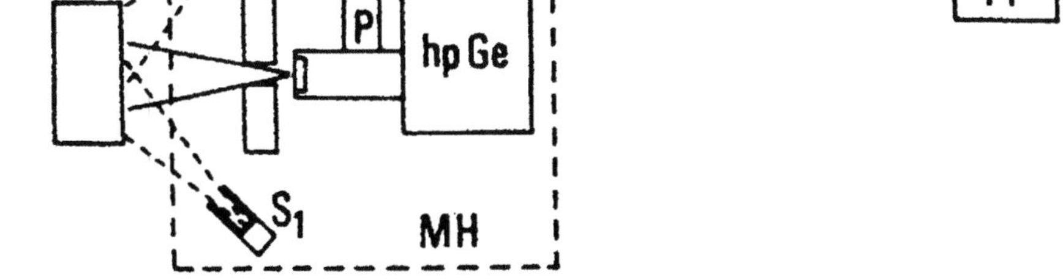

Figure 72. Photon scattering mineralometer (PSM): S(1) and S(2) are ^{241}Am point sources; hpGe = hyperpure Ge detector; MH = measuring head; μP = microcomputer; FD = floppy disk; Pr = printer; scattering angle = 135° (Courtesy: GE Gigante)

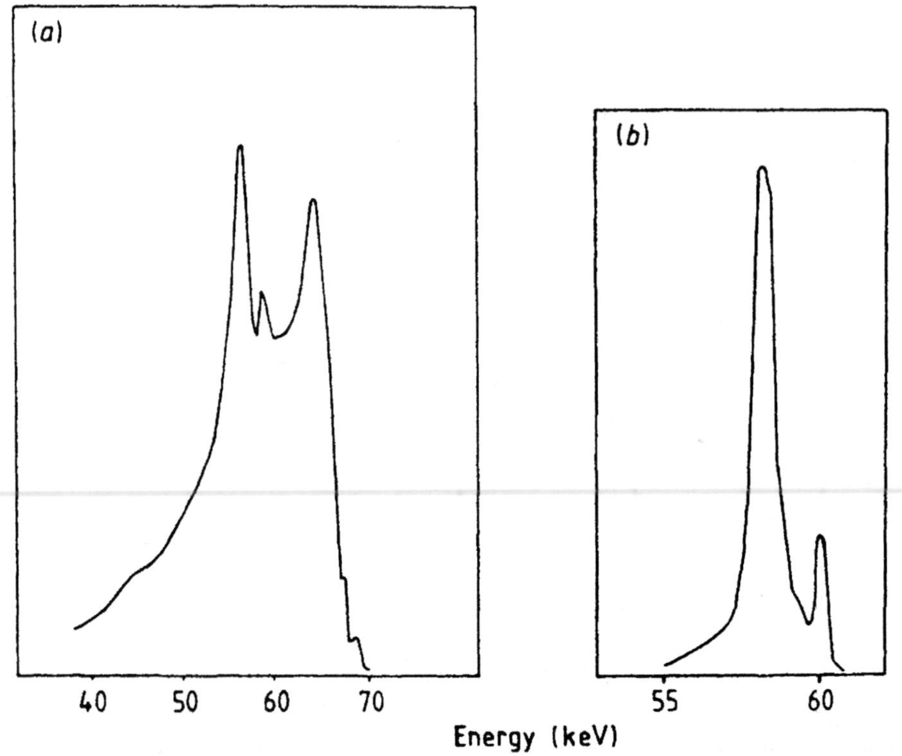

Figure 73. Scattered radiation spectra from a sample of dry vertebra using (a) tungsten-filtered x-ray beam and (b) ^{241}Am source with scattering angle = 50° (Courtesy: DJ Webster)

detector for increasing sensitivity. It was stated that the system would provide good in vivo precision and accuracy, provided that the trabecular bone thickness was greater than 2.0 cm. Since the amount of fat in bone varies by as much as 10%, it is expected that the coherent/Compton ratio R may decrease by 2.5% to 3% using this method. It was concluded that the backscatter geometry represents an increase in the relative sensitivity of the coherent/Compton method.

Webster and Lillicrap (1985) suggested the use of the x-ray tube for coherent/Compton-scatter measurements to assess trabecular bone mineral content. The disadvantage of the use of radionuclide sources is the reduced incident beam intensity, which reduces the detectable coherent- and Compton-scatter intensities and requires the use of longer measurement times. A 100 kVp x-ray beam (Philips mobile unit) filtered with 0.3 mm of tungsten was used in conjunction with a high-purity germanium detector. The characteristic x-rays from the tungsten anode and the tungsten filter were observed, in addition to the sharp K-absorption edge discontinuity (69.9 keV) in the incident energy spectrum. A continuous spectrum extending over the range of 30 to 70 keV was observed in the scatter spectra for various samples using a scattering angle of 50°. Because the coherent- and Compton-scatter peaks were not resolved, the expected energy ranges were sampled by setting appropriate energy windows. The coherent window was selected near the K-edge discontinuity, and a correction for overlap of Compton events into the coherent energy window was applied. The Compton energy window was chosen so as to reduce any contributions from the coherent scatter events.

A second method was used by Webster and Lillicrap, in which ^{241}Am (activity, 500 HB_q) was the radionuclide source. The results of measurements with the two methods were compared, since the incident beam energy of the radionuclide source (59.5 keV) was considered to be close to that of the filtered x-ray beam (70 keV). The coherent/Compton-scatter ratios were plotted as a function of the atomic number; the experimental values using the filtered x-ray beam method, and those obtained with the ^{241}Am method demonstrated good agreement with theoretical ratios determined for 70 keV incident photons using Hubbell's data (Hubbell et al., 1975). This data demonstrated an approximate Z-square dependence.

The effective atomic number of a sample of dry vertebra was determined using both techniques (figure 73). The filtered x-ray beam and ^{241}Am methods gave values of 10.0 ± 0.2 and 11.0 ± 0.5, respectively. Both values were close to the calculated effective atomic number 10.2 for dry bone. The effect of overlying soft tissue in bone studies was investigated, and it was concluded that a correction factor was necessary. It was determined, however, that the presence of multiple scattered photons in the scattered beam did not significantly influence the coherent/Compton-scatter ratios. The accuracy of the coherent/Compton-ratio method obtained using the filtered x-ray beam was similar to that obtained by the ^{241}Am method. The main advantage of the filtered x-ray beam method was the reduction in the measurement time by a factor of six.

7. ACTIVATION ANALYSIS METHODS

Total-body and partial-body neutron activation analysis (TBNAA; PBNAA) and partial-body proton activation analysis (PBPAA) have been used to measure total-body calcium. However, only a few laboratories are able to perform these procedures because of the requirements for the appropriate particle sources and the need to detect extremely low levels of activated elements within the human body. Total-body activation analysis systems are expensive and require significant expertise for operation. Partial-body systems involve somewhat less complication and expense.

Neutron activation methods were discovered following a reactor accident in 1957 in which a number of persons were irradiated with neutrons. The presence of activated ^{24}Na in the blood serum of these individuals provided the basis for the calculation of the whole-body radiation doses that they received. This experience demonstrated the potential for using small controlled doses of neutrons to investigate the elemental composition of the human body (Cohn, 1981).

The first application of neutron activation analysis in man (in vivo) was performed in 1964 (Anderson et al., 1964). In this study, the investigators measured total-body chlorine and sodium, and suggested that total-body calcium could also be determined by NAA. Measurement of the iodine content of the thyroid gland was investigated by Boddy (1966) and Lenihan et al. (1967). The estimation of total hydrogen content in humans was studied by Rundo and Bunce (1966). Chamberlain et al. (1968) published findings on the determination of total-body calcium and sodium. Palmer et al. (1968) demontrated the feasibility of in vivo measurements of total-body calcium and other elements by NAA. Comar et al. (1968) published the results of a study that investigated the method of partial-body NAA. Boddy (1978) published a bibliography on in vivo NAA that provides a review of the subject.

In the process of neutron activation, the nucleus absorbs a neutron, which places the resulting nucleus in an excited state (the binding energy and the kinetic energy of the incoming neutron are added the total energy of the nucleus). The nucleus returns to its equilibrium state by emitting gamma radiations, or it may emit protons, alpha particles, or neutrons. The energies of the gamma photons emitted by the isotope produced by neutron irradiation are characteristic of the target element. The photon intensities are proportional to the amounts of the elements present within the body. The intensities are determined by an appropriate detector system (sodium iodide or germanium crystal detector), which is shielded to reduce background radiations that may interfere with the intensity determinations.

Whole-body counting of the skeleton following neutron activation and production of ^{49}Ca is generally considered to be an estimate of whole-body calcium. Prior to 1973, the direct proportionality of the number of counts under the ^{49}Ca photopeak had been demonstrated only in water-filled phantoms. Since these early studies, it has become possible to determine the absolute concentrations of calcium, sodium, chlorine, and phosphorus in the human body. In addition, the measurement of total-body calcium constitutes a direct measurement of bone mineral, since 99% of the body's calcium resides in bone.

Total-body calcium, as determined by neutron activation, is expressed in grams of calcium normalized to body size. For partial-body neutron activation, the volume of the hand is used for normalization. In measurements of the forearm, axial skeleton, and total skeletal calcium, the normalization factor is the cube of the subject's height. The *calcium bone index* (CaBI) has been defined as the ratio of the patient's calcium measurement to the mean value for normal subjects of the same body size based on height and arm span (Harrison et al., 1979).

PRINCIPLES OF MEASUREMENT

The ^{48}Ca (a stable isotope of natural calcium, 0.18 abundance) which resides in skeletal bones is converted into radioactive calcium (^{49}Ca) when placed in a neutron beam. The human body's sodium is converted into radioactive sodium (^{24}Na), chlorine into radioactive chlorine (^{38}Cl), and phosphorus into radioactive phosphorus (^{32}P) during neutron bombardment. Since ^{32}P is a beta emitter, these radiations are absorbed within the body and are not detectable outside the body. ^{24}Na, ^{38}Cl, and ^{49}Ca are short-lived gamma emitters. With the decay of ^{49}Ca, 3.1-Mev gamma rays are emitted; these photons penetrate the body tissues and are detected by a whole-body counter. The spectra of these gamma emitters are analyzed using a spectrometer system. The amount of ^{49}Ca is quantified by the measurement of the relative intensities of the spectral peaks that are characteristic for this radionuclide. By comparing the intensities emitted from the activated region of the body with the intensities emitted by a set of reference ^{49}Ca standards of known activity, it is possible to determine the concentration of the ^{49}Ca present the body. The radioactive calcium (^{49}Ca) activity is, then, a measure of the amount of stable calcium in the body, as determined by the whole-body counter.

Neutron activation analysis requires a source of neutrons (thermal neutron energy range). Neutron sources include the following: accelerators, reactors, alpha-neutron sources (^{241}Am-Be or ^{238}Pu-Be), and the fission source ^{252}Cf. The flux of neutrons may be provided by an array of sources positioned above and below the patient, exposing a given length of the body trunk or smaller areas. A weak neutron flux (neutrons per second per square centimeter) is adequate to induce measurable amounts of activity (on the order of 5 μCi) for axial skeletal studies.

Counting is done immediately following the activation because of the short half-life (8.8 min) of ^{49}Ca (figure 74). Radiations from this amount of activity may be separated from the normal levels of all radionuclides in the body, such as the radioactive potassium (^{40}K) in the body.

Nelp et al. (1970) described a NAA method in which a 60-inch cyclotron (University of Washington) provided a beam of 22-MeV deuterons directed onto a target of beryllium. This reaction (activation of ^{48}Ca, yielding ^{49}Ca) produced 4- and 12-MeV neutrons, which were collimated to a 3 foot × 7 foot irradiation field. For patient irradiation, a ¾-inch thick lucite helmet was used over the head and neck to moderate the neutrons prior to entry into the bone of the outer skull and cervical spine. Each arm was inserted to the level of the axilla into a 4.5-inch diameter lucite cylinder. The patient stood in a lucite boot, 6 inches thick and and 30 inches high. Both fixtures were filled with water to provide additional hydrogenous moderator for bones of the hands, forearms, and lower legs. The irradiation enclosure was a plywood box with 6-inch thick walls in which the patient was positioned as described. The patient support system was on a turntable, which was rotated 180°, providing equal neutron dose to the front and then the back of the patient. Calcium standards attached to the sides of the box were irradiated simultaneously with the patient. Exposure monitors were also included to determine the absorbed dose to the patient. The irradiation time was in the range 1 to 1.5 minutes.

A total-body counting system was used to assess the calcium levels. Four minutes following the irradiation, the patient was placed supine in an aluminum trough while an annular array of four unshielded NaI(Tl) crystals scanned from the head to the feet of the patient. The total-body count was performed in 12.5 minutes. The detector system was scanned at an exponentially decreasing speed because of the diminishing activity of the ^{49}Ca. The calcium standards

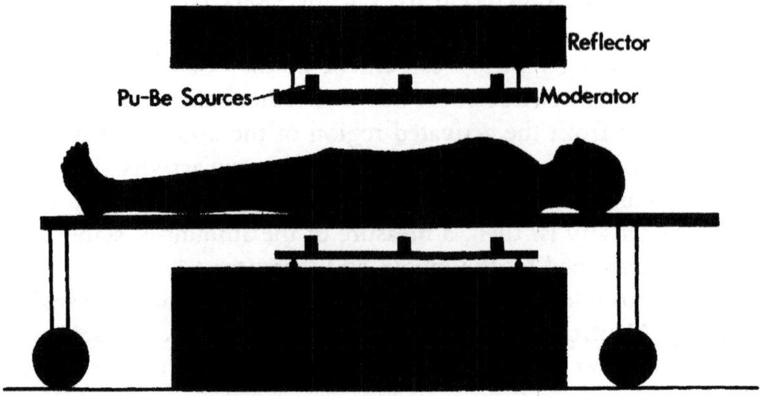

Figure 74. Neutron irradiation chamber for NAA studies (Courtesy: JE Harrison)

were counted for 10 minutes. The ratio of these two measurements represented an "index" of the patient's total body calcium. The maximum total-body radiation dose was determined as 2.1 rem. The precision of the measurement was estimated as 2.0%. It was suggested that serial changes of total-body calcium of 3% were detectable. Nelp et el. (1972) later quantitated body calcium in grams with an estimated 5.2% accuracy. This was done by irradiating cadavers and comparing the ratios of their induced ^{49}Ca activities with those of the calcium standards. The investigators determined the ^{49}Ca activity induced per gram of skeletal calcium by ashing and chemically analyzing the cadavers. The study also included the determination of the normal range of total-body calcium, and the decreased calcium levels of patients with known osteopenia were confirmed by NAA.

An early NAA system at Brookhaven National Laboratory consisted of a Texas-Nuclear generator that produced 14-Mev neutrons by the bombardment of tritium with deuterons (Cohn and Dombrowski, 1971). Patients were exposed bilaterally to maximize the uniformity of the neutron flux, and a polyethylene moderator was used on the front and back of the body. The uniformity as measured in a phantom was ±5%. The distance from the target to the patient was 1.5 m, and the exposure time was 5 minutes. Patients were immediately transported to a 54-detector whole-body counter following irradiation. Two 15-minute counts were taken on each subject, beginning at 6 and 23 minutes postirradiation. Analysis of the gamma spectrum was performed in which the levels of ^{49}Ca, ^{24}Na, ^{38}Cl, ^{13}N, and ^{28}Al were determined by comparison with known concentrations of these elements in an Alderson phantom to the partially-moderated 14-MeV neutron beam. It was found that the measured activities of Ca, Na, and Cl in patients could be converted to absolute grams of each element with an accuracy of ±4%; however, deviations in size and shape from the phantom resulted in a decrease in accuracy. The precision of the measurement in the same patient was better than ±4%. The determinations of N and P were found to be less accurate than those for Ca, Na, and Cl.

The Brookhaven 54-detector whole-body counter and its associated computer facility are described in the literature (Cohn et al., 1969). High spectral resolution, high sensitivity, relative invariance of response to distributions of radioactivity and body size, and the ability to detect rapidly moving short-lived radionuclides were characteristics of the system. The counter room was shielded with walls of 122 cm of concrete lined with 10 cm steel, 0.032 cm lead, and 0.16 cm aluminum. A patient bed was supported between two banks of detectors, one above and one below. Each bank consisted of 27 uncollimated NaI(Tl) matched crystal detectors arranged in a 3 × 9 array. The detector arrays and the bed could be moved independently. With this system, a 10-second whole-body count was possible. The minimum detectable activity was on the order of 0.15 nCi. Calibration of the counter was accomplished through the use of an Alderson phantom or, alternatively, it was based upon measurements of injected amounts of ^{42}K or ^{40}K in human subjects. Empirical corrections were made for tissue absorption and for geometrical efficiency of the detector arrays. A computer accumulated the data and analyzed the resulting spectra. The system had an eightfold greater sensitivity than a previous counting system that used a standard chair geometry (Cohn, 1965).

In later studies at Brookhaven National Laboratory (Cohn, 1972), the first patient irradiation facility using radioactive alpha/neutron sources was implemented. The irradiator consisted of 14 neutron sources, each containing 50 Ci of (80% enriched ^{238}Pu-Be). The average neutron energy was about 5 MeV. The sealed sources had diameters of 3.81 cm and lengths of 3.81 cm. The sources were raised from a shielded storage vault below the patient and positioned 26 to 31 cm above and below the patient; the longitudinal separation (along the patient axis) between the sources was 28.6 cm. The exposure cell in which the patient was located was shielded with a 3-foot thick concrete barrier. The cell was lined with bismuth (7.6 cm thickness) to provide a reflector of neutrons. Sheets of 0.64 cm borated polyethylene were placed between the concrete walls and the bismuth for absorbing neutrons. A fairly uniform broad beam of neutrons was produced, with an average neutron yield of 2.0×10^6 n/s/Ci of ^{238}Pu. The uniformity of the neutron flux within the patient was determined by using neutron dosimeters placed in a patient-simulation phantom. The thermal neutron flux density from front-to-back of the patient was determined as ±8%; the variation in flux density along the midline axis from the center of the lower head to the feet was ±4%. The incident flux along the front surface of the phantom was ±10%, excluding the head. The patient was exposed to neutrons for 5 minutes in the cell and then transported to the whole-body counting room. The counting time was 15 minutes. The absolute calibration of the Brookhaven counter was determined by exposing an Alderson phantom containing known concentrations of the individual elements of the human body. The maximum radiation dose to the patient when using this Pu-Be source system was 0.277 rem. The accuracy and the precision of the method was ±1%, as determined by studies in a phantom. This 5 MeV Pu-Be NAA system had the advantage of giving only 45% of the minimum dose required by the 14 MeV neutron generator system. In addition, the Pu-Be system consisted of an inherent simplicity for obtaining a uniform neutron flux.

Kennedy et al. (1982) designed a neutron irradiation system in which the neutron beam from a cyclotron was used to optimize the uniformity of activation of calcium in the human body. The mean neutron energy resulting from the reaction of 15-MeV deuterons on a beryllium target was 6.5 MeV. The human subject was positioned inside an enclosure containing polyethylene sheets for moderating the neutron beam to minimize the thermal neutron flux within the patient. The variation in the neutron flux was ±7% across a 24 cm phantom, and ±13% across a limb phantom 12.5 cm in diameter. Two successive 22-second neutron irradiations were performed for each patient, the second of which was delivered following the 180° rotation of the patient in the enclosure (target-to-subject distance, 5.4 m). The total radiation dose at the level of the pelvis was 1.68 mGy (dose equivalent, 13.2 mSv) and was nearly constant with depth through the patient.

Following irradiation (about 6 minutes), the patient was transferred to a whole-body counter containing four 15-cm diameter × 10-cm thick sodium iodide detectors, two above and two below the couch. The upper and lower counters were separated by a distance of 40 cm. Four 5-minute scans were performed in which spectra were collected over the energy range 0 to 4 MeV on a multichannel analyzer. Five standard spectra measured with phantoms were fitted, including those for calcium, sodium, chlorine, phosphorus, and potassium, using least squares fitting routines. A 3.1% correction was applied to the calcium content because of the interference resulting from the presence of ^{37}S. The interference resulting from ^{38m}K and ^{24}Na were negligible. The reproducibilities (coefficients of variation) of the measurements of the various elements, obtained from 13 irradiations of a phantom were ±1.7% for calcium, ±2.2% for sodium, ±4.3% for chlorine, and ±4.3% for phosphorus. Using a phantom consisting of a human skeleton, the reproducibility was 1.8% for calcium and 2.1% for sodium.

Kennedy et al. (1982) incorporated several necessary corrections into the determinations of absolute calcium content. These corrections were for subject height, thickness of the subject and body fat, and separation of the walls of the enclosure. The absolute calibration for calcium was found by the equation:

$$\text{TBCa} = \text{measured calcium} \times \text{height correction} \times \text{depth correction} \times \text{fat correction} \times \text{wall correction.}$$

These investigators presented normal ranges for the measured total-body calcium in 40 volunteers in which the coefficients of variation were 6.2% for men and 6.6% for women.

A neutron activation method was developed in which the activated ^{37}Ar in the lung (air) was measured upon expiration by the subject. ^{37}Ar is produced by the bombardment of ^{40}Ca, which resides in bone (Palmer, 1973). The ^{37}Ar leaves the bone and is excreted from the body through the lungs in the expired air. The amount of released ^{37}Ar has been found to be proportional to the calcium content of the body. Although the initial study by Palmer was done in animals, the method was thought to be potentially applicable in the study of human bone diseases. A 14 MeV neutron generator was used in the initial animal studies. The Auger electrons resulting during the decay of ^{37}Ar and the low-energy photons emitted when the L and M levels are filled provided a total energy release of 2.82 keV per disintegration. A proportional counter was sufficient for counting the ^{37}Ar expired by animals. In dogs, about 88% of the ^{37}Ar was excreted within 60 minutes following neutron irradiation for a period ranging from 5 to 10 minutes. The argon was easily separated from oxygen, carbon dioxide, and water vapor, although a waiting period prior to counting was required for the decay of interfering ^{41}Ar. The precision of the method was within ±2%, which was considered acceptable for many studies of changes in total-body calcium. The radiation dose (in rats) was about 11 rads for each determination. Although radionuclide sources such as ^{238}Pu and ^{252}Cf have been tested as irradiation sources, the 14 MeV neutron generator was recommended for calcium activation in humans because of the better uniformity. The advantage of the ^{37}Ar method is that fewer and less expensive facilities and equipment are needed, since it eliminates the need for the whole-body counter. Modern IVNAA methods, however, provide reduced radiation dose and equivalent accuracy. In addition, the results of this method have been variable due to the retention of ^{37}Ar in fat and bone.

PARTIAL-BODY NAA

Partial-body neutron activation analysis has been used for the determination of the calcium content of the hand (Catto et al., 1973) and of the spine (McNeill et al., 1973). The precision error associated with local measurements is on the order of 3% to 5% and the radiation dose ranges from 300 to 3000 mrem. Although it might be expected that spinal neutron activation techniques would be superior to other methods, present experience does not confirm this. Further, it has been shown that neutron activation of the spine does not provide a better discrimination of osteoporosis than other techniques of bone measurement on the appendicular skeleton. The measurement of spinal calcium in normals and osteoporotics correlated well (r = 0.92) with measurements of the radius bone mineral using photodensitometry (Meema et al., 1977).

McNeill et al. (1973) measured total-body calcium with an in vivo neutron activation technique that was applied preferentially to the trunk of the body. Sequential measurements of osteoporotic and osteomalacic patients were performed. The IVNAA system at the University of Toronto utilized 12 Pu-Be sources, each of 5 Ci and with a neutron flux of approximately 1.2×10^7 n/s. The sources were placed symmetrically above and below the trunk with a source-to-skin distance of about 12 cm for all patients. The neutron chamber was shielded with 18 inches to concrete, and patients were irradiated for 20 minutes. The patients were positioned on a wooden board above the sources, using the sternal notch as a reference point. The wooden board (4-cm thick) acted as a premoderator for the fast neutron beam; a similar wooden board was positioned above the patient. In addition, thick hydrogenous reflectors increased the neutron flux above and below the patient. The whole body counting system consisted of four fixed NaI(Tl) crystals, which viewed approximately one-third of the total bone of a 6-foot man. A 20-minute count was performed starting 3 minutes after the end of the irradiation. The 3.1 MeV photopeak of ^{49}Ca was analyzed and corrections were made for spectral overlap from ^{24}Na and ^{38}Cl. The radiation dose received by the patient was about 0.4 rem, of which greater than 90% was due to neutrons, and the remaining dose was from gamma rays from the Pu-Be sources and from the induced radioactivity. Measurements using human volunteers showed a reproducibility of 6.4% (1 SD); the reproducibility in a skeletal phantom was 4.8%. The study revealed significant changes in treated patients (calcium supplement) and decreases of total-body calcium in the untreated patients. It was suggested that by making measurements of the trunk rather than the whole body, small changes in bone calcium could be detected that may be less readily detected by total body IVNAA.

Total-body calcium measurements by NAA are currently being used as the reference standards for other techniques, such as dual-photon absorptiometry of the total skeleton. A potential advantage of the NAA method is its ability to measure all the trabecular bone in the body. It has been said, however, that since trabecular bone constitutes only 20% of the skeleton, the method lacks the precision to detect small changes in trabecular bone mass (Aitken, 1984). Other disadvantages of the method include the inevitable measurement of calcium in the gut, extraosseous calcium deposits, and calcium in nonfunctional parts of the skeleton (osteophytes). The presence of developing osteophytes contributes to the measurement of total-body calcium and may be erroneously interpreted as an increase in functional bone mass.

PRECISION AND ACCURACY (NAA)

The precision and accuracy available with the neutron activation analysis method is comparable to that of the single-photon and dual-photon bone mineral analysis techniques. One of the major sources of imprecision in activation analysis results from the nonuniformity of the neutron flux density that occurs in human subjects. Because neutrons entering the body lose energy by reacting with hydrogen, there is an initial buildup of thermal neutrons near the surface and a decrease in the neutron flux with depth. The uniformity of the neutron flux decreases with decreasing incident neutron energy. Thus, low-energy neutron beams such as those produced by ^{252}Cf (average energy, 2.3

MeV) are not suitable for total-body irradiation. ^{252}Cf is, however, useful for partial-body applications such as the forearm. Delivering a uniform neutron flux to elements concentrated within a organ (such as calcium in the skeleton) is more difficult than for homogeneously distributed elements such as N, Na, and Cl (Cohn, 1981). Moderators made of polypropylene or polyethylene are used to establish the maximum buildup of the neutron flux, which provides a more uniform flux throughout the irradiated patient volume. Moderators, however, absorb neutrons and reduce the intensity available for activation within the patient. Bilateral irradiation of the patient provides a more uniform neutron flux, and this technique has been used in most NAA centers. The best uniformity is achieved with moderated 14 MeV neutrons, although the radiation dose is higher than for lower energy neutrons (Cohn, 1981).

In addition, the uniformity of the detection system response influences the absolute determination of induced ^{49}Ca. Various counting systems have been designed for use in the NAA centers. At the University of Washington (Seattle) an annular array of four NaI(Tl) detectors that scan across the body (Palmer et al., 1968) has been used. The Scottish Universities (SURRC) system uses two NaI(Tl) detectors (above and below the patient) and a motorized bed for scanning. The University of Birmingham system uses four detectors in fixed geometry. The Brookhaven National Laboratory system uses a matrix of 54 NaI(Tl) detectors arranged above and below the patient, and the entire body is counted at once. The irradiation chamber and the counting chambers must ensure reproducible geometries in order to accurately measure absolute amounts of an element within the human body. It is equally important that the background radiation is reduced to a minimum, since a high background count rate reduces the accuracy and precision of the NAA method.

The precision of neutron activation analysis (PBNAA) measurements in the forearm of patients or cadavers was given as 2.6%, with a coefficient of variation of 12% for the normal range of calcium (Wahner et al., 1984). For partial-body activation of the hand, the precision and accuracy for measurements in bone phantoms was given as 2.4% to 5.0% and 3.2%, respectively. The coefficient of variation after normalization of the calcium content of the hand in a normal population was 9% to 14%. The precision of neutron activation analysis measurements in the hand of patients or cadavers was 2.4% (Wahner et al., 1984).

In the spine, the precision of NAA measurements in patients or cadavers was given as 3% to 5%, whereas the precision in phantoms and bone specimens was in the range of 2% to 4%. In NAA of the torso, the precision in patients or cadavers was given as 6.4%, whereas the precision in phantoms and bone specimens was 4.8%. For the torso, the accuracy of NAA was not given, although the coefficient of variation (after normalization) was stated as 10% to 13% for the normal range (Wahner et al., 1984).

Total-body neutron activation analysis can be performed with a precision of approximately 2% in patients or cadavers, and a precision in phantoms and bone specimens of 1% to 3.5%. Zanzi has given the precision for total-body calcium determinations in phantoms as ±1%, the precision in serial measurements of a female population was found to be ±1.7% when a correction was made for normal aging changes in their total-body calcium. The accuracy errors ranged from 1% to 8%. However, another source has suggested that the errors of precision and accuracy were about 2% to 5% (Williams et al., 1978). Other sources have given the accuracy of total-body calcium measurements in patients or cadavers as 5.2%, whereas the accuracy in phantoms and excised bones was 4% to 4.5%. The coefficient of variation between actual and measured calcium in normal individuals (after normalization) was 6.5% to 7%. These values were stated for in vivo studies and for studies using excised bones and bone-equivalent phantoms (Wahner et al., 1984; Smith, 1982).

Nicoll et al. (1987) compared the in vivo precision of total-body calcium and total-body sodium determinations by NAA. Using a cyclotron as the neutron source, Chamberlain et al. (1968) found that the precision of the TBCa measurement in a cadaver was 2% to 3% for a dose equivalent of 15 mSv. Spinks et al. (1977) and Nelp et al. (1970), using the cyclotron as the neutron source, reported a precision of 2% for cadaver TBCa measurements. Kennedy et al. (1982, 1983), again using the cyclotron, reported precisions of 1.8% for TBCa measurements and 2.1% for TBNa measurements in a phantom irradiated with a neutron dose of 13 mSv.

Using neutron generators, Cohn et al. (1970), Boddy et al. (1973), Burkinshaw (1985), and Sharafi et al. (1983) found precisions for TBCa measurements in the range of 1.7% to 3.6% using phantoms. The precision for the TBNa measurement was 1.9% (Sharafi et al., 1983). Cohn et al. (1972, 1976) later reported a precision of 1.1% for TBCa measurements and 2.8% for TBNa measurements in a phantom.

Although longitudinal studies using TBNAA have demonstrated changes in total-body minerals resulting from disease or treatment (Eastell et al., 1985; Gruber et al., 1984), the long-term in vivo precision of TBNAA based on patient measurements has only been recently reported in the literature. Nicoll et al. (1987) reported on a recent study of the long-term precision in patients in which three or four measurements of TBCa and TBNa were made at 6-month intervals in 156 patients. The measured values were corrected for patient height, body thickness, and fat layer and for the air gap in the irradiation chamber, using methods developed by Kennedy et al. (1982, 1983). The in vivo precision for the TBCa measurements was 2.9% over the 18-month period, whereas the precision for the phantom TBCa measurement was 1.8%. The in vivo precision for the TBNa measurements was 3.6% over the 18-month period, as compared with a 2.1% precision in phantom studies over a 3-month period.

CLINICAL MEASUREMENTS

The first clinical applications of in vivo neutron activation analysis (INNAA) were demonstrated in the early 1970s. Total-body calcium measurements became useful in the investigation of metabolic bone diseases, and studies were obtained in normal subjects. Further studies have concentrated on the assessment of osteoporosis and the effects of various therapeutic agents on this disease.

It is questionable whether the total-body calcium measurement is the most specific approach to the diagnosis of osteoporosis, since only 20% of total-body skeletal bone is trabecular bone. Neutron activation of the trunk of the body includes the spine and hips, and the total-body calcium determination does not account for the possible different rates of bone loss at these two sites in osteoporosis (Riggs et al., 1982). In addition, neutron activation of the hand and forearm may not provide information beyond that obtainable by single- and dual-photon absorptiometry methods.

Chesnut et al. (1977) reported on the efficacy of treatments for osteoporosis. In the study, the total-body calcium (TBCa) was measured by NAA before and after treatments. In the procedure, the patient and a liquid calcium comparator standard were exposed to a uniform 4 to 12 MeV neutron flux (200 mrad total body dose) over a 1.5-minute period. The neutron beam was generated by bombardment of a beryllium target with a beam of cyclotron-produced 22 MeV deuterons.

Immediately following the irradiation, the patient and the comparator standard were counted in a whole-body counter. The ratio of counts of the patient versus the counts of the standard served as an index of TBCa. The precision of the method was ±2%. The absolute TBCa in grams was obtained by comparison of the ratio to a previously established cadaver standard of similar body form. The accuracy of the absolute TBCa determination was found as ±5.2%. The TBCa value provided, in effect, a measure of total bone mass.

Harrison et al. (1977) performed clinical studies in patients with renal failure in order to assess their bone calcium status. The procedure determined the calcium bone index (CaBI), which relates the calcium in a patient to that in a normal person of the same height. Calcium of the trunk and upper thighs (about one-third of the total-body calcium for most adults) was measured in the study using the Toronto neutron activation facility (McNeill et al., 1973). Patients also received skeletal surveys including radiographs of both hands, thoracic and lumbar vertebrae, pelvis, and skull. The hand radiographs were made using industrial film (Meema and Schatz, 1970).

The determination (PBNAA) of body calcium in the central skeleton showed a fair correlation ($r = 0.76$) with the bone mineral mass of the radius as measured by x-ray photodensitometry. Corrections were made for variations in the body thickness. The corrected ^{49}Ca count was then normalized for body size using the previously validated formula for the calcium bone index:

$$\text{CaBI} = \frac{\text{corrected } ^{49}\text{Ca count} - 17}{207 \cdot [\text{ht(m)}]^3}$$

The CaBI was defined as a comparison between the corrected Ca count found for an individual and that predicted for a normal young adult of the same height. The CaBI depends on the "true" height, which may be reduced in osteoporotic subjects because of spinal compression fractures. The mean normal value for this index based on 25 subjects was 1.02 ± 0.096 (1 SD). The reproducibility of the technique was ±5.5% (1 SD). The long-term drift in the efficiency of the counting system was determined using KCl phantoms and was found to be 3% over a 4-year period.

It was later demonstrated (figure 75) by Harrison that, for volunteers under the age of 55, the calcium bone index (CaBI) values have a spread of ±25% (2 SD) around the mean value of 1.0 for normal subjects, with little difference between men and women. The spread of the normal data was partially a result of the overall precision of the procedure (5%). Patients with osteoporosis demonstrated, on the average, 30% lower CaBI values, with a mean value of 0.7 and a spread of ±20%. Differences between male and female osteoporotic patients were not statistically significant. However, 75% of the patients with fractures demonstrated CaBI values below the normal range, with only 25% overlap into the low normal range (Harrison et al., 1984).

Normal men showed an insignificant decrease in their calcium bone index (CaBI) with advancing age (3% per decade after age 50). However, women have demonstrated an 8% decrease in CaBI per decade, which is consistent with data obtained by other densitometry techniques (Harrison et al., 1984).

Ott et al. (1983) investigated total-body calcium measurements by neutron activation analysis in normal and osteoporotic populations. The study was implemented to find a discriminator of significant bone mass loss for identifying individuals at risk in the population. Bone mineral content by SPA was also evaluated. A cyclotron provided the neutron beam for activation as described previously (Nelp et al., 1970). The gamma emissions from Ca^{49} were detected and analyzed in a whole-body counter, and the results were converted to grams by simultaneously counting standards, which were calibrated with chemically-analyzed cadavers of various body sizes. The accuracy of the method was ±5.2%. The site of the SPA measurement was taken as one-tenth of the forearm length proximal to the tip of the styloid, which contained both cancellous and cortical bone. The results demonstrated a wide range of TBCa values in normal individuals. Using multiple linear regression analysis, the TBC (predicted) was determined based upon the height of each subject. The ratio TBCa/TBC (predicted) was determined. The results indicated that TBCa offers greater detectability for osteoporosis than the regional bone mass (BMC) measurements. However, the study indicated a high false negative rate in the osteoporotic population.

Aloia et al. (1985) studied osteoporotic women by neutron activation analysis and single-photon absorptiometry of the radius (figure 76). Total-body neutron activation was performed using a uniform exposure to a beam of partially moderated fast neutrons. The induced activities were determined in

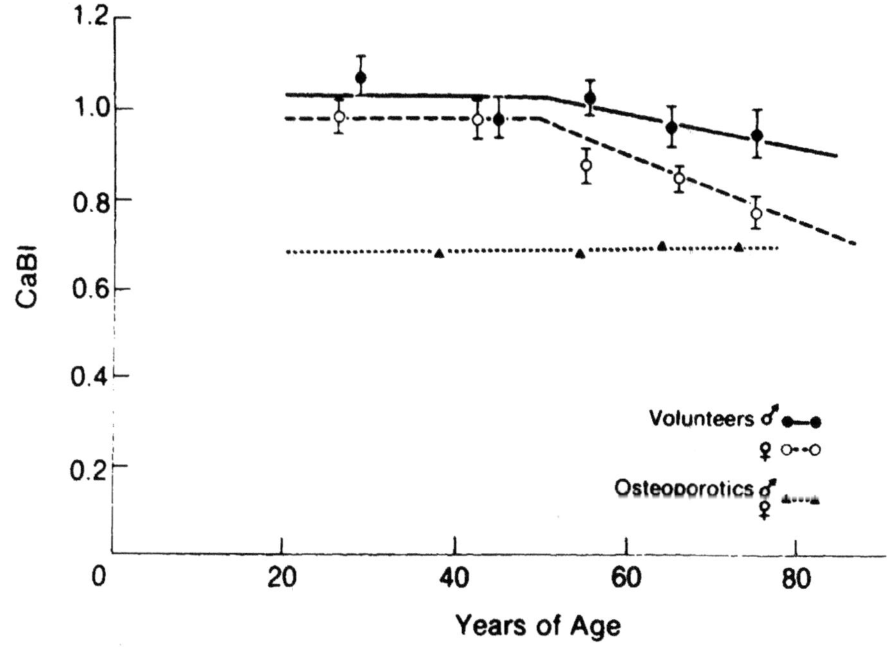

Figure 75. Mean CaBI values as a function of age for volunteer men, volunteer women, and for osteoporotic patients; error bars representing 1 standard error of the mean (Courtesy: JE Harrison)

the 54 detector whole-body counter (Brookhaven National Laboratory, New York). The precision error as determined by anthropomorphic phantoms was ±1.1%. The radiation dose for each activation was 0.28 rem.

In this study, the bone mineral content and width of the radius were determined in each subject. Measurements were performed at the 8 cm radius site. The stated accuracy of the Norland Instruments system was ±5%, and the precision was ±2.5%. The relationship between bone mineral content (radius) and total-body calcium was highly correlated (r = 0.75). It was shown that both the total-body calcium levels and the bone mineral content values of the radius were significantly lower as compared to normal values.

TBNAA has been used for the investigation of the effects of various drug therapy regimens in patients. In studies of the treatment of osteoporosis with calcitonin, it was found that the results of bone mineral measurements of the radius were not in agreement with the results of neutron activation analysis (Aloia, 1985). A bank of 14 Ci encapsulated ^{238}Pu, Be sources were used, exposing the patient to a uniform broad beam of partially moderated fast neutrons. The accuracy and precision in phantoms was ±1%. The sensitivity of the system was given as four times greater than any other activation system in clinical use for counting total-body calcium. The bone mineral content (BMC) and bone width (BW) were determined with the Norland Instruments SPA device.

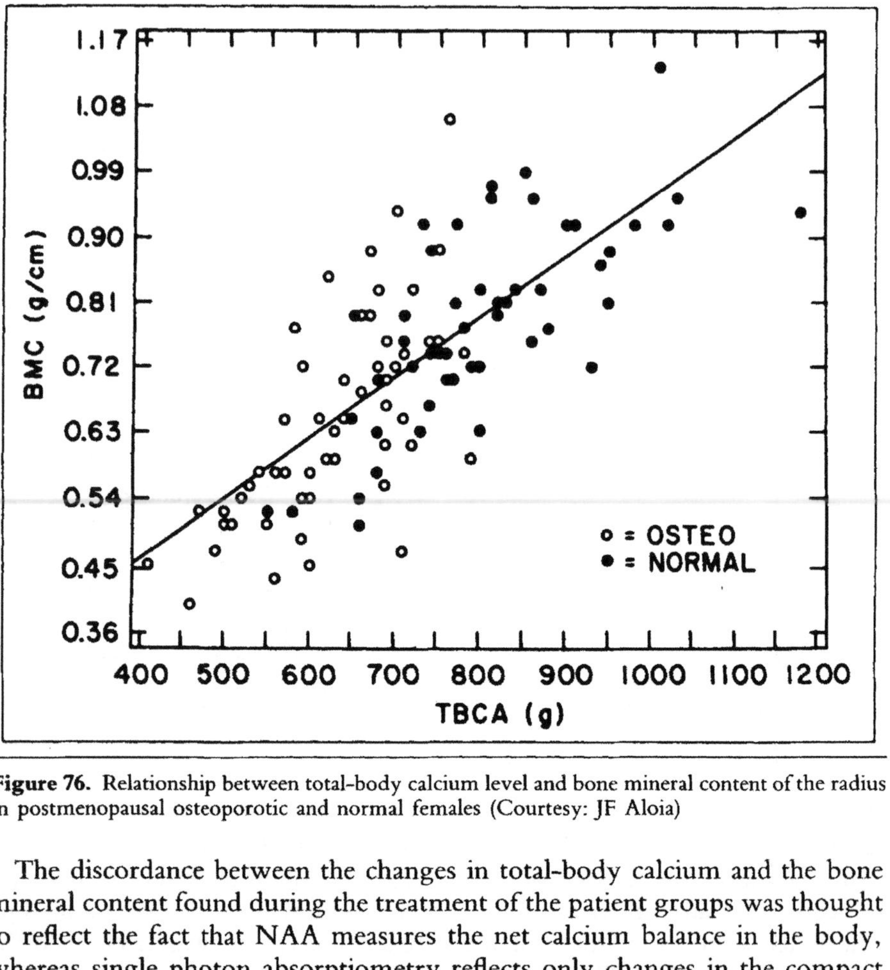

Figure 76. Relationship between total-body calcium level and bone mineral content of the radius in postmenopausal osteoporotic and normal females (Courtesy: JF Aloia)

The discordance between the changes in total-body calcium and the bone mineral content found during the treatment of the patient groups was thought to reflect the fact that NAA measures the net calcium balance in the body, whereas single photon absorptiometry reflects only changes in the compact bone of the radius. It was concluded that there is a necessity to measure both regional and total bone mass in patients with metabolic bone disease.

Cohn et al. (1986) performed clinical studies for identifying women at risk for developing osteoporosis. Total-body neutron activation analysis (TBNAA) was performed in the subjects, as well as single-photon and dual-photon absorptiometry. Previous efforts to quantify calcium in individuals were made by use of the calcium ratio: measured total-body calcium (TBCa)/predicted body calcium. This qualitative method, which normalizes TBCa for skeletal size, was found to provide merely a threshold value for distinguishing normal women from women at risk. The variance associated with the calcium ratio was quite large.

Cohn introduced a *multiple logistic regression* (MLR) model to discriminate women at risk of osteoporosis on the basis of their calcium deficit. The method was a statistical technique used to quantify the probability of an individual being at risk. Cohn stated that the TBNAA technique made it possible to measure directly total-body calcium (TBCa) and, hence, to infer skeletal mass with high accuracy and precision. In these subjects, AP and lateral radiographs of the lumbar vertebrae were obtained. TBNAA was performed with the neutron exposure provided by an array of fourteen 50 Ci encapsulated ^{238}Pu, Be neutron sources. The subjects were uniformly exposed to a beam of partially moderated fast neutrons. The absolute levels of the induced ^{49}Ca were counted in the Brookhaven whole-body counter. From the data, the absolute levels of calcium were calculated. The accuracy and precision of the method were determined as ±1% for total body calcium in an anthropomorphic phantom, and 2.5% in women studied over a 4 to 5 year period. The threshold value of the ratio $TBCa/(H)^{1/2}$ for the presence of osteoporosis in these females subjects was approximately 57.4 $g/(cm)^{1/2}$.

Reid et al. (1986) reported the results of an 18-month longitudinal study of total-body calcium in patients with rheumatoid arthritis and those with primary generalized osteoarthrosis. The method used was that described by Kennedy et al. (1982), which showed an in vivo precision of 2.9% over the 18-month period. The mean annual rate of bone loss in 24 patients with rheumatoid arthritis treated with nonsteroidal anti-inflammatory drugs alone was 3.4%. The mean annual rate of loss of TBCa in 19 patients with primary generalized osteoarthrosis was 1.6%.

Williams et al. (1986) performed in vivo total-body calcium content (TBCa) measurements using TBNAA in the study of patients with Cushing's syndrome. The method has been described by Spinks et al. (1977). The patients were irradiated with fast neutrons generated from a beryllium target bombarded by deuterons accelerated in the MRC cyclotron at Hammersmith Hospital, London. The patients were in the upright position in a polyethylene enclosure to ensure uniform irradiation; the total dose to the front and back was 0.1 rad. Following irradiation, the patient was rapidly transferred to the whole-body counter consisting of ten 15 cm diameter × 10 cm thick NaI(Tl) detectors surrounding a horizontal couch. The gamma radiation of the ^{49}Ca photopeak (3.1 MeV) was counted for 20 minutes, and corrections were made for interference from ^{24}Na and ^{37}S. The TBCa was estimated by comparison with a phantom of known calcium content irradiated and counted under the same conditions as the patient.

The precision of the measurement of ^{49}Ca counts was 3%, and the coefficient of variation of the measurement of total-body calcium content (in grams) was 7.5%. The "predicted" TBCa was calculated by the formulae of Kennedy et al. (1982). TBCa was found to be a useful index of bone mass, since 98% of body calcium resides in the skeleton. The method was thought to be well established, reproducible, and noninvasive; and it involved only a small radiation dose. It was noted that TBCa measurements may be relatively insensitive to changes affecting mainly trabecular bone, which comprises only 20% of total skeletal mass.

RADIATION DOSE TO PATIENT (NAA)

In general, the radiation dose associated with NAA ranges from 300 to 3000 mrem, although higher doses are possible with the use of fast neutrons (Mazess, 1979). The radiation doses have been studied by Maziere et al. (1979). The radiation dose to the hand during partial body neutron activation of the hand was estimated as 2 to 15 rem. NAA of the forearm delivered approximately 6 rem to the skin and 1.7 rem to bone of the forearm. The radiation dose to the spine in NAA delivers 6 rem to the skin of the patient and 0.7 rem to the spinal skeleton. The radiation dose to the total body in NAA of the total body was in the range of 0.3 to 2.1 rem.

PROTON ACTIVATION ANALYSIS (PAA)

The use of proton activation has been investigated for in vivo partial-body calcium determinations (Eilbert, 1977). Studies with phantoms were performed using the 160 MeV Harvard cyclotron. PAA offers several advantages over the NAA method: (1) Proton beam collimation is simpler to accomplish than in NAA, providing a beam that remains parallel to within 1 to 2 mm spread in tissues. (2) Protons have a sharp, finite end of range, which allows tissue sparing beyond the irradiated bone. (3) Extremely uniform activation of calcium is assured (exceeding the uniformity possible with PBNAA) using range modulation. (4) PAA requires about 10 times less rem dose than PBNAA for the same accuracy, since protons have a lower RBE than neutrons and ^{40}Ca is in higher natural abundance than the ^{48}Ca used as the target for PBNAA. The nuclear reaction that was used for proton energies in excess of 25 MeV is:

$$^{40}Ca + p \rightarrow {}^{38}K + 2p + n$$

This reaction is followed by the decay of ^{38}K as described:

$$^{38}K \rightarrow {}^{38}Ar + \beta + \alpha$$

The maximum cross section for this reaction is 77 mb at a proton energy of 40 MeV. The half-life of ^{38}K is 7.71 minutes, and it emits photons at 2.17 MeV (100% abundance) and 511 keV (200% abundance from positron annihilation). The proton flux was determined by the use of an ionization chamber, and the 2.17 MeV gamma rays were detected with a NaI(Tl) detector system. The calcium content was determined based on these measured data. The high energy of the emitted gamma rays ensures their transmission and ultimate detection outside the body. The measurement of the activity of ^{38}K in vivo is complicated by the presence of two interfering radionuclides, ^{14}O (half-life: 70.5 s; energy: 2.31 MeV) and ^{34m}Cl (half-life: 32.2 min; energy: 2.13 and 3.30 MeV). Background radiation is present in the photopeak region as a result of radium and thorium chain activities in construction materials and cosmic rays. The activity of ^{38}K was determined by separating the interfering isotopes by decay curve analysis. The ^{14}O activity disappears rapidly, removing the interference and allowing an accurate determination of ^{38}K activity. The statistical error of the method was 1.9%.

The precision for PAA was found to be dependent on the calcium content present and the administered radiation dose. The reproducibility was investigated using calf vertebrae in a simulated in vivo geometry; 2.6% reproducibility was found using a radiation dose to the phantom in 1 to 2 minutes of 2.44 rad. Higher radiation doses were found to improve the reproducibility to 0.3%. A high correlation coefficient ($r = 0.998$) was observed between ^{38}K activity and calcium content using a phantom containing calcium nitrate solutions. The suggested in vivo procedure required the alignment of the patient with the proton beam using an x-ray tube aligned with the beam axis. For in vivo measurements, empirical corrections were required for (1) the ^{38}K produced from common potassium contained in soft tissues (on the order of 10%) and (2) diffusion of ^{38}K out of the bony region viewed by the detectors during the study period (on the order of 1% of the total activity).

MUONIC X-RAY EXCITATION

A method developed at the Los Alamos Meson Physics Facility in Los Alamos, New Mexico (Hutson, 1976) has taken advantage of the fact that x-rays are emitted when negative muons are captured in a material that is irradiated with a muon beam (Daniel, 1969; Rosen, 1971). Negative muons are negatively charged particles having a mass of 105.7 MeV and a mean life of 2.2×10^{-6} seconds. Detection of the x-rays provides quantitative information about the elemental composition of the material. This technique is potentially useful in clinical diagnosis and medical research (figure 77).

A muon beam (5 cm × 10 cm) was produced by bombarding a carbon target with protons of energy greater than about 300 MeV (from a high-energy linear accelerator), causing nuclear interactions which produced negative pions. The pions decay (with very short mean life) into negative muons, which were collected and focused into a beam by a system of magnets. The Fermi-Teller "Z-law" was used to deduce the composition of the tissues, which was based on the total numbers of x-rays emitted when the muons were stopped in the samples. Various animal tissues were used in this work, including frozen samples of bovine bone removed from the cancellous bone of the tibia. The samples were placed in the muon beam, and the muonic x-rays were detected by an intrinsic germanium detector placed at an angle of 90° to the beam axis. Chemical analyses were also performed on the samples.

This x-ray analysis method was found to be capable of detecting the presence of carbon, nitrogen, oxygen, phosphorus, and calcium in bone. The sensitivity of the method was thought to be great enough to detect the less

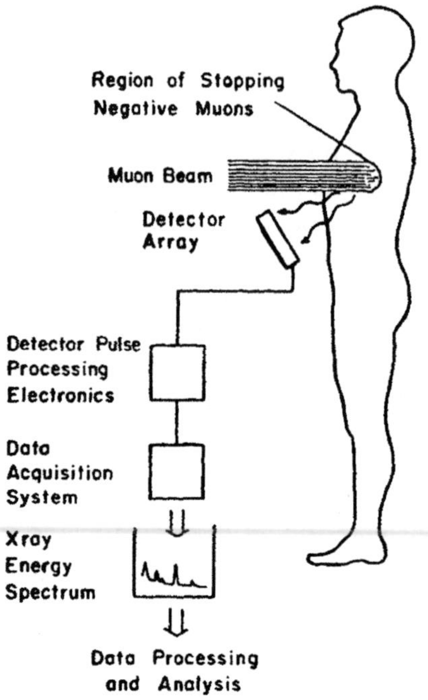

Figure 77. Muonic x-ray detection system for elemental analysis of selected regions of tissue within the human body (Courtesy: RL Hutson)

abundant elements down to the 0.05% abundance level with an accuracy of 10% ±5% in less than 5 minutes of irradiation. It was believed that, for the more abundant elements, an accuracy of 1% could be obtained. The radiation dose to a 100 cc volume of tissue was estimated to be 2 to 3 rad. It was concluded that muons may be used for the detection of bone mineral depletion in localized areas that may not be amenable to neutron activation or photon absorptiometry. However, the cost of routine clinical diagnostic studies using muonic x-rays is thought to be prohibitive.

8. CLINICAL APPLICATIONS AND COMPARISON OF METHODS

The development of the noninvasive radiological methods in densitometry has enhanced the diagnosis and monitoring of osteoporosis and other bone-related diseases. These methods have progressed over the years from the qualitative to the quantitative, providing the medical community with important additional information regarding the assessment of bone disease. We have seen that these methods have unique characteristics that delineate their suitability and advantages for a particular application. However, the physical measurement parameters associated with each method are characterized by specific limitations upon their applicability, precision, and accuracy in the clinical environment.

Densitometry measurements of peripheral bones correlate only moderately ($r = 0.6–0.7$) with vertebral parameters, as shown by both noninvasive techniques and direct analysis, although the intercorrelation among peripheral bone measurements is very good ($r = 0.95$) (Mazess, 1979). Measurements of the peripheral skeleton are the least sensitive and may not extrapolate well to the central skeleton in metabolic bone disorders; but the sensitivity is increased by doing multiple measurements (Mazess, 1979). Radiogrammetry, photodensitometry, and single-photon absorptiometry are not useful for the axial skeleton and, therefore, may be of limited clinical use in the assessment of those metabolic bone diseases that involve greater proportions of trabecular bone (Kimmel, 1984).

The use of radiographs in the assessment of osteoporosis has been shown to be less than satisfactory for all but the most general evaluations of this bone disease. The *biconcavity index* for the spinal vertebrae is a convenient index for clinical use, but this method is not well correlated with the true vertebral density. In addition, the biconcavity index has not demonstrated a good correlation with the presence of compression fractures and is therefore not a useful indicator for the diagnosis of osteoporosis.

The use of other qualitative indices derived from radiographs, including the Singh Index of femoral trabecular patterns and the calcaneal trabecular index, have been shown to have large precision errors in clinical studies. Indirect measures such as the trabecular pattern of the femoral neck are quite unreliable (15% to 30% error) (Mazess, 1979). These qualitative methods are poorly correlated with bone measurements at these sites, and thus they are not generally applied throughout the medical community, although they may offer some benefits in large population studies or in research.

Radiogrammetry, the assessment of the cortical thickness or cortical area of peripheral bones, consistently underestimates the skeletal bone loss by about 20% to 30%. Radiogrammetry is subject to large inaccuracy errors, because it does not take into account the intracortical porosities that are often present. Radiogrammetry should, therefore, be used together with absorptiometry, since absorptiometry reflects the actual bone mass and it accounts for the presence of intracortical porosities (Mazess, 1979).

In peripheral bones, measurements by radiogrammetry or photodensitometry (or total bone by radiokinetic or balance methods) seem to have prohibitively large errors of accuracy. Radiographic photodensitometry is subject to 5% to 10% errors (Mazess, 1979). Radiographic photodensitometry has shown limited success in the measurement of the cortical regions of the phalanges and the metacarpals, following some improvement of the in vivo precision of this method (3% to 4%). However, photodensitometry is not useful in areas of the skeleton that consist of large tissue cover. The accuracy of the method for appendicular regions has also been limited by 5% to 15% errors. Videodensitometry, however, has improved the precision and accuracy of the method to better than 2% errors.

Single-photon absorptiometry using a highly collimated beam of gamma rays has provided a method, that reduces the problems associated with scattered radiation and has improved the spatial resolution of bone mineral assessments. Further improvements in the precision of SPA have resulted from the design of systems that provide rectilinear scans for better localization of the bone site. Prior to the development of newer commercial devices, the accuracy of bone mineral content measurements using the single-photon absorptiometry method was questioned (Goldsmith and Cohn, 1977; Mazess, 1977). Mazess (1977) found that a 4% calibration error produced lower bone mineral content values. It was concluded that the BMC error inherent to the calibration of the commercial system was 4% to 6% in either direction. The use of single-photon absortiometry in studies of individual patients was thought to lead to falsely high or low appendicular bone mineral content values, unless these inherent calibration errors were eliminated from the measurement. Rustgi et al. (1980) investigated the accuracy of the Norland-Cameron Bone Mineral Analyzer, which has been in wide use over the years. In studies of human cadaver radii and ulnae, the instrumental bone mineral content values for a commercially available SPA system were found to be on the average about 6.5% higher than the bone ash values. In addition, it was found that the bone mineral densities (BMD) calculated from the measured BMC were also higher than the bone mineral densities obtained from ashing.

Because the SPA method is limited to the peripheral skeleton, the value of bone mineral assessments in some patient populations is reduced. The method has been primarily used in the radial midshaft, although studies have been done on areas containing more trabecular bone, such as the distal radius and the os calcis. The single-photon absorptiometry method, performed in the midradius (cortical bone), is less sensitive in the assessment of osteoporosis; 10 to 20% of patients with osteoporosis have values below the fifth percentile of normals (Wahner, 1985). A strong intercorrelation between these sites and other trabecular bone sites is desired and could be very meaningful. However, studies have shown that the SPA measurements may not provide a clinically useful prediction of bone status at sites other than the site of the measurement itself. SPA measurements of the os calcis (trabecular bone) have been suggested as the more useful measurement, although this site may be more important for assessing longitudinal changes than for the diagnosis of bone diseases (Mazess, 1983).

Wahner et al. (1985) performed measurements of the bone mineral content (BMC) in the femoral neck of cadavers using the two methods: SPA and DPA. The ^{125}I SPA bone mineral content values (g/cm) were highly correlated ($r = 0.99$) with DPA bone mineral content values (g/cm) in the femoral neck. These results support the usefulness of SPA as a physical method when it is applied to other than appendicular sites.

Stellon et al. (1985) have compared the results of three methods for determining bone loss: (1) metacarpal cortical/total area ratio (CA/TA), (2) single-photon absorptiometry (^{241}Am), and (3) bone histomorphometry. In a population consisting of 36 patients with chronic active hepatitis treated with corticosteroids, the study confirmed that measurements of the appendicular skeleton (radiogrammetry and single-photon absorptiometry) correlate poorly with those of the axial skeleton (iliac crest biopsy). No significant correlation was found between the trabecular bone volume (TBV) and either the cortical/total area ratio (CA/TA) or the normalized bone mineral content (BMC/BW) at the metaphysis or diaphysis of the radius. However, significant correlations were found between the cortical bone sites (metacarpal and diaphysis of the radius).

The use of single-photon measurements of the radius in screening procedures can identify abnormalities in some cases, but these measurements do not exclude the possibility of abnormalities in normal individuals. Kruse et al.

(1975) have shown that subjects with normal radius BMC values may well be osteoporotic. In conclusion, Mazess et al. (1984) found the following: (1) radius measurements indicate total skeletal state and spinal state with moderate accuracy (approx. 10%) in normal subjects, (2) the accuracy for either total-body or spinal state is poorer for osteoporotic subjects than for normal subjects, and (3) trabecular bone must be measured in order to diagnose or monitor bone disease. Radius BMC/BW may also overestimate the bone mineral content in patients with renal osteodystrophy (Mazess et al., 1984).

In a recent study, four measurements of bone mineral were performed and the results were compared in order to determine the method that best predicted the risk of postmenopausal fracture in women (Wasnich et al., 1985). Bone mineral measurements were performed at four skeletal sites: (1) os calcis, (2) proximal radius, (3) distal radius, and (4) lumbar spine. The single-photon method was used for the os calcis and radius, while the dual-photon method was used for the spine. The os calcis bone mineral content measurement was found to be the best predictor of nonspine fracture risk and the best overall indicator of spinal fracture risk. This result was unexpected, since the dual-photon absorptiometry measurements of the spine may be expected to yield the best assessments of fracture risk. The number of spinal bone mineral measurements in this study was smaller than for the other sites, and this may partially explain the result. Although the os calcis bone mineral content was found to yield a better estimate of fracture risk in the spine, there is conflicting evidence for the correlation between bone mineral content of the os calcis and that of the spine.

Mazess (1979) has stated that spinal measurements are not desirable for the determination of normal aging changes or in diseases where spinal changes proceed at the "normal" slow rate, but they are indicated where rapid spinal changes are evident. With regard to monitoring, it is clear that direct spinal measurements offer the greatest advantage. The major need in monitoring changes in the skeleton is a precise spinal measurement or multiple measurements (Mazess, 1979).

Dual-photon absorptiometry has provided yet another improvement in the methods of bone densitometry. The measurement of two photon energies simultaneously eliminates the need to have a constant thickness of soft tissue cover above the bone of interest, as is required by the SPA method. The dual energy ^{153}Gd source must be replaced on an annual basis because of the physical decay and consequent loss of incident intensity, which reduces the beam penetrability and the statistical precision of the transmission measurements. The long-term precision of the DPA method is 2% to 3%, which is adequate for monitoring fracture sites in the skeleton. Although the accuracy for measurements of the bone mineral density in vertebral samples has been assessed as 2% to 5%, suitable studies for assessing the in vivo accuracy of DPA have not been published. The long-term machine drift was evaluated in a later study as measured with a phantom and was found to be 1% to 2% per year (Lunar Radiation Corp, Madison, Wisconsin). However, replacement of the radiation source was found to produce 2% to 5% changes. The average coefficient of variation of the phantom bone mineral content using DPA was 2.9% (Ott et al., 1986).

Radius measurements at both the midshaft and the distal sites (and even trabecular bone measurements of the os calcis or from CT of the limbs) cannot accurately predict the mineral density at critical fracture sites, such as the proximal femur and spine (Mazess and Cameron, 1985; Mazess et al., 1984; Hangartner et al., 1983). The 95% confidence interval in normal subjects for prediction of the spinal values from radius measurements or os calcis measurements is about 0.25 g/cm^2 for area density or about 50 mg/cc for volumetric density (at mean densities of 1.00 g/cm^2 or 150 mg/cc, respectively). This uncertainty is too great for using appendicular sites as a clinical indicator of the spine. About 35% of subjects (under 70 years of age) with osteopenia are missed using appendicular measurements such as SPA of the radius. However, the appendicular skeleton may be extremely useful in pediatric patients and as a low-cost mass screening tool in elderly adults, in which the appendicular bone loss more closely approximates that of the spine of these individuals (Mazess and Cameron, 1985). Therefore, the above mentioned appendicular measurement methods are not suitable for diagnosing osteoporosis, and an axial measurement should be used.

In a later study, it was demonstrated in cadaver specimens that dual-photon absorptiometry accurately indicates bone mass and bone density and is only slightly affected by either the surrounding tissue or the fat changes in the bone marrow (Wahner et al., 1985). In clinical practice, the spinal bone mineral content is measured at L1–L4 with dual-photon absorptiometry (DPA) in patients with osteoporosis and compared with age-matched and sex-adjusted normal ranges. The DPA technique identifies abnormal bone mass in patients, but the broad range of normal values makes it impossible to distinguish small increases or losses of bone mass. Some studies have shown that only about 60% to 70% of patients with osteoporosis have bone mineral content values (areal densities) below the fifth percentile of normal (Wahner, 1985).

Although the DPA method has the advantage of providing measurements of the central skeleton, as opposed to SPA, dual-photon absorptiometry does not separate trabecular from cortical bone within the vertebrae or femoral neck. The measured bone mineral density (g/cm^2) is derived from the presence of both compact and trabecular bone tissue at these sites. This disadvantage prevents the discrimination between bone diseases that affect trabecular and compact bone in different ways and at different rates.

Munk-Jensen et al. (1986) investigated the predictive value of bone mass measurements of the forearm for assessing the bone mass in other parts of the skeleton. The bone mineral densities of the second, third, and fourth lumbar vertebrae were measured with the dual-photon absorptiometer (^{153}Gd source). Bone mineral density of the distal forearm was also measured with a single-photon absorptiometer (^{125}I source). In a study of 150 normal postmenopausal women, measurements were performed at 6-month intervals. The standard error of the estimate (SEE) of lumbar BMD from forearm BMD was 11% at the initial measurement and at 6 months. The correlation coefficients were 0.53 and 0.52 at the respective times of measurement. It was concluded that the estimation of lumbar BMD from the forearm BMD is inaccurate in normal postmenopausal women. It was suggested that studies of bone mass, including investigations on osteoporosis, should consist of more than one bone site, preferably the forearm (predominantly cortical bone) and the lumbar spine (predominantly trabecular bone).

Riggs et al. (1981) compared the measurements of the lumbar spine using dual-photon absorptiometry with measurements of the distal and midradius in populations of normal and osteoporotic individuals. The dual-photon system (^{153}Gd) developed from a commercial Ohio-Nuclear rectilinear scanner was used to assess the bone mineral density (g/cm^2) of the lumbar spine (L1–L4). The single-photon system (^{125}I) was used to scan the midradius and the distal radius (10% of the radius length) of the nondominant arm; three scans were made at each forearm site. The BMC (g/cm) of the radius was determined with coefficients of variation of 3% for the midradius and 3% to 5% for the distal radius. The authors suggested that the data showed a disproportionate loss of trabecular bone from the axial skeleton as opposed to the appendicular skeleton and further suggested that this loss is a distinguishing characteristic of spinal osteoporosis. In addition, it was found that the ninetieth percentile for vertebral BMD for patients with nontraumatic vertebral fractures is the threshold below which the risk of nontraumatic fractures increases. It was concluded that direct spinal measurements of bone mineral density are greatly superior to appendicular measurements for evaluating the severity of spinal osteoporosis.

Dual-photon absorptiometry can provide local spinal measurements with relatively good precision (3%) (Mazess, 1979). In a study that compared the single-photon and dual-photon absorptiometry methods, Mazess et al. (1984) used a rectilinear scanning device consisting of a dual-photon source (^{153}Gd) for the determination of the areal density (bone mineral content per unit area, BMD) and the total-body bone mineral per unit area (TBBM/area). The measurements were performed in 72 normal females (aged 20 to 80 years) and 13 normal males (aged 20 to 61). In addition, 18 older females (aged 50 to 74) with confirmed osteoporosis, 11 adult osteoporotic males taking corticosteroids, and 20 patients with renal osteodystrophy were scanned. In this study, a direct-readout single-photon absorptiometer was used for measurement of the bone mineral content (BMC in g/cm) of the radius at the standard site one-third of the forearm length proximal to the styloid process of the ulna. The BMC data was normalized by dividing by the bone width displayed on the bone mineral analyzer system (BMC/BW).

In the normal subjects there were moderate correlations between the SPA and DPA measurement sites. In normal males and females, there were relatively small errors (6% to 10%) in estimating the status of the total skeleton or of the subregions including the spine, from BMC measurements of the radius. Previous studies have indicated this result (Mazess et al., 1972; Cohn et al., 1975; Manzke et al., 1975; Horsman et al., 1970; Horsman et al., 1983).

Since radius measurements in normal subjects have been shown to be well correlated (r = 0.95) with the density of iliac crest samples, it is believed that single-photon abosorptiometry of the radius is useful in epidemiological studies of normal populations. However, such measurements are not appropriate for clinical management of metabolic bone diseases in individual patients because of the inability of the SPA method to assess trabecular bone changes. TBBM/area values reflected the spinal BMD better than the radius BMC/BW values in both normal and patient populations. It was concluded that the widely used noninvasive measurements that assess primarily compact bone (single-photon absorptiometry, photodensitometry, radiogrammetry) are far less useful in osteoporosis than measurements that assess trabecular bone changes. Total body measurements provided little if any better discrimination of abnormalities than other measurements of compact bone. Total body measurements provide a "complete picture" but are not as sensitive (Mazess, 1979).

Several investigators have shown that subjects with fractures are well separated (2 SD) from controls on the basis of their lumbar spine bone mineral. However, subjects with fractures of the femoral neck have not demonstrated as clear a separation from normal controls (Mazess, 1983). Fracture thresholds have been defined by many investigators. The fracture threshold for the spine is defined as the bone mineral value below which the values of 90% of all patients with one or more spinal compression fractures are found. This threshold value was determined as 0.98 g/cm^2 for L2–L4 in both sexes, and as two standard deviations below the mean areal density value of the general population at maximal bone mass (Riggs et al., 1981). It should be noted that because normal subjects fall below the fracture threshold in advanced age, it is difficult to distinguish between the age-related bone loss and the loss due to a pathologic condition. The fracture index is useful, however, in the evaluation of women under 50 years and men under 60 years of age. Melton et al. (1985) have shown that the risk of fracture can be predicted on the basis of bone mineral measurements.

The method of neutron activation analysis in the determination of skeletal bone mass has had the distinct disadvantage of high cost and limited availability. The requirements for a neutron irradiation facility and a total-body counter, along with other disadvantages, prevent the broad clinical application of these methods. Neutron activation methods have, in the past, been associated with patient radiation doses greater than 3 rem. These doses may be comparable with the doses from QCT, although much smaller volumes of tissue are irradiated with CT methods. There have also been problems in obtaining a uniform neutron flux and uniformity in the detection of the emitted radiations. In addition, the presence of ectopic calcifications (calcification not present in the skeleton itself) causes errors, especially in elderly patients or in those with bone diseases. The precision error of the NAA method is 3% to 5%, and the accuracy error is at least 5% (Mazess, 1983).

Partial-body neutron activation techniques using Pu-Be sources have been successfully used for activation of the trunk, including the spine (University of Toronto). The radiation dose associated with this procedure is about 500 mrem, a much more reasonable level by comparison to TBNAA. PBNAA methods using the radionuclide source ^{252}Cf have also been used for calcium determination of the spine, but with radiation doses similar to those of TBNAA. Local (partial-body) neutron activation analysis for calcium provides 5% precision but is restricted to only a few laboratories (Mazess, 1979).

Cohn et al. (1986) have shown, through the development of the multiple logistic regression (MLR) model, that NAA is useful for the discrimination of women at risk of osteoporosis on the basis of their calcium deficit. Using the model with data obtained from three types of measurements (TBNAA, DPA, and SPA), it was shown that the bone density measurement (DPA) placed more women in the normal category than did the total calcium data obtained by NAA. The bone density data from the distal radius (SPA) represented the least sensitive predictor of women at risk.

The study showed that the measurement of TBCa is more sensitive than either DPA of the spine or SPA of the distal radius in determining women at risk for osteoporosis. However, the MLR model using TBCa data identified only 87% of the true osteoporotic patients, leaving 13% false negatives; other factors besides the loss of calcium were implicated in determining spinal fracture. The correlation between BMC at the distal radius and TBCa models was high, indicating that BMC of the distal radius is a satisfactory mass screening technique for determining women potentially at risk. It is noted that Ott et al. (1983) found in an earlier study that the ratio TBCa/TBCa (predicted) provided a better discriminator of osteoporosis than the wrist BMC. Reid et al. (1986) confirmed the usefulness of the measurement of TBCa in assessing treatment programs for osteoporosis. The precision of the TBCa method was 2.9%.

Quantitative computed tomographic methods have provided densitometry with an innovation not previously available. Commercial CT scanners with the appropriate BMD software are capable of providing high-resolution images in addition to quantitative bone mineral content data. The major advantage of QCT is the ability of the method to separate trabecular and compact bone. Although the complete separation may be limited by the partial volume effect that is common to all CT methods, a clear delineation between the two bone types present in the vertebrae is possible with this method. Although the major disadvantage of QCT has been the associated radiation dose, new scanning procedures have reduced patient doses below 500 mrem.

Nordin et al. (1983) indicated that the radiation dose associated with QCT may be reduced to less than 1 rem per vertebral scan. The radiation dose is less for DPA than for QCT: 15 mrads for DPA and at least 20 times that dose for QCT (Powell, 1984). With regard to commercially available CT scanners (head and body units), the cost, accessibility, and radiation dose (2 rem) from CT scans were factors that made peripheral bone CT measurements less feasible than absorptiometry, which is lower in cost and radiation dose (10 mrem) to the patient (Mazess, 1979).

QCT measurements have been suggested as perhaps a more sensitive method than DPA in the spine, since QCT can measure the purely trabecular bone in the centrum of the vertebrae, whereas the total spinal bone (including the compact bone of the vertebrae) is measured with DPA. QCT may be more appropriate, since it is thought that at menopause women lose twice as much bone in the anterior centrum as in the entire vertebra and seven times more than in compact one (Mazess and Whedon, 1983). However, since DPA offers lower radiation dose than QCT and is less affected by the presence of vertebral crush fractures, DPA may be the preferred bone mineral method, especially for serial studies in young subjects (Sambrook et al., 1985).

Although computed tomography offers fairly reliable measurements of peripheral bone mass with a precision of about 3%, large accuracy errors in the QCT method (greater than 30%) have been reported in the literature for in vitro experiments on spinal (trabecular) bone. It has been suggested that errors arise when significant amounts of marrow fat are present in the vertebrae, leading to errors of 3% to 10% in the CT bone mineral values (Mazess, 1983). In addition, QCT measurements may be falsely lowered by 20% to 25% in the elderly osteoporotic persons because of marrow fat concentrations, which are increased with age. Under carefully controlled conditions of measurement, however, the QCT method gives good precision (3%).

Dual-energy QCT has been suggested as a means of reducing the errors introduced by changes in the amount of marrow fat present (a 10% change in fat gives a 5% error for single-energy CT). Dual-energy CT methods can reduce the magnitude of this error caused by fat, but at the expense of an increased radiation dose (Kimmel, 1984). However, dual-energy CT methods have not been broadly applied in clinical practice. Some x-ray manufacturers have developed systems that are capable of switching between two different energies (kVp's), but technical difficulties have resulted in a seriously reduced precision for bone mineral measurements. However, most investigators now favor the dual-energy CT method because its precision on the newer generation of scanners has been improved to match that of the single-energy technique (Black et al., 1985).

The ^{125}I gamma CT method has the limitation of being confined to measurements of the peripheral skeleton. However, the method has the advantages of separating trabecular from compact bone, producing a high-resolution image and providing measurements having good long-term precision. The low radiation dose ^{125}I CT scanner of P. Ruegsegger (Institute for Biomedical Engineering, Zurich, Switzerland) has demonstrated high precision (less than 0.3%) for bone mineral determinations in the appendicular skeleton. Ruegsegger demonstrated a high correlation (r = 0.9) between peripheral sites (tibia and radius) with each other and with spinal mineral.

When comparing the QCT and DPA methods, some authors have found that the precision (reproducibility) is approximately 1.5% to 3% for both methods. The accuracy of in vitro measurements of vertebral specimens for both QCT and DPA is approximately 5% to 10%, although it may be poorer in the elderly population (Genant and Cann, 1984). It has been stated that vertebral compressions, hypertrophy of articular facets, discogenic sclerosis, or marginal osteophytosis and extraosseous calcification, which are common in the elderly population, cannot be excluded in vertebral DPA measurements and may result in poorer accuracy and precision.

The QCT method is said to have shorter scan times than the DPA method; the scan time required for QCT is on the order of 10 to 15 minutes per patient, whereas the scan time for DPA is 30 to 40 minutes. Other logistical problems must be addressed when considering the advantages and disadvantages of each method. The cost for adding QCT to an existing CT scanner is about $500 to $1000, whereas the cost for a DPA unit is between $30K and $60K and requires a dedicated space and technologist training.

Widely differing correlations have been reported between measurements of spinal bone mineral made with QCT and DPA in apparently similar groups of patients. Sambrook et al. (1985) compared the DPA and QCT methods for the measurement of spinal bone mineral in a population of 44 human subjects, including normals and patients with vertebral crush fractures. QCT was performed in the lumbar vertebrae (L2, L3, or L4) using a General Electric 8600 whole-body scanner. The bone mineral densities were based upon calibrations of K_2HPO_4 solutions simultaneously scanned, as in the method of Cann and Genant. Measurements were made in the largest circular area of trabecular bone that could be found within the cortical envelope of an intact vertebra. The results were expressed in mg/cc of trabecular bone. The anteroposterior and transverse diameters of the vertebral bodies were measured, and the cross-sectional area (CSA) of the vertebral body was calculated using the formula for the area of an ellipse. The authors found a moderately good correlation (r = 0.80) between QCT and DPA values of the spine when these methods were applied in the same subject and to the same vertebra. The DPA and QCT methods showed a reasonable correlation in the cross-sectional study, but there remains the need to assess their usefulness by comparative longitudinal studies for predicting bone loss.

Some of the possible reasons for the differences in correlation found between QCT and DPA may be found in the methods of edge detection used, the comparison of nonsimilar quantities, and the presence of bone irregularities in some of the measurements. In addition, the method of correcting BMC to a density value involves the use of an approximate rather than the true volume. QCT measures only trabecular bone in the vertebral body, whereas DPA measures both cortical and trabecular components of the vertebrae. In addition, in osteoporotic patients, regional demineralization of trabecular bone in the vertebral body may result in more striking abnormalities in QCT measurements than in DPA of the whole vertebra (Powell et al., 1983). However, because of the suggested increases of the vertebral marrow fat content in osteoporotic patients, the apparent deficit of bone mineral may be exaggerated much more severely in QCT measurements than in DPA measurements (Mazess, 1984). The repositioning errors associated with the use of CT densitometry (and x-ray tube sources), even with 1.0 cm slices, may exceed 10% (Mazess, 1979) unless special positioning techniques and bone-edge detection routines are used.

Chesnut et al. (1983) compared bone mass measurements by three methods (SPA, CT, DPA) to the total-body calcium (TBCa) determination by neutron activation analysis. The TBCa method measures total skeletal mass: 80% compact bone, 20% trabecular bone. Data on postmenopausal osteoporotic females resulted in the following correlations.

	r	*p value*	*n*
CT (spine) vs. TBCa	0.44	< 0.05	18
SPA (radius) vs. TBCa	0.57	< 0.05	26
DPA (spine) vs. TBCa	0.95	< 0.001	5
CT (spine) vs. SPA (radius)	0.41	NS	20

These data show that the strongest correlation ($r = 0.95$) resulted from the use of the dual-photon absorptiometry method, although the number of determinations was limited (five). It is interesting to note that previous studies have shown good correlations between the DPA and QCT measurements in the spinal vertebrae, but it is apparent that this study reflects a poor correlation between QCT values and TBCa values for osteoporotic subjects. This implies that further investigations of the two methods is required in both normal and osteoporotic populations.

Bone mass has recently been investigated in a population of postmenopausal women using four techniques: SPA, DPA, QCT, and TBNAA (Ott et al., 1986). The bone mineral content was measured by single-photon absorptiometry (Norland-Cameron Bone Mineral Analyzer, Model 178) using an ^{125}I source. The radius was measured at two sites, one-tenth and one-fifth the length of the forearm proximal to the styloid process. Each site was scanned twice, and the mean value was recorded. The precision was 2% to 3% in normal subjects. In this study, TBNAA was performed to measure the total-skeletal calcium in grams. The subjects were counted in the total-body counter at the University of Washington. Using cadavers, the precision was 2%. The long-term precision using a phantom was 2% over a 10-year period. The dual-photon method (DPA) was used in the lumbar vertebrae and consisted of a modified Ohio-Nuclear scanner and a ^{153}Gd source. The average coefficient of variation in normal subjects over a 3-year period was 3.9%. The QCT measurements in the study were performed on two computed tomography units (GE 8800 and GE 9800 scanners). The precision as determined in an anthropomorphic phantom was 3.5% for the GE 8800 unit and 4.8% for the GE 9800.

A difference of 15% was found between the BMC values measured on the two CT units; the values from the GE 8800 were adjusted (increased) by 15% in order to intercompare the results on both machines for longitudinal studies. Although some reports have stated that the results from one CT scanner could be compared to normal values from another unit (Genant et al., 1983), Ott and coworkers found considerable variability in the QCT measurements when different CT scanners were used, even when using the same calibration phantom. This finding supports the idea that inherently different results are obtained on different CT scanners and that it is inappropriate to assume that the direct intercomparison of BMC values can be made.

In this clinical study, women receiving two treatment regimens were compared by performing measurements at an interval of 1 year. The changes in the DPA and QCT bone mineral values were significantly lower than the baseline values after 1 year. However, the changes observed using one technique did not show significant correlations with the changes observed using the other methods. This study demonstrated that the precisions of these methods, as used in the clinical setting, were not sufficient to show correlations after only 1 year of treatment. It was suggested that multiple measurements over a prolonged period of time might overcome the errors in reproducibility.

The scattering methods provide the only direct determination of the physical density of bone. The major disadvantage is the fact that this density represents both the bone tissue and the marrow components. However, none of the previously discussed methods separates marrow composition from compact and trabecular bone. Additionally, the CT methods, in which compact and trabecular bone are separated, similarly share the problem of the presence of variable marrow composition. Several Compton-scatter imaging systems, unlike the fixed-point Compton-scatter devices, have been found to require relatively high radiation doses (5 to 10 rem) for the production of clinically diagnostic images.

The fixed-point Compton-scatter methods have not received the attention that imaging methods have received, possibly because of the complexities associated with the detection and analysis of Compton-scattered radiation. Fixed-point Compton-scatter devices require lower radiation doses (300 to 500 mrem) as compared with the imaging devices. The Compton-backscatter method has been suggested as a clinically simple method for bone densitometry in the spinal vertebrae. However, technical problems, such as the appropriate correction for multiple scattering, have prevented the further improvement of the precision and accuracy of the method.

The electron densities of tissues can be determined by the extent of Compton-scattering produced by the incident radiation. The fixed-point Compton-scatter method can be used for the accurate in vivo measurement of the electron density of bone tissues within the human body. However, at the present time, the method has not been performed on humans in vivo, except in the peripheral skeleton. Compton-scattering measurements of bone density have been done in trabecular areas of the distal radius and calcaneous, but not in the spine (Mazess, 1979). Some investigators, however, are studying the feasibility of the Compton-scattering method for vertebral measurements.

Scattering methods, like all densitometry methods, do not measure the density of bone mineral alone, but of all tissue components within the defined scattering volume. Although the scattering volume may be confined to the trabecular region of the vertebrae or other bones, corrections for attenuation by the surrounding cortical bone must be determined. In addition, the detected single-scattered photons include those scattered from marrow fat and other components within the vertebrae. Dual-energy Compton-scattering methods may eliminate the need for attenuation corrections, but these methods remain to be tested in the clinical environment. The Compton-scattering method is subject to two sources of error, for which corrections can be applied: (1) effects of overlying tissues and (2) multiple-scattering. The errors can be minimized by the use of high-energy incident radiation sources, but at the expense of increased radiation doses.

The statistical precision of the Compton-scattering methods is typically 1%, and the reproducibility precision error is 3% to 5%. The precision and accuracy errors for phantoms and for in vitro specimens is 1%. The radiation dose for the various Compton-scattering geometries ranges from 200 to 2000 mrem and is small for low-energy sources and high for sources such as ^{137}Cs.

The coherent/Compton-scatter ratio method provides a reliable measurement, having similar precision and accuracy as the Compton-scatter method. However, a high-resolution germanium detector is required for the measurement. The coherent/Compton ratio method has been used by M. Greenfield (Univ. of California, Los Angeles) and others for in vivo measurements of both the distal radius and the os calcis, but the accuracy has been found to be affected by multiple scattering and other factors. The precision of the method has been reported as 4% in vivo. Large changes in marrow composition, which result from prolonged patient immobilization, have been recognized as a problem for these noninvasive bone measurements. The coherent/Compton-scatter methods may, however, represent an improvement in accuracy and precision over more conventional scattering methods while providing a reduced radiation dose.

All of the methods presented here are noninvasive (except histomorphometry) but expose the patient to radiation risks. Radiogrammetry and photodensitometry involve minimal radiation exposure, with negligible bone marrow or gonadal radiation dosage. The single-photon absorptiometric method delivers a radiation dose of 2 to 5 mrad to the limb (usually the forearm). The body dose from SPA is negligible, because there is virtually no scattered radiation. The dual-photon absorptiometry method delivers a radiation dose of 5 to 15 mrad. The radiation dose to the ovaries is less than 2 mrad, and the bone marrow dose is less than 0.2 mrad. However, when spinal radiographs are taken for the purpose of localization of the measurement site, this additional radiation dose must be considered. The radiation dose from the quantitative computed tomography method is significantly greater; a 10 cm region of the upper abdomen receives 200 to 250 mrad, which is one-tenth the dose required for a standard lumbar CT. The gonadal dose from QCT is less than 10 mrad. It should be noted that some institutions have reported surface radiation doses up to 10 times greater, while others have reported half the doses stated above. Total-body neutron activation analysis requires higher radiation doses, on the order of 300 to 5000 mrad. Partial-body neutron activation analysis requires proportionately smaller doses. By comparison, a routine chest radiograph delivers an exposure of 20 to 40 mrad (Kimmel, 1984).

The treatment of bone disease in the elderly is a challenging and important field for further clinical research. The geriatric patient represents a patient with complex characteristics resulting from poor vitamin D intake, poor nutrition, reduced exposure to sunlight, and reduced physical activity, all of which may contribute to osteoporosis or osteomalacia. In addition, the normally expected changes in endocrinology and bone physiology that are associated with aging interact with all these factors. The noninvasive bone measurement methods discussed in this book offer the promise of important data in the years to come. It is, therefore, important that research support continue and increase at a time when the elderly population in the U.S. is increasing in number.

In considering all the methods represented here, it is not possible to choose a single measurement that provides the physician or researcher with complete information regarding the bone status of the skeleton. At the present time, there appears to be no single quantitative method that is capable of providing an unequivocal diagnosis or that is capable of precisely defining normal bone mineral content at all sites of the skeleton. Several of these methods, however, provide the ability for evaluating bone mass or bone mineral density at selected skeletal sites. Many of the methods are correlated with each other at some sites and not at other sites. Some methods are not intercorrelated well enough for use at multiple sites. We are, therefore, required to select the appropriate densitometry method for the appropriate skeletal measurement site. However, by using several of these appropriately chosen methods for each patient evaluation, we may increase our diagnostic abilities in the area of metabolic bone disease.

Bone densitometry methods, therefore, must still be classified as experimental, although useful, indicators of the presence of bone disease. Densitometry may also be useful for monitoring skeletal changes that result from treatments for various bone-related diseases. Most of these densitometry methods are useful in longitudinal or population studies but have somewhat limited value on an individual patient basis. There is still a definite need for an inexpensive and accurate method of detecting skeletal changes in the axial and appendicular skeleton, which will allow the monitoring of the treatment for bone disorders. However, the utilization of the present methods within the clinical environment adds to our collective understanding of the meaning of densitometry data. As further improvements are made in the detection of radiation and in the use of the physical principles of densitometry, advances will lead to better accuracy, precision, and specificity in bone mineral measurements.

At the present time, two methods are commonly used for the accurate measurement of bone mineral content and follow-up of patients — dual-photon absorptiometry (DPA) and quantitative computed tomography; (QCT) (Kimmel, 1984). Both of these procedures may be used for evaluation of the central (axial) skeleton. The American College of Physicians recommends the dual-photon absorptiometry method (DPA) as the best procedure for the recognition and follow-up of patients with osteoporosis (Davies and Saha, 1985).

Recognizing that each densitometric method has specific limitations, the investigator and the clinician alike must carefully analyze these recommendations, seeking out the advantages and disadvantages of the methods and finding the method or combination of methods that best satisfy the needs of the clinic or the research study. Over the years, some bone densitometry methods have proved disappointing in their diagnostic capabilities. However, osteoporosis and other bone-related diseases are complex by their very nature, and it is therefore important to realize that the noninvasive measurement of bone characteristics must be progressively developed and perfected through the clinical use and improvement of its diagnostic potential. Progress in bone densitometry has been made over the years, and it is hoped that these radiological methods will continue to improve our diagnostic capabilities in bone disease.

REFERENCES

1. Abols Y, Genant HK, Rosenfeld D et al. Spinal bone mineral determination using computerized tomography in patients, controls, and phantoms. In: Mazess RB (ed). Proceedings of the 4th International Conference on Bone Measurement, NIH Pub. 80-1928. Washington, DC, US Government Printing Office, 1980, p 297.
2. Adams P, Davies GT, Sweetnam PM, Observer error and measurements of the metacarpal. Br J Radiol 42:192, 1969.
3. Aitken M. Osteoporosis in clinical practice. Wright, Bristol, 1984.
4. Aloia JF, Vaswani A, Atkins H, Zanzi I, Ellis K, Cohn SH. Radiographic morphometry and osteopenia in spinal osteoporosis. J Nucl Med 18:425, 1977.
5. Aloia JF, Ellis K, Zanzi I, and Cohn SH. Photon absorptiometry and skeletal mass in the treatment of osteoporosis. J Nucl Med 16:196, 1975.
6. Aloia JF, Cohn SH, Vaswani A, Yeh JK, Yuen K and Ellis K. Risk factors for postmenopausal osteoporosis. Am J Med 78:95, 1985.
7. Aloia JF, Vaswani A, Kapoor A, Yeh JK and Cohn SH. Treatment of osteoporosis with calcitonin, with and without growth hormone. Metabolism 34(2):124, 1985.
8. Als OS, Gotfredsen A and Christiansen C. The effect of glucocorticoids on bone mass in rheumatoid arthritis patients. Arthritis Rheum 28(4):369, 1985.
9. Alwens W. Spatrachitis, osteomalazie, senile osteoporose, hungerosteopathie. In: Bergmann G, Staehelin R (eds). Handbuch der Inneren Medizin. Springer, Berlin, p 584, 1926.
10. Albright F, Smith PH, Richardson AM. Postmenopausal osteoporosis: its clinical features. JAMA 116:2465, 1941.
11. Am College of Physicians, Position Paper. Ann Int Med 100:908, 1984.
12. Anderson J, Osborne SB, Tomlinson RWS, Newton D, Rundo J, Salmon L and Smith JW. Neutron activation analysis in man in vivo. Lancet 2:1201, 1964.
13. Andresen J and Nielsen HE. Metacarpal bone mass in normal adults and in patients with chronic renal failure. Acta Radiol 22(6):715, 1981.
14. Andresen J and Nielsen HE. Interrelationship between metacarpal bone mass and bone mineral content in nondialyzed and dialyzed patients with chronic renal failure. Clin Orthop 166:104, 1982.

15. Anton HC. Width of clavicular cortex in osteoporosis. Br Med J 1:409, 1969.
16. Archer-Hall JA, Carpenter PB, Edwards JP and Francois PE. A new method of bone mineral estimation using a conventional x-ray set. Br J Radiol 46:375, 1973.
17. Armstrong WD and Singer L. Composition and constitution of the mineral phase of bone. Clin Orthop 38:179, 1965.
18. Arnold JS. Focal excessive endosteal resorption in aging and senile osteoporosis. In: Osteoporosis. Barzel US (ed). Grune and Stratton, New York, p 80, 1970.
19. Atkinson PJ and Weatherall JA. Variation on the density of the femoral diaphysis with age. J Bone Joint Surg 49-B:781, 1967.
20. Avioli LV. Osteoporosis. JAMA 252(6):799, 1984.
21. Baker PT, Schraer H and Yalman RG. The accuracy of human bone composition determined from reontgenograms. Photogram Engr 25:455, 1959.
22. Banks LM and Stevenson JC. Modified method of spinal computed tomography for trabecular bone mineral measurements. J Comput Assist Tomogr 10(3):463, 1986.
23. Banzer D, Schneider U, Wegener OH, Oeser H and Pleul O. Quantitative mineralsalzbestimmung im Wirbelkorper mittels computertermorgraphie. ROFO 130:77, 1979
24. Barnett E and Nordin BEC. The radiological diagnosis of osteoporosis: a new approach. Clin Radiol 11:166, 1960.
25. Battista JJ and Bronskill MJ. Compton-scatter tissue densitometry: calculation of single and multiple scatter photon fluences. Phys Med Biol 23(1):1, 1978.
26. Battista JJ, Santon LW and Bronskill MJ. Compton scatter imaging of transverse sections. Corrections for multiple scatter and attenuations. Phys Med Biol 22(2):229, 1977.
27. Battista JJ and Bronskill MJ. Compton scatter imaging of transverse sections: an overall appraisal and evaluation for radiotherapy planning. Phys Med Biol 26(1):81, 1981.
28. Bauer GC. The use of radionuclides in orthopedics. J Bone Joint Surg. 50A:1681, 1968.
29. Bell GH, Dunbar O, Beck JS and Gibb A. Variations in strength of vertebrae with age and their relation to osteoporosis. Calcif Tissue Res 1:75, 1967.
30. Black DM, Daniels AU, Dunn HK and Kruger RA. Computerized tomographic determination of vertebral density after total hip arthoplasty. Clin Orthop 198:259, 1985.
31. Blitz RM and Pelligrano ED. The chemical anatomy of bone. I. A comparative study of bone composition in sixteen vertebrates. J Bone Joint Surg 51A:456, 1969.
32. Bloom RA and Laws JW. Humeral cortical thickness as an index of osteoporosis in women. Br J Radiol 43:522, 1970.
33. Bloom RA, Pogrund H and Libson E. Radiogrammetry of the metacarpal: a critical reappraisal. Skeletal Radiol 10:5, 1983.
34. Boddy K. Proc. Symp. Bad Gastein, Urban and Schwarzenberg, Munich 7:377, 1966.
35. Boddy K, Holloway I and Elliot A. A simple facility for total body in vivo activation analysis. Int J Appl Radiat Isot 24:428, 1973.
36. Boddy K. Bibliography on in vivo activation analysis. Scottish Universities Res and Reactor Center (SURRC) 65:78, 1978.
37. Bohr H and Schaadt O. Bone mineral content of the femoral neck and shaft: relation between cortical and trabecular bone. Calcif Tissue Int 37:340, 1985.
38. Brassow F, Crone-Munzebrock W, Weh L et al. Correlations between breaking load and CT absorption values of vertebral bodies. Eur J Radiol 2:99, 1982.
39. Briancon D and Meunier PJ. Treatment of osteoporosis with fluoride, calcium and vitamin D. Orthop Clin North Am 12:629, 1981.
40. Burkinshaw L. Private communication, 1985.
41. Cameron JR, Mazess RB and Sorenson JA. Precision and accuracy of bone mineral determination by direct photon absorptiometry. Invest Radiol 3:141, 1968.
42. Cameron JR and Sorenson J. Measurement of bone mineral in vivo: an improved method. Science 142:230, 1963.
43. Cann CE. Low-dose CT scanning for quantitative spinal mineral analysis. Radiology 140:813, 1981.
44. Cann CE and Genant HK. Precise measurement of vertebral mineral content using computed tomography. J Comput Assist Tomogr 4(4):493, 1980.
45. Cann CE, Genant HK and Boyd DP. Vertebral mineral determination by CT: Clinical results and specimen studies. Proceedings of the 65th Scientific Assembly, Radiological Society of North America, Atlanta, Georgia. J Comput Assist Tomogr 3(6):847, 1979.

46. Cann CE, Genant HK, Kolb FO and Ettinger BE. Quantitative computer tomography for prediction of vertebral fracture risk. Metab Bone Dis Relat Res 5:1, 1984.
47. Cann CE, Genant HK and Young DR. Comparison of vertebral and peripheral mineral losses in disuse osteoporosis in monkeys. Radiology 134:525, 1980.
48. Catto GRD, McIntosh JAR, MacDonald AF and MacLeod M. Hemodialysis therapy and changes in skeletal calcium. Lancet 1:1150, 1973.
49. Catto GRD, McIntosh JAR and Macleod M. Partial body neutron activation analysis in vivo: a new approach to the investigation of metabolic bone disease. Phys Med Biol 18:508, 1973.
50. Cesareo R. Analysis of silver alloys by elastic and inelastic scattering of gamma rays. Nucl Instr Meth 179:545, 1981.
51. Chalmers J, Conacher WDH, Gardner DL et al. Osteomalacia — a common disease in elderly women. J Bone Joint Surg (Brit) 49B:403, 1967.
52. Chalmers J. Distribution of osteoporotic changes in the aging skeleton. Clin Endocrinol Metab 2:203, 1973.
53. Chalmers J and Ho KC. Geographical variatons in senile osteoporosis. The association with physical activity. J Bone Joint Surg 52-B(4):667, 1970.
54. Chamberlain MJ, Fremlin JH, Peters DK and Phillip H. Total body calcium by whole-body neutron activation: new technique for study of bone disease. Br Med. J.2:581, 1968.
55. Chesney RW, Mazess RB, Rose PG and Jax DK. Bone mineral status measured by direct photon absorptiometry in childhood renal disease. Pediatrics 60:864, 1977.
56. Chesney RW and Shore. The noninvasive determination of bone mineral content by photon absorptiometry. Am J Dis Child 136:578, 1982.
57. Chesney RW. Current clinical applications of vitamin D metabolite research. In: Clinical Orthopedics and Related Research. Urist MR (ed). JB Lippincott Co., Philadelphia, p 285, 1981.
58. Chesnut CH, Nelp WB, Baylink DJ and Denney JD. Effect of methandrostenolone on postmenopausal bone wasting as assessed by changes in total bone mineral mass. Metabolism 26:267, 1977.
59. Chesnut CH, Hanson JA, Kilcoyne RF, Murano R, Lewellen TK, Nelp WB, Mack L, Grahan MM and Hu B. Bone mass assessment at differing skeletal sites by multiple diagnostic parameters. Proceedings of the 30th Annual Mtg, J Nucl Med 24(5):P58, 1983.
60. Christiansen C, Rodbro P and Jensen GF. Bone mineral content in the forearm measured by photon absorptiometry. Scand J Clin Lab Invest 35:323, 1975.
61. Christiansen C and Rodbro P. Long-term reproducibility of bone mineral content measurements. Scand J Clin Lab Invest 37:321, 1977.
62. Christiansen C, Christiansen MS, Rodbro P, Hagen C and Transbol I. Effect of 1, 25-dihydroxy-vitamin D3 in itself or combined with hormone treatment in preventing postmenopausal osteoporosis. Eur J Clin Invest 11(4):305, 1981.
63. Clarke RL. A gamma ray scanner for diagnostic radiography. Chalk River, Ontario. AECL 2270, 1965.
64. Clarke RL and Van Dyk G. The use of Compton-scattered gamma radiatopn in diagnostic radiography. Medical Radioisotope Scintigraphy, IAEA Vienna STI/PUB 193, p 247, 1969.
65. Clarke RL and Van Dyk G. A new method for measurement of bone mineral content using both transmitted and scattered beams of gamma-rays. Phys Med Biol 18:532, 1973.
66. Clarke RL. Conference on Application of Optical Instrumentation in Medicine, Kansas City, 1974.
67. Clarke RL, Milne ENC and Van Dyk G. The use of Compton scattered rays for tomography. Invest Radiol 11:225, 1976.
68. Cockshott WP, Occleshaw CJ, Webber C, Walter SD and O'Brien K. Can a calcaneal morphologic index determine the degree of osteoporosis? Skeletal Radiol 12:119, 1984.
69. Cohn SH. In: Progress in Atomic Medicine. Vol. 1, Grune and Stratton, New York p 1, 1965.
70. Cohn SH, Dombrowski CS, Pate HR et al. A whole body counter with an invariant response to radionuclide distribution and body size. Phys Med Biol 14:645, 1969.
71. Cohn SH, Dombrowski CS and Fairchild RG. In vivo neutron activation analysis of calcium in man. Int J Appl Radiat Isot 21:127, 1970.
72. Cohn SH and Dombrowski CS. Measurement of total-body calcium, sodium, chlorine, nitrogen, and phosphorus in man by in vivo neutron activation analysis. J Nucl Med

12(7):499, 1971.

73. Cohn SH, Shukla KK, Dombrowski CS and Fairchild RG. Design and calibration of a "broad-beam" ^{238}Pu, Be neutron source for total-body neutron activation analysis. J Nucl Med 13:487, 1972.
74. Cohn SH, Ellis KJ, Wallach S, Zanzi I, Atkins HL and Aloia JF. Absolute and relative deficit in total-skeletal calcium and radial bone mineral in osteoporosis. J Nucl Med 15:428, 1974.
75. Cohn SH, Ellis KJ, Caselnova RC, Asad SN and Letteri JM. Correlation of radial bone mineral content and total body calcium in chronic renal failure. J Lab Clin Med 86:910, 1975.
76. Cohn SH, Vaswani A, Zanzi I, Aloia JF, Roginsky MS and Ellis KJ. Changes in body chemical composition with age measured by total-body neutron activation. Metabolism 25:85, 1976.
77. Cohn SH. Retrospect and Prospects. In: Non-invasive Measurements of Bone Mass and Their Clinical Application. Cohn SH (ed). CRC Press, Boca Raton, Florida, p 222, 1981.
78. Cohn SH, Aloia JF, Vaswani AN, Yuen K, Yasumura S and Ellis KJ. Women at risk for developing osteoporosis: determination by total body neutron activation analysis and photon absorptiometry. Calcif Tissue Int 38:9, 1986.
79. Colbert C, Mazess RB and Schmidt PB. Bone mineral determination in vitro by radiographic photodensitometry and direct photon absorptiometry. Invest Radiol 5:336, 1970.
80. Colbert C and Bachtell RS. Radiographic absorptiometry (photodensitometry). In: Non-invasive Measurements of Bone Mass and Their Clinical Application. Cohn SH (ed). CRC Press, Boca Raton, Florida, p 51, 1981.
81. Comar D, Riviere R, Raynaud C and Kellershon C. Radioaktive isotope in klinik and forschung. Urban and Schwarzenberg, Munich 8:186, 1968.
82. Compton AH. A Quantum theory of the scattering of X-rays by light elements. Phys Rev 21:483, 1923.
83. Conrad B. Theoretical concepts and experimental data in Compton densitometry. Prog Resp Res 11:33, 1979.
84. Custer RP. An atlas of the blood and bone marrow. WB Saunders, Philadelphia, 1974.
85. DaCosta M, DeLaney M and Goldsmith SJ. Reproducibility of dual-photon absorptiometry using a clinical phantom. Proceedings of the 32nd Annual Meeting. J Nucl Med 26(5):P23, 1985.
86. Dalen N and Jacobsen B. Bone mineral assay: Choice of measuring sites. Invest Radiol 9:174, 1974.
87. Dalen N and Lamke B. Grading of osteoporosis by skeletal roentgenology and bone scanning. Acta Radiol 15:177, 1974.
88. Daniel H. The muon as a tool for scanning the interior of the human body. Nuclearmedizin 8:311, 1969.
89. Davies R and Saha S. Osteoporosis. Am Fam Physician 32(5):107, 1985.
90. Dequeker J. Periosteal and endosteal surface remodeling in pathologic conditions. Invest Radiol 6:260, 1971.
91. Dequeker J. Bone loss in normal and pathological conditions. Leuven University Press, Leuven, Belgium, p 124, 1972.
92. Dequeker J, Gautama K and Roh YS. Femoral trabecular patterns in asymptomatic spinal osteoporosis and femoral neck fracture. Clin Radiol 25:243, 1974.
93. Dequeker, J. Problems in measuring amount of bone: reproducibility, variability, sequential evaluation. In: Bone Histomorphometry. Meunier PJ (ed), Second International Workshop. Armour Montagu, Paris, p 19, 1977.
94. Dequeker, J. Influence of sampling, sex, age, skeletal size on the variability of radiogrammatic bone mass values. In: Noninvasive Bone Measurements: Methodological Problems. Dequeker J, Johnston CL (eds). Proceedings of the Workshop on Noninvasive Bone Measurements, the XVI European Symposium on Calcified Tissue Research. IRL Press, Knokke, Belgium, p 107, 1982.
95. Dobbins JT, Mazess RB and Cameron JR. Scanning-slit X-ray videoabsorptiometry for measurement of bone-mineral content. Med Phys 8(4):563, 1981.
96. Dobbins JT, Pedersen PL, Mazess RB, Cameron JR, Hansen JL and Hefner LV. A scanning slit x-ray videoabsorptiometric technique for bone mineral measurement. Med Phys 11(5):582, 1984.
97. Dohring W. Quantitative analyses of regional pulmonary ventilation using Compton densito-

metry and computed tomography. Prog Resp Res 11:48, 1979.
98. Doyle FH, Gutteridge DH, Joplin GF and Fraser R. An assessment of radiological criteria used in the study of spinal osteoporosis. Br J Radiol 40:241, 1967.
99. Doyle FH. Involutional osteoporosis. In: Clinics in Endocrinology and Metabolism — Calcium Metabolism and Bone Disease. MacIntyre I (ed). WB Saunders, London, p 143, 1972.
100. Duke PR and Hanson JA. Compton scatter densitometry with polychromatic sources. Med Phys 11(5):624, 1984.
101. Dunnhill MS, Anderson JA and Whitehead R. Quantitative histological studies on age changes in bone. J Pathol 94:275, 1967.
102. Dunn WL, Wahner HW and Riggs BL. Measurement of bone mineral content in human vertebrae and hip by dual photon absorptiometry. Radiology 136:485, 1980.
103. Dunscombe PB, Datz DE and Stacey AJ. Some practical aspects of dual-energy CT scanning. Br J Radiol 57:82, 1984.
104. Dyson ED and Whitehouse WL. The composition of traebecular bone in children. In: Symposium Ossium, Jellifee AM, Strickland P (eds). ES Livingstone, Edinburgh, p 62, 1970.
105. Eastell R, Kennedy NS, Smith MA, Tothill P and Anderton JL. Changes in total body calcium after renal transplantation: effect of low-dose steroid regime. Nephron 40:139, 1985.
106. Eilbert RF, Koehler AM, Sisterson JM, Wilson R and Adelstein SJ. Partial body calcium determination in bone by proton activation analysis. Phys Med Biol 22(5):817, 1977.
107. Elias C, Heaney RP and Recker RR. Placebo therapy for postmenopausal osteoporosis. Calcif Tissue Int 37:6, 1985.
108. Ettinger B, Genant HK, Gordon GS and Cann CE. Bone determination in oophorectomized women. In: Proceedings of the CT Densitometry Workshop, San Francisco, Calif. J Comput Assist Tomogr 3(6):847, 1979.
109. Evans RA, McDonnell GD and Shibe M. Metacarpal cortical area as an index of bone mass. Br J Radiol 51:428, 1978.
110. Exner GU, Prader MD, Elsasser U, Ruegsegger P and Anliker M. Bone densitometry using computer tomography. Part I: Selective determination of trabecular bone density and other bone mineral parameters. Normal values in children and adults. Br J Radiol 52:14, 1979.
111. Farmer FT and Collins MP. A new approach to the determination of anatomical cross-sections of the body by Compton scattered gamma-rays. Phys Med Biol 16(4):577, 1971.
112. Farmer FT and Collins MP. A further appraisal of the Compton scattering method for determining anatomical cross-sections of the body. Phys Med Biol 19(6):808, 1974.
113. Faul DD, Couch JL, Cann CE, Boyd DP and Genant HK. Composition-selective reconstruction for mineral content in the axial and appendicular skeleton. In: Proceedings of the Second CT Densitometry Workshop, Zuos, Switzerland. J Comput Assist Tomogr 6:202, 1982.
114. Firooznia H, Rafii M, Golimbu C, Schwartz MS and Ort P. Computed tomography measurement of trabecular mineral content of the spine in women with hip fracture. 1986 (in press).
115. Firooznia H, Golimbu C, Rafii M, Schwartz MS and Alterman ER. Quantitative computed tomography assessment of spinal trabecular bone. I. Age related regression in normal men and women. J Comput Assist Tomogr 8:91, 1984.
116. Firooznia H, Golimbu C, Rafii M, Schwartz MS and Alterman ER. Quantitative computed tomography assessment of spinal trabecular bone. II. In: Osteoporotic women with and without vertebral fractures. J Comput Assist Tomogr 8:99, 1984.
117. Fish HR and Dons RF. Primary Osteoporosis. Am Fam Physician 31:216, 1985.
118. Fisher E and Hausser D. Kompaktadicke von rippen und schlusselbein. Med Klin (Munich) 65:1212, 1970.
119. Fogelman I. Osteoporosis, bone mineral measurements and photon absorptiomerty. Nucl Med Comm 6(7):373, 1985.
120. Fogelman I, Bessent RG, Turner JG, Citrin DL, Boyle IT and Greig WR. The role of bone scanning in osteomalacia. J Nucl Med 19:245, 1978.
121. Fogelman I, Bessent RG, Turner JG, Citrin DL, Boyle IT and Greig WR. The use of whole-body retention of Tc-99m diphosphonate in the diagnosis of metabolic bone disease. J Nucl Med 19:270, 1978.

122. Fogelman I, Citrin DL, Turner JG, Hay ID, Bessent RG and Boyle IT. Semi-quantitative interpretation of the bone scan in metabolic bone disease: definition and validation of the metabolic index. Eur J Nucl Med 4:287, 1979.
123. Fogelman I, Bessent RG, Cohen HN, Hart AM and Lindsay R. Skeletal uptake of diphosphonate: method for prediction of post-menopausal osteoporosis. Lancet 2:667, 1980.
124. Fox KM, Tobin JD and Plato CC. Longitudinal study of bone loss in the second metacarpal. Calcif Tissue Int 39:218, 1986.
125. Friedman AM, Oltman BG, Kastner J, Eckerman KF and Goodman LS. Use of ^{244}Cm and ^{145}Pm as sources for bone mineralization studies. J Nucl Med 15:335, 1974.
126. Frost HM. Treatment of osteoporosis by manipulation of coherent bone cell populations. Clin Orthop 143:227, 1979.
127. Garn SM. The earlier gain and the later loss of cortical bone in nutritional perspective. CC Thomas, Springfield, 1970.
128. Garn SM, Rohmann CG and Wagner B. Bone loss as a general phenomenon in man. Fed Proc 26:1729, 1967.
129. Garnett ES, Kennett TJ, Kenyon DB and Webber CE. A photon scattering technique for the measurement of absolute bone density in man. Radiology 106:209, 1973.
130. Genant HK, Cohn SH, Pozzi-Mucelli RS et al. Vertebral mineral determination by quantitative CT: clinical feasibility and normative data. Proceedings of the Third International Workshop on Bone and Soft Tissue Densitometry Using Computed Tomography. J Comput Assist Tomogr 7:554, 1983.
131. Genant HK, Boyd D, Rosenfeld D, Abols Y and Cann CE. Quantitative bone mineral analysis using computed tomography. In: Non-Invasive Measurement of Bone Mass and Clinical Applications, Cohn SH (ed). CRC Press, New York, p 121, 1981.
132. Genant HK, Ettinger B, Cann CE, Reiser U, Gordan GS, Kolb FO. Osteoporosis: assessment by quantitative computed tomography. Orthop Clin North Am 16(3):557, 1985.
133. Genant HK. Assessing osteoporosis: CT's quantitative advantage. Diagnostic Imaging (Aug), 1985.
134. Genant HK, Cann CE, Boyd DP, Kolb FO, Ettinger B, and Gordan GS. Quantitative computed tomography for vertebral mineral determination. Frame B and Potts JT (eds). Proceedings of the Henry Ford Hospital Symposium on Clinical Disorders of Bone and Mineral Metabolism. Excerpta Medica, New York, p 40, 1983.
135. Genant HK, Powell MR, Cann CE, Stebler B, Rutt BK, Richardson ML and Kolb. Comparison of methods for in vivo spinal bone mineral measurements. In: Osteoporosis. Christiansen C (ed). Proceedings of the Inter Symp on Osteoporosis, Copenhagen, p 94, 1984.
136. Genant HK and Cann CE. Medical Staff Conf on Osteoporosis. West J Med 140(1):103, 1984.
137. Genant HK, Cann CE, Ettinger B and Gordan GS. Quantitative computed tomography of verbal spongiosa: a sensitive method for detecting early bone loss after oophorectomy. Ann Intern Med 97:699, 1982.
138. Genant HK, Gordan GS and Hoffman PG, Jr. Osteoporosis: Part I. Advanced radiologic assessment using quantitative computed tomography. West J Med 139:75, 1983.
139. Genant HK and Boyd D. Quantitative bone mineral analysis using dual energy computed tomography. Invest Radiol 12:545, 1977.
140. Gigante GE and Sciuti S. A large-angle coherent Compton scattering method for measurement in vitro of trabecular bone mineral concentration. Med Phys 12(3):321, 1985.
141. Glover GH and Pelc NJ. Nonlinear partial volume artifacts in x-ray computed tomography. Med Phys 7:238, 1980.
142. Giuntini C, Guzzardi R, Pistolesi M, Mey M and Solfanelli S. Evaluation of a system for 90° Compton scattering in lung tomography. Prog Resp Res 11:76, 1979.
143. Gotfredsen A, Borg J, Christiansen C and Mazess RB. Total body mineral in vivo by dual photon absorptiometry. I. Measurement procedures. Clin Physiol 4:343, 1984.
144. Goldsmith NF and Cohn SH. Bone mineral data debated (letter). Am J Radiol 128:526, 1977.
145. Gordan GS. Medical Staff Conf on Osteoporosis. West J Med 140(1):102, 1984.
146. Greenspan M. Development of black mineral density and bone area norms. Radiological Research Laboratory, Yellow Springs, Ohio (unpublished report), 1978.
147. Greer FR, Lane J, Weiner S et al. An accurate and reproducible absorptiometric technique for determining bone mineral content in newborn infants. Pediatrics Res 17:259, 1983.

148. Griffiths HJ, Zimmerman RE, Bailey G and Snider R. The use of photon absorptiometry in the diagnosis of renal osteodystrophy. Radiology 109:277, 1973.
149. Grubb SA, Jacobson PC, Awbrey BJ, McCartney WH, Vincent LM and Talmage RV. Bone density in osteopenic women: a modified distal radius density measurement procedure to develop an "at risk" value for use in screening women. J Orthop Res 2(4):322, 1984.
150. Gruber HE and Brautbar N. Metabolic bone disease and the elderly: current approach to diagnosis and therapy. Nephron 38:76, 1984.
151. Gruber HE and Baylink DJ. The diagnosis of osteoporosis. J Am Geriat Soc 29:490, 1981.
152. Gryfe CI, Exton-Smith AN, Payne PR and Wheeler EF. Pattern of development of bone in childhood and adolescence. Lancet 1:523, 1971.
153. Gryfe CI, Exton-Smith AN and Stewart RJ. Determination of the amount of bone in the metacarpal. Age Aging 1:213, 1972.
154. Gupta SM. Assessment of osteodystrophy in patients with chronic renal failure. Aust NZ J Med 13:295, 1983.
155. Gupta S, Luna E, Belsky J, Gelfman N, Miller K and Davies T. Photon absorptiometry for non-invasive measurement of bone mineral content. Clin Nucl Med 9(8):435, 1984.
156. Guzzardi R, Mey M, Pistolesi M, Solfanelli S and Giuntini C. The 90° Compton scattering tomography of the lung. J Nucl Med All Sci 22(1):11, 1978.
157. Guzzardi R and Mey M. Further appraisal and improvements of 90° Compton scattering tomography of the lung. Phys Med Biol 26(1):155, 1981.
158. Guzzardi R, Mey M and Zito F. State-of-art of Compton tomography and application to objects recognition. In: Proceedings of the Seventh Annual Conference of the IEEE Engineering in Medicine and Biology Society, Chicago, Illinois, vol 2, p 943, 1985.
159. Hangartner TN and Overton TR. Quantitative measurement of bone density using gamma-ray computed tomography. J Comput Assist Tomogr (6):1156, 1982.
160. Hangartner TN, Overton TR and Regal WM. Comparison of trabecular bone density at axial and peripheral sites using computed tomography. In: Clinical Disorders of Bone and Mineral Metabolism, Frame D and Potts JT (eds). Excerpta Medica, Amsterdam, p 54, 1983.
161. Hangartner TN and Overton TR. Workshop on CT Technology for Bone Density Measurements, Alberta, Canada, 1984.
162. Hangartner TN, Overton TR, Harley CH, Van den Berg L and Crockford PM. Skeletal challenge: an experimental study of pharmacologically induced changes in bone density in the distal radius, using gamma-ray computed tomography. Calcif Tissue Int 37:19, 1985.
163. Hansson T, Roos B and Nachemson A. The bone mineral content and ultimate compressive strength of lumbar vertebrae. Spine 5:46, 1980.
164. Hansson T and Roos B. The influence of age, height and weight on the bone mineral coontent in lumbar vertebrae. Spine 5(6):545, 1980.
165. Hansson T and Roos B. The bone mineral content of the lumbar spine at the occurrence of the first vertebral crush fracture. Clin Orthop, 1986 (in press).
166. Hanson JE. In: Analysis of ^{153}Gd and of ^{125}I/^{241}Am sources. Proceedings of the Inter Conf Bone Min Meas, DHEW 75–683, Washington, DC, 1974.
167. Hanson JA, Moore WE, Figley MM and Duke PR. Compton scatter with polychromatic sources for lung densitometry. Med Phys 11(5):633, 1984.
168. Harding G, Strecker H and Tischler R. Philips Tech Rev 41:46, 1983.
169. Harding G. On the sensitivity and application possibilities of a noval Compton scatter imaging system. IEEE Trans Nucl Sci NS-29(3):1260, 1982.
170. Harding G and Tischler R. Dual-energy Compton scatter tomography. Phys Med Biol 31(5):477, 1986.
171. Harrison JE, McNeill KG, Meema HE, Oreopoulos D, Rabinovich S, Fenton S and Wilson DR. Partial body calcium measurements on patients with renal failure. Metabolism 26(3):255, 1977.
172. Harrison JE, McNeill KG, Hitchman AJ and Britt BA. Bone mineral measurements of the central skeleton by in vivo neutron activation analysis for routine investigation of osteopenia. Invest Radiol 14:27, 1979.
173. Harrison JE, Neutron activation studies and the effect of exercise on osteoporosis. J Medicine 15(4):285, 1984.
174. Hartsock RJ, Smith EB and Petty CS. Normal variations with aging of the amount of hematopoietic tissue in bone marrow from the anteroiliac crest; a study made from 177 cases of

sudden death examined by necropsy. Am J Clin Pathol 43:236, 1965.
175. Hazan G, Leichter I, Loewinger E and Weinreb A. The early detection of osteoporosis by Compton gamma ray spectroscopy. Phys Med Biol 22:1073, 1977.
176. Heaney RP. Estrogens and post-menopausal osteoporosis. Clin Obstet Gynecol 19:791, 1976.
177. Helela T. Age-dependent variations of the cortical thickness of the clavicle. Ann Clin Res 1:140, 1969.
178. Helela T. Combined cortical thickness and cortical index in various age groups. Ann Clin Res 2:420, 1970.
179. Hemmingsson A, Jung B, Ytterbergh C. Dual energy computed tomography: simulated monoenergetic and material-selective imaging. J Comput Assist Tomogr 10(3):490, 1986.
180. Heron JF, Sabatier JP, Bouvard G et al. Densitometrie osseuse femorale. Premiers resultats. J Fr Biophys Med Nucl 2:85, 1978.
181. Heuck F. and Schmidt E. Bestimmung des mineral gehaltes des knochen aus dem roentgenbild. Fortschr Roentgenstr 93:523, 1960.
182. Holder LE. Radionuclide bone imaging in the evaluation of bone pain. J Bone Joint Surg 64A:1391, 1982.
193. Holt RS, Kouris K, Cooper MJ and Jackson DF. Assessment of gamma ray scattering for the characterization of biological material. Phys Med Biol 28(12):1435, 1983.
184. Horsman A, Bulusu L, Bentley HB et al. Internal relationships between skeletal parameters in twenty-three male skeletons. In: Proc of Bone Meas Conf. Cameron JR (ed). US Atomic Energy Comm, Conf 700515. US Dept of Commerce, Springfield, Virginia, p 365, 1970.
185. Horsman A and Kirby PA. The geometric properties of the second metacarpal. Calcif Tissue Res 10:289, 1972.
186. Horsman A and Simpson M. The measurement of sequential changes in cortical bone geometry. Br J Radiol 48:471, 1975.
187. Horsman A, Reading DH, Connolly J, Bateman E, Glasglow W, and McLachlan MSF. Bone imaging using a gadolinum-153 source and a xenon-filled multiwire proportional counter as detector. Am J Roentgenol 126:1273, 1976.
188. Horsman A. Bone mass. In: Calcium, Phosphate and Magnesium Metabolism. Nordin BEC (ed). Churchill Livingstone, Edinburgh, p 357, 1976.
189. Horsman A, Nordin BEC, Gallagher JC, Kirby PA, Milner RM and Simpson M. Observations of sequential changes in bone mass in postmenopausal women: a controlled trial of oestrogen and calcium therapy. Calcif Tissue Res 22:217, 1977.
190. Horsman A, Simpson M, Kirby PA and Nordin BEC. Non-linear bone loss in oophorectomized women. Br J Radiol 50:504, 1977.
191. Horsman A, Burkinshaw L, Pearson D, Oxby CB and Milner RM. Estimating total body calcium from peripheral bone measurements. Calcif Tissue Int 35:135, 1983.
192. Horsman A and Currey JD. Estimating of mechanical properties of the distal radius from bone mineral content and cortical width. Clin Orthop 176:298, 1983.
193. Hosie CJ. Does bone measurement on the radius indicate skeletal status? (letter). J Nucl Med 25(10):1151, 1984.
194. Hospital Physicists' Association. Measurement of the performance characteristics of diagnostic x-ray systems used in medicine. Part III. The physical specifications of CT x-ray scanners. London: Hospital Physicists' Association, p 10, 1981.
195. Huang HK, O'Malley S, Kendrick M and Suarez F. A CT study of bone mineral changes in the lower extremities of human amputees. In: Proceedings of the 4th International Conference on Bone Measurement. Toronto. Am J Roentgenol 131:539, 1979.
196. Hubbell JH, Veigele WJ, Biggs EA, Brown RT, Cromer DT and Howerton RJ. Atomic form factors, incoherent scattering functions, and photon scattering cross sections. J Phys Chem Ref Data 4:471, 1975.
197. Huddleston AL, Agarwal SK, Friesen E and Bhaduri D. Assessment of bone density using the single-source Compton scattering technique. Appl Radiol 7:232, 1978.
198. Huddleston AL and Bhaduri D. Compton scatter densitometry in cancellous bone. Phys Med Biol 24(2):310, 1979.
199. Huddleston AL, Bhaduri D and Weaver JB. Geometrical considerations for Compton scatter densitometry. Med Phys 6(6):519, 1979.
200. Huddleston AL and Weaver JB. Dual-energy Compton-scatter densitometry. Int J Appl

Radiat Isot 34(7):977, 1983.
201. Huddleston AL and Sackler JP. The determination of electron density by the dual-energy Compton scatter method. Med Phys 12(1):13, 1985.
202. Huddleston AL, Posteraro RH, Sackler JP and Dunn SE. Determination of multiple- and single-scatter fractions in Compton-scatter densitometry. Appl Radiat Isot 37(11):1095, 1986.
203. Hutson RL, Reidy JJ, Springer K, Daniel H and Knowles HB. Tissue chemical analysis with muonic x-rays. Radiology 120:193, 1976.
204. ICRP Publ 23. Report of the Task Group on Reference Man, Oxford, Permagon, 1975.
205. Imamura K and Fujii M. Empirical beam hardening correction in the measurement of vertebral bone mineral content by computed tomography. Radiology 138:223, 1981.
206. Imamura K and Masamichi F. Empirical beam hardening correction in the measurement of vertebral bone mineral content by computed tomography. Radiology 138:223, 1981.
207. Isherwood I, Rutherford RA, Pullan BR and Adams PH. Bone-mineral estimation by computer-assisted transverse axial tomography. Lancet 2:712, 1976.
208. Iskrant AP and Smith RW Jr. Osteoporosis in women 45 years and over related to subsequent fractures. Public Health Rep 84:33, 1969.
209. Jackson WPU. Osteoporosis — commonest of all diseases. South African Med J 29:885, 1955.
210. Jacobson B. X-ray spectrophotometry in vivo. Am J Roentgenol 91:202, 1964.
211. Jawordki ZF. Proceedings of the First Workshop on Bone Morphometry. Univ of Ottawa Press, Ottawa, Canada, 1976.
212. Jensen GF, Christiansen C, Bosen J, Hegedus V and Transbol I. Epidemiology of postmenopausal spinal and long bone fracture. Clin Orthop 166:75, 1982.
213. Jensen PS, Orphanoudakis SC, Baron R, Lang R, Rauschkolb EN and Rasmussen H. Determination of bone mass by CT and correlation with qualitative histomorphometric analysis. Proceedings of CT Densitometry Workship. San Francisco, Calif. J Comput Assist Tomogr 3(6):847, 1979.
214. Jensen PS, Orphanoudakis SC, Rauschkold EN, Baroa R, Lang R and Rassmussen H. Assessment of bone mass in the radius by computed tomography. Am J Roentgenol 134:285, 1980.
215. Jhamaria NL, Lal KB, Udawat M, Banerji P and Kabra SG. The trabecular pattern of the calcaneum as an index of osteoporosis. J Bone Joint Surg 65B(2):195, 1983.
216. Johnell O. The clinical significance of osteoclast activity in man. MD thesis. University of Lund, 1980.
217. Johnston CC, Smith DM, Yu P-L and Deiss WP. In vivo measurement of bone mass in the radius. Metabolism 17:1140, 1968.
218. Johnston CC, Norton JA, Khairi RA and Longcope C. Age-related bone loss. In: Osteoporosis II. Barzel (ed). Grune and Stratton, New York, p 91, 1979.
219. Joseph PM and Spital RD. The exponential edge-gradient effect in x-ray computed tomography. Phys Med Biol 26:473, 1981.
220. Joseph PM and Spital RD. A method for correcting bone induced artifacts in computed tomography scanners. J Comput Assist Tomogr 2:100, 1978.
221. Karellas A, Leichter I, Craven JD and Greenfield MA. Characterization of tissue via coherent-to-Compton scattering ratio: sensitivity considerations. Med Phys 10(5):605, 1983.
222. Karjalainen P. A method for determination of the mineral content and mineral density of the distal radius using gamma-ray attenuation. Ann Clin Res 5:231, 1973.
223. Kaufman L, Gamsu G, Savoca C, Swann S, Murphy L, Hruska B, Palmer D and Ullman J. Measurement of absolute lung density by Compton-scatter densitometry. IEEE Trans Nucl Sci NS-23 (1):599, 1976.
224. Kennedy NS, Estell R, Ferrington CM, Simpson JD, Smith MA, Strong JA and Tothill P. Total body neutron activation of calcium: calibration and normalization. Phys Med Biol 27:697, 1982.
225. Kennedy NS, Eastell R, Smith MA and Tothill P. Normal levels of total body sodium and chlorine by neutron activation analysis. Phys Med Biol 28(3):215, 1983.
226. Kennett TJ, Garnett ES and Webber CE. An in vivo measurement of absolute bone density. J Can Assoc Radiol 23:168, 1972.
227. Kennett TJ and Webber CE. Bone density measured by photon scattering. II. Inherent sources of error. Phys Med Biol 21:770, 1976.

228. Kerr SA, Kouris K, Webber CE and Kennett TJ. Coherent scattering and the assessment of mineral concentration in trabecular bone. Phys Med Biol 25(6):1037, 1980.
229. Khairi MR, Cronin JH, Robb JA, Smith DM, Yu PL, Johnston CC. Femoral trabecular pattern index and bone mineral content measured by photon absorption in senile osteoporosis. J Bone Joint Surg 58:221, 1976.
230. Kimmel PL. Radiologic methods to evaluate bone mineral content. Health and Public Policy Committee, American College of Physicians. Ann Int Med 100:908, 1984.
231. Kivilaasko R and Palolampi E. On the density of the ulna and on the relationship between density and cortical thickness. Acta Anat 60:325, 1965.
232. Kissel L and Pratt RH. New predictions for Rayleigh scattering — 10 keV-10 MeV. Phys Rev Lett 40:387, 1978.
233. Klemm T, Banzer DH and Schneider U. Bone mineral content of the growing skeleton. Am J Roentgenol 126:1283, 1976.
234. Koehler PR, Anderson RE and Baxter B. The effect of computed tomography viewer controls on anatomical measurements. Radiology 130:189, 1979.
235. Kranedonk DH, Jurist JM and Lee HG. Femoral trabecular pattern and bone mineral content. J Bone Joint Surg. 54A:1472, 1972.
236. Krolner B and Pors Nielsen S. A scanning lumbar osteodensitometer using a 153-Gadolinium source. Proceedings of the 2nd Congress of the European Society of Nuclear Medicine. London, 1978.
237. Krolner B and Pors Nielsen S. Measurement of bone mineral content (BMC) of the lumbar spine. I. Theory and application of a new two-dimensional dual-photon attenuation method. Scand J Clin Lab Invest 40:653, 1980.
238. Krolner B, Pors Nielsen S and Lund B. Measurement of bone mineral content (BMC) of the lumbar spine. II. Correlation between forearm BMC and lumbar spine BMC. Scand J Clin Lab Invest 40:665, 1980.
239. Krolner B and Pors Nielsen S. Bone mineral content of the lumbar spine in normal and osteoporotic women: cross-sectional and longitudinal studies. Clin Sci 62(3):329, 1982a.
240. Krolner B and Pors Nielsen S. Long-term reproducibility of dual-photon absorptiometry of lumbar vertebrae (lumbar BMC). In: Non-invasive Bone Measurements: Methodological Problems. Dequeker J and Johnson CC (eds). IRL Press, Oxford, p 73, 1982b.
241. Krolner B, Tondevold E, Toft B, Berthelsen B and Pors Nielsen S. Bone mass of the axial and the appendicular skeleton in women with Colles fracture: its relation to physical activity. Clin Physiol 2:147, 1982c.
242. Krolner B. Seasonal variation of lumbar spine BMC in normal women. Calcif Tissue Int 35:145, 1983.
243. Krolner B. Lumbar spine bone mineral content by photon beam absorptiometry. Dan Med Bull 32(3):153, 1985.
244. Kruse HP, Kuhlencordt F, Ringe JD. Correlation of clinical, densitometric and histomorphometric data in osteoporosis. In: Calcified Tissues. Pors NS and Hjorting-Hansen E (eds). FADL Publishing, Copenhagen, p 457, 1976.
245. Lachman E. Osteoporosis: the potentialities and limitations of its roentgenologic diagnosis. Am J Radiol 74:712, 1955.
246. Lacy JL. Bone density determinations with the multiwire gamma camera and I-125 X-rays. Proceedings of the 31st Annual Mtg, Los Angeles, Calif J Nucl Med 25(5):P104, 1984.
247. Lahtinen T, Vaananen A and Karjalainen P. Effect of intraosseous fat on the measurements of bone mineral of distal radius. Calcif Tissue Int 32:7, 1980.
248. Lale PG. The examination of internal organs using gamma-ray scatter with possible extension to megavoltage radiography. Phys Med Biol 4:159, 1959.
249. Lale PG. The examination of internal tissues by high energy scattered x-radiation. Radiology 90:510, 1968.
250. Lampmann LE, Duursma SA and Ruys JH. CT Densitometry in Osteoporosis. Martinus Nijhoff, Boston, p 41, 1984.
251. Landin L and Nilsson BE. Forearm bone mineral content in children. Acta Paediatr Scand 70:919, 1981.
252. Landin L and Nilsson BE. Bone mineral content in children with fractures. Clin Orthop 178:292, 1983.
253. Lange S, Weiss T, Gahl G and Golde G. Knochendichtemessung mit dem computertomo-

graphen. ROFO 129:66, 1978.
254. Larsson S, Bergstrom M, Dahlqvist I, Israelsson A and Lagergren C. A method for determining bone mineral content using Fourier image reconstruction and dual source technique. J Comput Assist Tomogr 2(3):347, 1978.
255. Leichter I, Karellas A, Craven JD and Greenfield MA. The effect of the momentum transfer on the sensitivity of a photon scattering method for the characterization of tissue. Med Phys 11(1):31, 1984.
256. Lenihan JJ, Comar D, Riviere R and Kellershon C. Estimation of thyroid iodine in vivo by activation analysis. Nature 214:1221, 1967.
257. Lewis AF. Fracture of neck of the femur: changing incidence. Br Med J 283:1217, 1981.
258. Lindquist O, Bengtsson C, Hansson T and Jonsson R. Changes in bone mineral content of the axial skeleton in relation to aging and the menopause. Scand J Lab Invest 43:333, 1983.
259. Ling SS, Rustgi S, Karellas A, Craven JD, Whiting JS, Greenfield MA and Stern R. The measurement of traebecular bone mineral density using coherent and Compton scattered photons. Med Phys 9:208, 1982.
260. Lukert BP. Diagnosis and management of osteoporosis. Compr Ther 10(12):8, 1984.
261. Madsen M, Peppler W and Mazess RB. Vertebral and total body bone mineral content by dual photon absorptometry. In: Calcified Tissue. Pors-Nielsen S and Hjorting-Hansen E (eds). FADL. Forlag, Copenhagen, 1976.
262. Madsen M, Peppler W and Mazess RB. Vertebral and total body bone mineral by dual photon absorptiometry. Calcif Tissue Res 21 (suppl):361, 1976.
263. Madsen M. Vertebral and peripheral bone mineral content by photon absorptiometry. Invest Radiol 13:185, 1977.
264. Manzke E, Chestnut CH III, Wergedal JE, Baylink DJ, Nelp WB. Relationship between local and total bone mass in osteoporosis. Metabolism 24:605, 1975.
265. Marschall A, Weissberger RG, Zamenhof SA and Neer RN. CT scanning for the measurement of bone mineral in the human spine. J Comput Assist Tomogr 2:253, 1978.
266. Mazess RB. Bone density in Sadlermiut Eskimo. Human Biol 38:42, 1966.
267. Mazess RB, Cameron JR and Sorenson JA. Determining body composition by radiation absorption spectrometry. Nature 228:771, 1970.
268. Mazess RB, Ort M, Judy P and Mather W. Absorptiometric bone mineral determination using ^{153}Gd. Proceedings of Bone Meas. Conf. (Conf. 700515). Cameron JR (ed). US Atomic Energy Commission, p 308, 1970.
269. Mazess RB. Estimation of bone and skeletal weight by direct photon absorptiometry. Invest Radiol 6:52, 1971.
270. Mazess RB and Cameron JR. Growth of bone in school children: comparison of radiographic morphometry and photon-absorptiometry. Growth 36:77, 1972.
271. Mazess RB, Cameron JR and Miller H. Direct readout of bone mineral content using radionuclide absorptiometry. Int J Appl Radiat Isot 23:471, 1972.
272. Mazess RB and Cameron JR. Bone mineral content in normal US whites. Proceedings of the International Conf. on Bone Mineral Measurement, Mazess RB (ed). Publication 75-683, US Dept of HEW, p 228, 1974.
273. Mazess RB, Hanson J, Kan W, Madsen M, Pelc N, Wilson CR and Witt RM. Progress in dual photon absorptiometry of bone. Proceedings of the Symposuim on Bone Mineral Determinations. Schmelling P (ed). Aktiebologet Atomenergi, Studsvik, Sweden 489:40, 1974.
274. Mazess RB, Wilson CR, Hanson J, Kan W, Madsen M, Pelc N, and Witt R. Progress in dual photon absorptiometry of bone. Proceedings of the Symposium on Bone Mineral Determinations AE-489. Schmeling P (ed). Aktiebologet Atomenergi, Studsvik, Sweden 2:40, 1974.
275. Mazess RB. Bone mineral data debated (letter). Am J Roentgenol 128:527, 1977.
276. Mazess RB. Bone mineral in Vilcabamba, Equador. Am J Roentgenol 130:671, 1978.
277. Mazess RB. Non-invasive measurement of bone. In: Osteoporosis II. Barzel US (ed). Grune and Stratton, New York, p 5, 1979.
278. Mazess RB. Measurement of skeletal status by noninvasive methods. Calcif Tissue Int 28:89, 1979.
279. Mazess RB and Wilson CR. Spinal bone measurement by CT and by dual photon absorptionmetry. Proc of CT Densitometry Workshop, San Francisco, Calif, J Comput Assist Tomogr 3(6):847, 1979.
280. Mazess RB. Advances in total body and regional bone mineral by dual-photon absorptio-

metry. Proceedings of the Inter Symp on Osteoporosis, Jerusalem, Israel, 1981.
281. Mazess RB, Peppler WW, Harrison JE and McNeill KG. Total body bone mineral and lean body mass by dual photon absorptiometry. Calcif Tissue Int 33:365, 1981.
282. Mazess RB. On aging bone loss. Clin Orthop Rel Res 165:239, 1982.
283. Mazess RB and Whedon DG. Immobilization and bone. Calcif Tissue Int 35:265, 1983.
284. Mazess RB. Errors in measuring trabecular bone by computed tomography due to marrow and bone composition. Calcif Tissue Int 35:148, 1983.
285. Mazess RB. Noninvasive methods for quantitating trabecular bone. In: The osteoporotic syndrome. Detection, prevention, and treatment. Avioli LV (ed). Grune and Stratton, New York, p 85, 1983.
286. Mazess RB, Peppler WW, Chesney RW, Lange TA, Lindgren U and Smith E Jr. Total body and regional bone mineral by dual-photon absorptiometry in metabolic bone disease. Calcif Tissue Int 36:8, 1984.
287. Mazess RB, Peppler WW, Chesney RW, Lange TA, Lindgren U and Smith E Jr. Does bone measurement on the radius indicate skeletal status? J Nucl Med 25:281, 1984.
288. Mazess RB, Peppler WW and Gibbons. Total body composition by dual-photon (Gd-153) absorptiometry. Am J Clin Nutr 40:834, 1984.
289. Mazess RB. Does bone measurement on the radius indicate skeletal status? J Nucl Med 25(10):1151, 1984.
290. Mazess RB and Cameron JR. Densitometry of appendicular bone in osteoporosis (letter). JAMA 254(14):1906, 1985.
291. Maziere B, Kuntz D, Comar D and Ryckewaert A. In vivo analysis of bone calcium by local neutron activation of the hand: results in normal and osteoporotic subjects. J Nucl Med 20:85, 1979.
292. McBroom RJ, Hayes WC, Edwards WT. (abstract) Proc. of the 30th Annual Meeting of the Orthopedics Research Society, Atlanta, 1984.
293. McNeill KG, Thomas BJ, Sturtridge WC and Harrison JE. In vivo neutron activation analysis for calcium in man. J Nucl Med 14:502, 1973.
294. Meema HE. The occurrence of cortical bone atrophy in old age and in osteoporosis. J Can Assoc Radiol 13:27, 1962.
295. Meema HE and Meema S. Measurable roentgenologic changes in some peripheral bones in senile osteoporosis. J Am Geriatr Soc 11:1170, 1963.
296. Meema HE and Meema S. The relationship of diabetes mellitus and body weight to osteoporosis in elderly females. Can Med Assoc J 96:132, 1967.
297. Meema HE and Meema S. Cortical bone mineral density versus cortical thickness in the diagnosis of osteoporosis. J Am Geriatr Soc 17:120, 1969.
298. Meema HE and Schatz DL. Simple radiologic demonstration of cortical bone loss in thyrotoxicosis. Radiology 97:9, 1970.
299. Meema HE and Meema S. Comparison of microradioscopic and morphometric findings in the hand bones with densitometric findings in the proximal radius in thyrotoxicosis and in renal osteodystrophy. Invest Radiol 7:88, 1972.
300. Meema HE and Meema S. Improved roentgenologic diagnosis of osteomalacia by microradioscopy of hand bones. Am J Roentgenol 125:925, 1975.
301. Meema HE, Taves DR and Oreopoulos DG. Comparisons between x-ray photodensitometric and gamma-ray absorptiometric findings of bone mineral measurements, and the evidence of their convertibility. Invest Radiol 11:550, 1976.
302. Meema S and Meema HE. Improved recognition of bone loss by concurrent measurements in the second metacarpal and radius. Proc First Workshop Bone Morphometry. Jowordki ZF (ed). Univ. of Ottawa Press, Canada, p 48, 1976.
303. Meema HE, Harrison JE, McNeill KG and Oreopoulos DG. Correlations between peripheral and central skeletal mineral content in chronic renal failure patients and in osteoporotics. Skeletal Radiol 1:169, 1977.
304. Meema HE and Meema S. Compact bone mineral density of the normal human radius. Acta Radiol [Oncol] 7(4):342, 1978.
305. Meema HE and Meema S. Radiogrammetry. In: Non-Invasive Measures of Bone Mass and their Clinical Application. Cohn SH (ed). CRC Press, Cleveland, p 31, 1981.
306. Meindock H, Rapoport A, Oreopoulos OG, Rabinovich S, Meema HE and Meema S. Quantitative radionuclide scanning in metabolic bone disease. Nucl Med Commun 6:141, 1985.

307. Melton LJ, Wahner HW, Richelson LS, O'Fallon WM, Dunn WL and Riggs BL. Bone-density — specific fracture risk: a population-based study of the relationship between osteoporosis and vertebral fracture (abstract) J Nucl Med 26:24, 1985.
308. Meunier PJ, Courpron P, Edouard C et al. Physiological senile involution and pathological rarefaction of bone. Quantitative and comparative histological data. Clin Endocrinol Metab 2:239, 1973.
309. Meunier PJ, Courpron P, Giroux JM, Edouard C, Bernard J and Vignon G. Bone histomorphometry as applied to research on osteoporosis and the diagnosis of hyperosteoidosis states. In: Calcified Tissues. Pors Nielsen S and Hjorting-Hansen E (eds). FADL, Copenhagen, p 354, 1976.
310. Meunier PJ. Bone Histomorphometry: Second International Workshop. Armour Montagu, Paris, 1977.
311. Meunier PJ. Bone biopsy in diagnosis of metabolic bone disease. In: Hormonal control of calcium metabolism. Cohn DV (ed). Excerpta Medica, Amsterdam, p 109, 1981.
312. Meunier PJ, Courpron P, Edouard C et al. Bone histomorphometry in osteoporosis. In: Osteoporosis II. Barzel US (ed). Grune and Stratten, New York, p 27, 1979.
313. Minton SD, Steichen JJ and Tsang RC. Bone mineral content in term and preterm appropriate-for-gestational-age infants. J Pediatrics 95:1037, 1979.
314. Mirell SG, Anderson GW and Blahd WN. A tomographic brain imaging system using Compton scattered gamma rays. Proceedings of the IAEA Symp on Medical Radionuclide Imaging. IAEA-SM-210/70, Los Angeles, Calif, 1976.
315. Mirell SG, Hopkins JM, Winston MA and Blahd WH. Bone mineral absorptiometry with a dual source irradiator and a scintillation camera. Clin Nucl Med 10:P16, 1985.
316. Moore R and Wahner H. The measurement of bone mineral. Appl Radiol 6(3):140, 1974.
317. Morgan DB, Spiers FW, Pulvertaft CN and Fourman P. The amount of bone in the metacarpal and the phalanx according to age and sex. Clin Radiol 18:101, 1967.
318. Morgan DB. The metacarpal bone: a comparison of the various indices for assessment of the amount of bone and for the detection of loss of bone. Clin Radiol 24:77, 1973.
319. Muller A, Ruegsegger P and Seitz P. Optimal CT settings for bone evaluations. Phys Med Biol 30(5):401, 1985.
320. Munk-Jensen N, Pors-Nielsen S and Obel E. Bone loss from lumbar vertebrae and distal forearm in early postmenopausal women. Calcif Tissue Int 39(S):A51, 1986.
321. Murty RC. Effective atomic numbers of heterogeneous materials. Nature 207:398, 1965.
322. Naor E, DiSegni V, Robin G, Makin M and Menczel J. Intra-observer variability in the determination of the metacarpal cortical index. Br J Radiol 45:213, 1972.
323. Nelp WB, Palmer HE and Murano R. Measurement of total body calcium (bone mass) in vivo with the use of total body neutron activation analysis. J Lab Clin Med 76:152, 1970.
324. Nelp WB, Denney JD, Murano R, Hinn GM, Williams JL, Rudd TG and Palmer HE. Absolute measurement of total body calcium (bone mass) in vivo. J Lab Clin Med 79(3):430, 1972.
325. Newton-John HF and Morgan DB. The loss of bone with age, osteoporosis and fractures. Clin Orthop 71:229, 1970.
326. Nicoll JJ, Tothill P, Smith MA, Reid D, Kennedy NS and Nuki G. In vivo precision of total body calcium and sodium measurements by neutron activation analysis. Phys Med Biol 32(2):243, 1987.
327. Nickoloff EL and Feldman F. Bone mineral assessment with dual energy computerized tomography (CT) imaging (unpublished).
328. Nilas L, Norgaard H, Podenphant J, Godfredsen A and Christiansen C. Bone composition in the distal forearm. Scand J Clin Invest (in press).
329. Nilas L, Borg J, Godredsen A and Christiansen C. Comparison of single- and dual-photon absorptiometry in postmenopausal bone mineral loss. J Nucl Med 26:1257, 1985.
330. Nordin BE. International patterns of osteoporosis. Clin Orthop 45:17, 1966.
331. Nordin BE. Clinical significance and pathogenesis of osteoporosis. Br Med J 1:571, 1971.
332. Nordin BE, Robertson A and Crowe A. The use of CT scanning for the diagnosis of osteoporosis. Proc Symp Clin Disorders Bone Mineral Metab. Excerpta Medica (in press).
333. Nordin BE, Need AG, Morris HA and Horowitz M. New approaches to the problems of osteoporosis. Clin Ortho p 200:181, 1985.
334. Nordin BE, Robertson A, Seamark RF, Bridges A, Philcox JC, Need AG, Horowitz M, Morris HA and Deam S. The relation between calcium absorption, serum dehydroepiandro-

sterone, and vertebral mineral density in postmenopausal women. J Clin Endocrinol Metab 60(4):651, 1985.
335. Odeblad E and Norhagen A. Measurements of electron densities with the aid of the Compton scattering process. Acta Radiol 45:161, 1956.
336. Olkkonen H and Karjalainen PA. A ^{170}Tm gamma scattering technique for the determination of absolute bone density. Br J Radiol 48:594, 1975.
337. Olkkonen H, Puumalainen P, Karjalainen P and Alhava EM. A coherent Compton scattering method for measurement of trabecular bone mineral density in the distal radius. Invest Radiol 16:491, 1981.
338. Orphanoudakis SC, Jensen PS, Rauschkolb EN, Lang R and Rasmussen H. Bone mineral analysis using single-energy computed tomography. Invest Radiol 14:122, 1979.
339. Ott SM, Murano R, Lewellen TK, Nelp WB and Chesnut CH. Total body calcium by neutron activation analysis in normals and osteoporotic populations: a discriminator of significant bone mass loss. J Lab Clin Med 102(4):637, 1983.
340. Ott SM, Kilcoyne RF and Chesnut III CH. Longitudinal changes in bone mass after one year as measured by different techniques in patients with osteoporosis. Calcif Tissue Int 39:133, 1986.
341. Pak CYC. Postmenopausal osteoporosis. In: Menopause, Buchsbaum HJ (ed). Springer-Verlag, New York p 36, 1983.
342. Palmer HE, Nelp WB, Murano R and Rich C. The feasibility of in vivo neutron activation analysis of total body calcium and other elements of body composition. Phys Med Biol 13:269, 1968.
343. Palmer HE. Feasibility of determining total-body calcium in animals and humans by measuring Ar-37 in expired air after neutron irradiation. J Nucl Med 14:522, 1973.
344. Peppler WW and Mazess RB. Total body bone mineral and lean body mass by dual-photon absorptiometry. Calcif Tissue Int 33:353, 1981.
345. Piper DG and Preuss LE. Gamma ray scattering for density determinations. Proceedings of the ERDA X and Gamma Ray Symp, Conf-760539, Ann Arbor, Michigan, 1976.
346. Pistolesi M, Solfanelli S, Guzzardi R, Mey M and Giuntini C. Chest tomography by gamma camera and external gamma source: concise communication. J Nucl Med 19(1):94, 1978.
347. Pitt M. Osteopenic bone disease. Orthop Clin North Am 14:65, 1983.
348. Posner I and Griffiths HJ. Comparison of CT scanning with photon absorptiometric measurement of bone mineral content in the appendicular skeleton. Invest Radiol 12:542, 1977.
349. Powell MR. Medical Staff Conference on Osteoporosis. West J Med 140(1):102, 1984.
350. Preuss LE, Piper DG, Bugenis C. Bone mineral (apatite) assay by photon scattering — A survey of sources and experimental evaluation. In: Advances in X-ray Analysis. Pickles WJ (ed). Plenum Press, New York, 18:545, 1975.
351. Preuss LE and Schmonsees W. ^{109}Cd for compositional analysis of soft tissue. Int J Appl Rad Isot 23:9, 1972.
352. Pullan BR and Roberts TE. Bone mineral measurement using an EMI scanner and standard methods: a comparative study. Br J Radiol 51:24, 1978.
353. Puumalainen P, Uimarihuhta A, Alhava E and Olkkonen H. A new photon scattering method for bone mineral density measurements. Radiology 120:723, 1976.
354. Puumalainen P, Olkkonen H, Sikanen P. Assessment of fat content of liver by a photon scattering technique. Int J Appl Radiat Isot 28:785, 1977.
355. Puumalainen P, Sikanen P and Olkkonen H. Measurement of stable iodine content of tissue by coherently and Compton scattered photons. Nucl Instr Meth 163:261, 1979.
356. Puumalainen P, Uimarihuhta A, Olkkonen H and Alhava EM. A coherent/Compton scattering method employing an X-ray tube for measurement of traebecular bone mineral content. Phys Med Biol 27:425, 1982.
357. Reed GW. Studies on bone mineralization (abstract). Brit Empire Cancer Campaign Annual Report 38:489, 1960.
358. Reed GW. The assessment of bone mineralization from the relative transmission of ^{241}Am and 137^{Cs} radiations (abstract). Phys Med Biol 11:174, 1966.
359. Reed GW and Atkinson PJ. Studies on bone mineralization (abstract). British Empire Cancer Campaign Annual Report 43:465, 1965.
360. Reich NE, Seidelmann RE, Tubbs RR, MacIntyre WJ, Meaney TF, Alfidi RJ and Pepe RG. Determination of bone mineral content using CT scanning. Am J Roentgenol 127:593, 1976.

361. Reid DM, Kennedy NS, Smith MA, Nicoll J, Brown N, Tothill P and Nuki G. Bone loss in rheumatoid arthritis and primary generalized osteoarthrosis: effects of corticosteroids, suppressive antirheumatic drugs and calcium supplements. Br J Rheumatol 25:253, 1986.
362. Reiser U and Genant HK. New water and bone equivalent solid phantom materials used for calibration in quantitative computed tomography. Radiology (special edition) 153(P):301, 1984.
363. Reiss KH and Schuster W. Quantitative measurements of lung function in children by means of Compton backscatter. Radiology 102:613, 1972.
364. Revak CS. Mineral content of cortical bone measured by computed tomography. J Comput Assist Tomogr 4:34, 1980.
365. Richardson ML, Genant HK, Cann CE, Ettinger B, Gordan GS, Kolb FO and Reiser UJ. Assessment of metabolic bone disease by quantitative computer tomography. Clin Orthop 195:224, 1985.
366. Richelson LS, Heinz WW, Melton III LJ and Riggs BL. Relative contributions of aging and estrogen deficiency to postmenopausal bone loss. N Engl J Med 311(20):1273, 1984.
367. Rickers H, Nielsen AH, Smith Pedersen R and Rodbro P. Bone mineral loss during maintenance hemodialysis. Acta Med Scand 204:263, 1978.
368. Rickers H, Balslev I, Foltved H and Rodbro P. Bone mineral content before and after intestinal bypass operation in obese patients. Acta Med Scand 209:203, 1981.
369. Riggs BL. Osteoporosis: a disease of impaired homeostatic regulation? J Clin Min Elec Metab 5:265, 1981.
370. Riggs BL, Wahner HW, Dunn WL, Mazess RB, Offord KP and Melton LJ. Differential changes in bone mineral density of the appendicular and axial skeleton with aging: relationship to spinal osteoporosis. J Clin Invest 67:328, 1981.
371. Riggs BL, Wahner HW, Seeman E, Offord KP, Dunn WL, Mazess RB, Johnson KA and Melton LJ. Changes in bone mineral density of the proximal femur and spine with aging. J Clin Invest 70:716, 1982.
372. Riggs BL, Seeman E, Hodgson SF, Taues DR and O'Fallon WM. Effect of the fluoride/calcium regimen of vertebral fracture occurance in postmenopausal osteoporosis. N Engl J Med 306:446, 1982.
373. Roberts CC, Chan GM, Folland D et al. Adequate bone mineralization in breast-fed infants. J Pediatr 99:192, 1981.
374. Roberts JG, DiTomasso E and Webber CE. Photon scattering measurements of calceneal bone density. Invest Radiol 17(1):20, 1982.
375. Roh YS. Evaluation of bone mass and bone remodeling in vivo and its clinical application in osteoarthrosis and osteoporosis. PhD Thesis, Catholic Univ. of Louvain, Belgium, 1973.
376. Roos B, Rosengren B and Skoldbron H. Determination of bone mineral content in lumbar vertebrae by a gamma-ray technique. Proceedings of Bone Measurement Conference (Conf. 700515). Cameron JR (ed). Washington, DC, Atomic Energy Commission 243, 1970.
377. Roos B. Dual photon absorptiometry in lumbar vertebrae. Thesis. Akademisk Avhaling, Goteborg, Sweden, 1974.
378. Roos B and Skoldborn H. Dual photon absorptiometry in lumbar vertebrae. I. Theory and method. Acta Radiol Ther Phys 13:266, 1974.
379. Roos B. Dual photon absorptiometry in lumbar vertebrae. II. Precision and reproducibility. Acta Radiol 14(3):291, 1975.
380. Roos BO, Hansson TH, Skoldborn H. Dual photon absorptiometry in lumbar vertebrae. Evaluation of the baseline error. Acta Radiol Oncol Radiat Phys 19:111, 1980.
381. Rosen L. Relevance of particle accelerators on national goals. Science 173:490, 1971.
382. Rosenfeld D, Genant HK, Abols Y and Boyd DF. Analysis of multiple-energy, computed tomography for the measurement of bone mineral content. Proc Fourth Int Conf Bone Mineral Measurement. Mazess RB (ed). NIH Publ 80–1938, p 284, 1980.
383. Roy RR and Reed RD. Interactions of photons and leptons with matter. Academic Press, New York, 1968.
384. Ruesegger P, Dambacher MA, Ruegsegger E, Fischer JA and Anliker M. Bone loss in premenopausal and postmenopausal women. J Bone Joint Surg 66-A(7):1015, 1984.
385. Ruegsegger P, Elsasser U, Anliker M, Gnehm H, Kind H and Prader A. Quantification of bone mineralization using computed tomography. Radiology 121:93, 1976.
386. Ruff CB and Hayes WC. Bone mineral content in the lower limb. Relationship to cross-

sectional geometry. J Bone Joint Surg 66-A(7):1024, 1984.
387. Rundo J and Bunce LJ. Estimation of the total hydrogen content of the human body. Nature (London) 210:1023, 1966.
388. Rustgi SN, Siegel JA, Braunstein M, Craven JD and Greenfield MA. Accuracy of bone mineral data. Am J Roentgenol 135:275, 1980.
389. Rutherford RA, Pullan BR and Isherwood I. Measurement of effective atomic number and electron density using an EMI scanner. Neuroradiology 11:15, 1976.
390. Rutherford RA, Pullan BR and Isherwood I. Calibration and response of an EMI scanner. Neuroradiology 11:7, 1976.
391. Rutherford RA, Pullan BR and Adams PH. Bone mineral estimation by computer assisted transverse axial tomography. Lancet 2:712, 1976.
392. Rutt B and Foster A. Split-filter computed tomography: a simple technique for dual energy scanning. J Comput Assist Tomogr 4:501, 1980.
393. Sabatier JP, Heron JF, Petiot JF, Sabatier N and Dronne JJ. Clinical usefulness of a bone mineral measurement method on the femoral shaft. Calcif Tissue Int 34:21, 1982.
394. Sambrook PN, Bartlett C, Evans R, Katz D and Reeve J. Measurement of lumbar spine bone mineral: a comparison of dual photon absorptiometry and computed tomography. Br J Radiol 58:621, 1985.
395. Sandrick JM and Judy PF. Effects of the polyenergetic character of the spectrum of ^{125}I on the measurement of bone mineral content. Invest Radiol 8:143, 1973.
396. Saville PD. Changes in bone mass with age and alcoholism. J Bone Joint Surg 47A:492, 1965.
397. Schaadt O and Bohr H. Loss of bone mineral in axial and peripheral skeleton in aging, prednisone treatment and osteoporosis. In: Non-invasive bone measurements, methodological problems. Dequeker JV and Johnston CC (eds). IRL Press, Oxford, Washington DC, p 207, 1982.
398. Schatzler HP. Basic aspects on the use of elastic and inelastic scattered gamma radiation for the determination of binary systems with effective atomic numbers of less than 10. Int J Appl Radiat Isot 30:115, 1979.
399. Schneider R. Radiologic methods of evaluating generalized osteopenia. Orthop Clin North Am 15(4):631, 1984.
400. Schneider VS, Hinderling T, Vogel JM and Rambaut P. CT I-125 gamma-ray densitometry (CT scanner): Noninvasive measurement of trabecular bone mineral. Proceedings of CT Densitometry Workship, San Francisco, J Comput Assist Tomogr 3(6): 847, 1979.
401. Seeman E, Wahner HW and Offord KP. Differential effects of endocrine dysfunction on the axial and the appendicular skeleton. J Clin Invest 69:1302, 1982.
402. Sharafi A, Pearson D, Oxby CB, Oldroyd B, Krupowicz DW, Brooks K and Ellis RE. Multi-element analysis of the human body using neutron activation. Phys Med Biol 28(3):203, 1983.
403. Shimmins J, Smith DA, Aitken M, Anderson JB and Gillespie FC. The accuracy and reproducibility of bone mineral measurements "in vivo." Clin Radiol 23:47, 1972.
404. Shrimpton PC. Electron density values of various human tissues: in vitro Compton scatter measurements and calculated ranges. Phys Med Biol 26:907, 1981.
405. Siegelman SS. The radiology of osteoporosis. In: Osteoporosis. II. Barzel US (ed). Grune and Stratten, New York, p 68, 1970.
406. Sinaki M. McPhee MC, Hodgson SF, Merritt JM and Offord KP. Relationship between bone mineral density of spine and strength of back extensors in healthy postmenopausal women. Mayo Clin Proc 61:116, 1986.
407. Singh M, Nagrath AR and Maini PS. Changes in trabecular pattern of the upper end of the femur as an index of osteoporosis. J Bone Joint Surg 52A:437, 1970.
408. Singh M, Riggs BL, Beabout JW and Jowsey J. Femoral trabecular-pattern index for evaluation of spinal osteoporosis. Ann Intern Med 77:63, 1972.
409. Singh M. Femoral trabecular pattern index for grading osteoporosis. Proceedings First Workship on Bone Morphometry. Jaworski ZFG (ed). Univ of Ottawa Press, Canada, p 86, 1976.
410. Smith MA. Neutron activation analysis: choice of site, precision and accuracy. In: Noninvasive Bone Measurements: Methodological Problems. Dequeker J and Johnston CC (ed). IRL Press, Oxford, p 77, 1982.
411. Smith DM, Johnston CC Jr and Yu PL. In vivo measurements of bone mass. JAMA 219:325, 1972.

412. Smith DM, Khairi MRA and Johnston CC Jr. The loss of bone mineral with aging and its relationship to risk of fracture. J Clin Invest 56:311, 1975.
413. Smith MA and Tothill P. The crossover correction in dual photon absorptiometry with ^{153}Gd. Phys Med Biol 27(12):1515, 1982.
414. Smith HW, DeSmet AA and Levine EL. Measurement of cortical thickness in a human cadaver fermur. Clin Orthop 169:269, 1982.
415. Smith RW and Walker RR. Femoral expansion in aging women: implications for osteoporosis and fractures. Science 145:156, 1964.
416. Smith RW and Frame B. Concurrent axial and appendicular osteoporosis. N Engl J Med 273:73, 1965.
417. Spinks TJ, Bewley DK, Ranicar ASO and Joplin GF. Measurement of total body calcium in bone disease. J Radioanal Chem 37:345, 1977.
418. Stalp JT and Mazess RB. Determination of bone density by coherent Compton scattering. Med Phys 7(6):723, 1980.
419. Stein H, Sabato S, Leichter I, Nir D and Weinreb A. A new method of measuring bone density in the lower tibia of normal and postinjury limbs. Clin Orthop Rel Res 174:181, 1983.
420. Stellon AJ, Davies A, Compston J and Williams R. Bone loss in autoimmune chronic active hepatitis on maintenance corticosteroid therapy. Gastroenterology 89:1078, 1985.
421. Stichen B, Kaplan B, Edwards N and Sangh RC. Bone mineral content in fullterm infants measured by direct photon-absorptiometry. Am J Roentgenol 126:1284, 1976.
422. Stonestrom JP, Alvarez RE and Macovski A. IEEE Trans Biomed Eng 28:128, 1981.
423. Stonestrom JP and Macovski A. A framework for spectral artifact corrections in X-ray CT. IEEE Trans Nucl Sci 23:1453, 1976.
424. Thomsen K, Gotfredsen A and Christiansen C. Is postmenopausal bone loss an age-related phenomenon? Calcif Tissue Int 39:123, 1986.
425. Tofts PS. Definitions of effective energy in computed tomography. Phys Med Biol 26:313, 1981.
426. Tothill P. Density distribution studies using Compton scattered radiation and scintillation detectors. Proceedings of the 4th International Conference on Medical Physics, Ottawa, Canada, 32:26.7, 1976.
427. Tothill P, Smith MA and Sutton D. Dual photon absorptiometry of the spine with a low activity source of gadolimium-153. Br J Radiol 56:829, 1983.
428. Trotter M, Broman GE and Peterson RR. Densities of bones of white and Negro skeletons. J Bone Joint Surg 42A:50, 1960.
429. Van Gerven DP, Armelagos GJ and Batley MH. Roentgenographic and direct measurement of femoral cortical involution in a prehistoric Mississippian population. Am J Phys Anthropol 31:23, 1969.
430. Verly JG and Bracewell RN. Blurring in tomograms made with x-ray beams of finite width. J Comput Assist Tomogr 3:662, 1979.
431. Virtama P, Gastrin G and Telkka A. Biconcavity of the vertebrae as an estimate of their bone density. Clin Radiol 13:128, 1962.
432. Virtama P and Helela T. Radiographic measurements of cortical bone. Acta Orthop Scand Suppl 293, 1969.
433. Virtama P. Geographic differences in thickness of cortical bone — comparison between a Welsh and Finnish population. Skeletal Radiol 1:29, 1976.
434. Vogel JM. Bone mineral measurement: Skylab experiment M-078. Acta Astronautica 2:129, 1975.
435. Vogel JM and Wittale MW. Bone mineral content changes in Skylab astronauts. Am J Radiol 126:1296, 1976.
436. Vogel JM, Cline JW, Harrison JF, Ulloa GA and McDonald RJ. Microcomputer based dual energy photon absorptiometric bone mineral analyzer (VCH). IEEE Trans Nucl Sci 26:576, 1979.
437. Wahner HW, Lawrence Riggs B and Beabout JW. Diagnosis of osteoporosis: usefulness of photon absorptiometry at the radius. J Nucl Med 18:432, 1977.
438. Wahner HW and Dunn WL. A new instrument for determination of bone mineral in the lumber spine. Nucl Med Commun 1:211, 1980.
439. Wahner HW, Dunn WL and Riggs BL. Noninvasive bone mineral measurements. Sem Nucl Med 13(3):282, 1983.
440. Wahner HW, Dunn WL, Thorsen HC, Griffin P and Hockert NL. Bone mineral measure-

ments: review of various techniques. In: Nuclear Medicine: Quantitative Procedures. Wahner HW (ed). Little, Brown and Co, Boston/Toronto, p 107, 1983.
441. Wahner HW. Bone mineral measurements: a new clinical tool. J Nucl Med 25(3):383, 1984.
442. Wahner HW, Dunn WL and Lawrence Riggs B. Assessment of bone mineral. Part 1. J Nucl Med 25:1134, 1984.
443. Wahner HW, Dunn WL and Riggs BL. Assessment of bone mineral. Part 2. J Nucl Med 25:1241, 1984.
444. Wahner HW. Assessment of metabolic bone disease: review of new nuclear medicine procedures. Mayo Clin Proc 60:827, 1985.
445. Wahner HW, Dunn WL, Mazess RB, Towsley M, Lindsay R, Markhard L and Dempster D. Dual-photon Gd-153 absorptiometry of bone. Radiology 156:203, 1985.
446. Wasnich RD, Ross PD Heilbrun LK and Vogel JM. Prediction of postmenopausal fracture risk with use of bone mineral measurements. Am J Obstet Gynecol 153:745, 1985.
447. Watt DE. Optimum photon energies for the measurement of bone mineral and fat fractions. Br J Radiol 48:265, 1975.
448. Weaver J and Chalmers J. Cancellous bone: its strength and changes with aging and an evaluation of some methods for measuring its mineral content. I. Age changes in cancellous bone. J Bone Joint Surg 48A:289, 1966.
449. Webber CE and Kennett TJ. Bone density measured by photon scattering: I. A system for clinical use. Phys Med Biol 21:760, 1976.
450. Webber CE and Garnett ES. Density of os calcis and limb dominance. J Anat 121(1):203, 1976.
451. Webster DJ and Lillicrap SC. Coherent/Compton scattering for the assessment of bone mineral content using heavily filtered x-ray beams. Phys Med Biol 30:531, 1985.
452. Weissberger MA, Zamenhof RG, Aronow S and Neer RM. Computed tomography for the measurement of bone mineral in the human spine. J Comput Assist Tomogr 2:253, 1978.
453. West RR and Reed GW. The measurement of bone mineral in vivo by photon beam scanning. Br J Radiol 43:886, 1970.
454. West RR. The estimation of total skeletal mass from bone densitometry measurement using 60 keV photons. Br J Radiol 46:599, 1973.
455. Williams B. Compton Scattering, McGraw-Hill, New York, 1977.
456. Williams ED, Boddy K, Harvey I and Haywood JK. Calibration and evaluation of a system for total body in vivo activation analysis using 14 MeV neutrons. Phys Med Biol 23:405, 1978.
457. Williams G, Spinks TJ, Freemantle C, Sandler L and Joplin GF. Total body calcium measurements using neutron activation analysis in Cushing's syndrome. Calcif Tissue Int 39:145, 1986.
458. Wilson CR, Ritman EL and Sturm RE. Roentgen video-absorptiometry. Phys Med Biol 19:256, 1974.
459. Wilson CR and Madsen M. Dichromatic absorptiometry of vertebrae bone mineral content. Invest Radiol. 12:180,1977.
460. Wilson JR, James C and Volz DJ. Quantitative computed tomography. Proceedings of the 4th International Conference on Bone Measurement, Toronto, Canada, 1978.
461. Witt RM, Mazess RB and Cameron JR. Standardization of bone mineral measurements. Proceedings of Bone Measurement Conference of Atomic Energy Commission Conf. 700515, p 303, 1970.
462. Witt RM and Mazess RB. Photon absorptiometry of soft-tissue and fluid content: the method and its precision and accuracy. Phys Med Biol 23:620, 1978.
463. Woodward HQ. The composition of human cortical bone: effect of age and of some abnormalities. Clin Orthop 37:187, 1964.
464. Wooten WW. Bone densitometry. The two photon technique and fat content of the bone. Thesis. University of California, Los Angeles, 1971.
465. Yalcintas MG and Nalcioglu O. A method for dose determination in computerized tomography. Health Phys 37:543, 1979.
466. Yano K, Wasnich RD, Vogel JM and Heilburn LK. Bone mineral measurements among middle-aged and elderly Japanese residents in Hawaii. Am J Epidemiol 119:751, 1984.
467. Yoneda Y and Chikaura Y. Scattering tomography. Jpn J Appl Phys 21(1):L31, 1982.
468. Zimmerman RE, Lanza RC, Tanaka T, Bolon GG, Griffiths HJ and Judy PF. A new detector

for absorptiometric measurement. Am J Roentgenol 126:1272, 1976.
469. Zito F, Mey M and Guzzardi R. Detector specifications and imaging implications in Compton scattering tomography. Proceedings of the World Congress on Medical Physics and Biomedical Engineering, Hamburg, 19.36, 1982 (abstract).

INDEX

GPSR Compliance

The European Union's (EU) General Product Safety Regulation (GPSR) is a set of rules that requires consumer products to be safe and our obligations to ensure this.

If you have any concerns about our products, you can contact us on ProductSafety@springernature.com

In case Publisher is established outside the EU, the EU authorized representative is:

Springer Nature Customer Service Center GmbH
Europaplatz 3
69115 Heidelberg, Germany

Batch number: 10755292

Printed by Printforce, the Netherlands